Cardiac Potassium Channel Disorders

Editors

MOHAMMAD SHENASA
STANLEY NATTEL

CARDIAC ELECTROPHYSIOLOGY CLINICS

www.cardiacEP.theclinics.com

Consulting Editors
RANJAN K. THAKUR
ANDREA NATALE

June 2016 • Volume 8 • Number 2

ELSEVIER

1600 John F. Kennedy Boulevard • Suite 1800 • Philadelphia, Pennsylvania, 19103-2899

http://www.theclinics.com

CARDIAC ELECTROPHYSIOLOGY CLINICS Volume 8, Number 2
June 2016 ISSN 1877-9182, ISBN-13: 978-0-323-44609-9

Editor: Lauren Boyle
Developmental Editor: Susan Showalter

Cardiac Electrophysiology Clinics (ISSN 1877-9182) is published quarterly by Elsevier Inc., 360 Park Avenue South, New York, NY 10010-1710. Months of issue are March, June, September, and December. Subscription prices are $205.00 per year for US individuals, $318.00 per year for US institutions, $225.00 per year for Canadian individuals, $359.00 per year for Canadian institutions, $285.00 per year for international individuals, $384.00 per year for international institutions and $100.00 per year for US, Canadian and international students/residents. To receive student/resident rate, orders must be accompanied by name of affiliated institution, date of term, and the signature of program/residency coordinator on institution letterhead. Orders will be billed at individual rate until proof of status is received. Foreign air speed delivery is included in all Clinics subscription prices. All prices are subject to change without notice. **POSTMASTER:** Send address changes to Cardiac Electrophysiology Clinics, Elsevier Health Sciences Division, Subscription Customer Service, 3251 Riverport Lane, Maryland Heights, MO 63043. **Customer Service: 1-800-654-2452 (US and Canada). From outside of the US and Canada, call 314-477-8871. Fax: 314-447-8029. E-mail: JournalsCustomerService-usa@elsevier.com (for print support); JournalsOnlineSupport-usa@elsevier.com (for online support).**

Reprints. For copies of 100 or more of articles in this publication, please contact the Commercial Reprints Department, Elsevier Inc., 360 Park Avenue South, New York, NY 10010-1710. Tel.: 212-633-3874; Fax: 212-633-3820; E-mail: reprints@elsevier.com.

Cardiac Electrophysiology Clinics is covered in *MEDLINE/PubMed (Index Medicus).*

Contributors

CONSULTING EDITORS

RANJAN K. THAKUR, MD, MPH, MBA, FACC, FHRS
Professor of Medicine and Director, Arrhythmia Service, Thoracic and Cardiovascular Institute, Sparrow Health System, Michigan State University, Lansing, Michigan

ANDREA NATALE, MD, FACC, FHRS
Texas Cardiac Arrhythmia Institute, St. David's Medical Center; Dell Medical School, University of Texas, Austin, Texas; MetroHealth Medical Center, Case Western Reserve University School of Medicine, Cleveland, Ohio; Division of Cardiology, Stanford University, Stanford, California; Electrophysiology and Arrhythmia Services, California Pacific Medical Center, San Francisco, California; Division of Cardiovascular Diseases, Scripps Clinic, La Jolla, California

EDITORS

MOHAMMAD SHENASA, MD
Heart and Rhythm Medical Group, Department of Cardiovascular Services, O'Connor Hospital, San Jose, California

STANLEY NATTEL, MD
Professor of Medicine and Paul-David Chair in Cardiovascular Electrophysiology, University of Montreal; Cardiologist and Director, Research Center; Editor-in-Chief, *Canadian Journal of Cardiology*, Montreal Heart Institute, Montreal; Department of Pharmacology and Therapeutics, McGill University, Montreal, Quebec, Canada; Faculty of Medicine, Institute of Pharmacology, University Duisburg-Essen, Essen, Germany

AUTHORS

ARNON ADLER, MD
Department of Cardiology, Tel Aviv Sourasky Medical Center, Sackler School of Medicine, Tel Aviv University, Tel Aviv, Israel

VINCENT ALGALARRONDO, MD, PhD
Department of Medicine, Research Center, Montreal Heart Institute, University of Montreal; Department of Pharmacology and Therapeutics, McGill University, Montreal, Quebec, Canada; Faculty of Medicine, Institute of Pharmacology, University Duisburg-Essen, Essen, Germany

AHMAD S. AMIN, MD, PhD
Department of Clinical and Experimental Cardiology, Heart Centre, Academic Medical Center, University of Amsterdam, Amsterdam, The Netherlands

JASON G. ANDRADE, MD
Department of Medicine, Université de Montréal and Montreal Heart Institute, Montreal, Québec, Canada; Heart Rhythm Services, Department of Medicine, University of British Columbia, Vancouver, British Columbia, Canada

RISHI ARORA, MD
Bluhm Cardiovascular Institute, Northwestern University Feinberg School of Medicine, Chicago, Illinois

HAMID ASSADI, MD
Heart and Rhythm Medical Group, Department of Cardiovascular Services, O'Connor Hospital, San Jose, California

MOHAMED BOUTJDIR, PhD
Research and Development Service, VA New York Harbor Healthcare System; Departments of Medicine, Cell Biology and Pharmacology, SUNY Downstate Medical Center, Brooklyn, New York; Department of Medicine, NYU School of Medicine, New York, New York

PIER LEOPOLDO CAPECCHI, MD
Department of Medical Sciences, Surgery and Neurosciences, University of Siena, Siena, Italy

LEI CHEN, PhD
Associate Research Scientist, Department of Pharmacology, College of Physicians and Surgeons of Columbia University, New York, New York

DAWOOD DARBAR, MD
Professor of Medicine and Pharmacology, Chief of Cardiology, Division of Cardiology, Department of Medicine, University of Illinois at Chicago, Chicago, Illinois

DOBROMIR DOBREV, MD
Institute of Pharmacology, West German Heart and Vascular Center, University Duisburg-Essen, Essen, Germany

NABIL EL-SHERIF, MD
Research and Development Service, VA New York Harbor Healthcare System; Departments of Medicine, Cell Biology and Pharmacology, SUNY Downstate Medical Center, Brooklyn, New York

ANNE M. GILLIS, MD, FRCPC, FHRS
Professor of Medicine, Department of Cardiac Sciences, Libin Cardiovascular Institute of Alberta, University of Calgary, Calgary, Alberta, Canada

SHAHRIAR HEIDARY, MD
Heart and Rhythm Medical Group, Department of Cardiovascular Services, O'Connor Hospital, San Jose, California

ROBERT S. KASS, PhD
Professor and Chairman, Department of Pharmacology, College of Physicians and Surgeons of Columbia University, New York, New York

JOHN ALVIN KPAEYEH Jr, MD
Fellow of Cardiovascular Disease, Division of Cardiology, Department of Medicine, Tourville Arrhythmia Center, Medical University of South Carolina, Charleston, South Carolina

FRANCO LAGHI-PASINI, MD
Department of Medical Sciences, Surgery and Neurosciences, University of Siena, Siena, Italy

PIETRO ENEA LAZZERINI, MD
Department of Medical Sciences, Surgery and Neurosciences, University of Siena, Siena, Italy

MARK McCAULEY, MD, PhD
Assistant Professor, Division of Cardiology, Department of Medicine, University of Illinois at Chicago, Chicago, Illinois

STANLEY NATTEL, MD
Professor of Medicine and Paul-David Chair in Cardiovascular Electrophysiology, University of Montreal; Cardiologist and Director, Research Center; Editor-in-Chief, *Canadian Journal of Cardiology*, Montreal Heart Institute, Montreal; Department of Pharmacology and Therapeutics, McGill University, Montreal, Quebec, Canada; Faculty of Medicine, Institute of Pharmacology, University Duisburg-Essen, Essen, Germany

JEANNE M. NERBONNE, PhD
Departments of Internal Medicine and Developmental Biology, Washington University Medical School, St Louis, Missouri

COLIN G. NICHOLS, PhD
Carl Cori Professor, Department of Cell Biology and Physiology; Director, Center for the Investigation of Membrane Excitability Diseases, Washington University School of Medicine, St Louis, Missouri

URSULA RAVENS, MD
Department of Pharmacology and Toxicology, Medical Faculty Carl Gustav Carus, Institut für Pharmakologie und Toxikologie, TU Dresden, Dresden, Germany

DAN M. RODEN, MD
Professor of Medicine, Pharmacology, and Biomedical Informatics; Assistant Vice-Chancellor for Personalized Medicine; Director, Oates Institute for Experimental Therapeutics, Vanderbilt University School of Medicine, Nashville, Tennessee

KEVIN J. SAMPSON, PhD
Associate Research Scientist, Department of Pharmacology, College of Physicians and Surgeons of Columbia University, New York, New York

MICHAEL C. SANGUINETTI, PhD
Professor, Department of Medicine, Nora Eccles Harrison Cardiovascular Research and Training Institute, University of Utah, Salt Lake City, Utah

FATEMAH SHENASA, BS
Heart and Rhythm Medical Group, Department of Cardiovascular Services, O'Connor Hospital, San Jose, California

HOSSEIN SHENASA, MD
Heart and Rhythm Medical Group, Department of Cardiovascular Services, O'Connor Hospital, San Jose, California

MOHAMMAD SHENASA, MD
Heart and Rhythm Medical Group, Department of Cardiovascular Services, O'Connor Hospital, San Jose, California

LASSE SKIBSBYE, PhD
Danish Arrhythmia Research Centre, Faculty of Health and Medical Sciences, University of Copenhagen, Copenhagen, Denmark

RAFIK TADROS, MD
Department of Medicine, Université de Montréal and Montreal Heart Institute, Montreal, Québec, Canada

TODD T. TOMSON, MD
Bluhm Cardiovascular Institute, Northwestern University Feinberg School of Medicine, Chicago, Illinois

SHARATH VALLABHAJOSYULA, MD
Clinical Research Coordinator in Cardiology, Division of Cardiology, Department of Medicine, University of Illinois at Chicago, Chicago, Illinois

SAMI VISKIN, MD
Department of Cardiology, Tel Aviv Sourasky Medical Center, Sackler School of Medicine, Tel Aviv University, Tel Aviv, Israel

NIELS VOIGT, MD
Institute of Pharmacology, West German Heart and Vascular Center, University Duisburg-Essen, Essen, Germany

JOHN MARCUS WHARTON, MD
Frank P. Tourville Professor of Medicine; Director, Cardiac Electrophysiology, Division of Cardiology, Department of Medicine; Director, Tourville Arrhythmia Center, Medical University of South Carolina, Charleston, South Carolina

ARTHUR A.M. WILDE, MD, PhD
Department of Clinical and Experimental Cardiology, Heart Centre, Academic Medical Center, University of Amsterdam, Amsterdam, The Netherlands; King Abdulaziz University, Princess Al-Jawhara Al-Brahim Centre of Excellence in Research of Hereditary Disorders, Jeddah, Kingdom of Saudi Arabia

WEI WU, PhD
Postdoctoral Fellow, Department of Medicine, Nora Eccles Harrison Cardiovascular Research and Training Institute, University of Utah, Salt Lake City, Utah

Contents

Atrial fibrillation (AF) is associated with increased morbidity and mortality. Atrial-selective potassium (K^+) channel blockers may represent a novel therapeutic target. The best validated atrial-specific ion currents are the acetylcholine-activated inward-rectifier K^+ current $I_{K,ACh}$ and ultrarapidly activating delayed-rectifier K^+ current I_{Kur}. Two-pore domain and small-conductance Ca^{2+}-activated K^+ channels and Kv1.1 channels may also contribute to the atrial repolarization. We review the molecular and electrophysiologic characteristics of atrial-selective K^+ channels and their potential pathophysiologic role in AF. We summarize currently available K^+ channel blockers focusing on the most important compounds.

Dofetilide is a class III antiarrhythmic agent with a selective blockade of rapid component of delayed rectifier potassium current (I_{Kr}). Dofetilide was found to be safe in patients after myocardial infarction and those with congestive heart failure and left ventricular systolic dysfunction (ejection fraction of less than 35%). An important adverse effect of dofetilide is its potential proarrhythmic risk of ventricular tachyarrhythmias, mostly torsades de pointes. Because dofetilide has about an 80% renal excretion, dose adjustment is required in patients with impaired renal function. Dofetilide should not be given or discontinued if the QTc is greater than 500 ms.

Sotalol is effective for treating atrial fibrillation (AF), ventricular tachycardia, premature ventricular contractions, and supraventricular tachycardia. Racemic (DL) sotalol inhibits the rapid component of the delayed rectifier potassium current. There is a near linear relationship between sotalol dosage and QT interval prolongation. However, in dose ranging trials in patients with AF, low-dose sotalol was not more effective than placebo. Orally administered sotalol has a bioavailability of nearly 100%. The only significant drug interactions are the need to avoid or limit use of concomitant drugs that cause QT prolongation, bradycardia, and/or hypotension.

Dronedarone is the newest antiarrhythmic drug approved for the maintenance of sinus rhythm in patients with nonpermanent atrial fibrillation (AF). It is a multi-channel blocker with diverse electrophysiologic properties. Dronedarone decreases the incidence of AF recurrence and the ventricular rate during recurrence. Dronedarone decreases rates of cardiovascular hospitalizations in patients with paroxysmal and persistent AF. Dronedarone increases mortality in patients with permanent AF and those with moderate-severe heart failure, and should thus be avoided in these populations. Dronedarone is less effective than amiodarone but also has less toxicity. Direct comparison with other antiarrhythmic drugs is not available.

Ranolazine: Electrophysiologic Effect, Efficacy, and Safety in Patients with Cardiac Arrhythmias

467

Mohammad Shenasa, Hamid Assadi, Shahriar Heidary, and Hossein Shenasa

Ranolazine is currently approved as an antianginal agent in patients with chronic angina (class IIA). Ranolazine exhibits antiarrhythmic effects that are related to its multichannel blocking effect, predominantly inhibition of late sodium (late I_{Na}) current and the rapid potassium rectifier current (I_{Kr}), as well as I_{Ca}, late I_{Ca}, and I_{Na-Ca}. It also suppresses the early and delayed after depolarizations. Ranolazine is effective in the suppression of atrial and ventricular arrhythmias (off-label use) without significant proarrhythmic effect. Currently, ongoing trials are evaluating the efficacy and safety of ranolazine in patients with cardiac arrhythmias; preliminary results suggest that ranolazine, when used alone or in combination with dronedarone, is safe and effective in reducing atrial fibrillation. Ranolazine is not currently approved by the US Food and Drug Administration as an antiarrhythmic agent.

Proarrhythmic and Torsadogenic Effects of Potassium Channel Blockers in Patients

481

Mark McCauley, Sharath Vallabhajosyula, and Dawood Darbar

The most common arrhythmia requiring drug treatment is atrial fibrillation (AF), which affects 2 to 5 million Americans and continues to be a major cause of morbidity and increased mortality. Despite recent advances in catheter-based and surgical therapies, antiarrhythmic drugs continue to be the mainstay of therapy for most patients with symptomatic AF. However, many antiarrhythmics block the rapid component of the cardiac delayed rectifier potassium current (I_{Kr}) as a major mechanism of action, and marked QT prolongation and pause-dependent polymorphic ventricular tachycardia (torsades de pointes) are major class toxicities.

Guidelines for Potassium Channel Blocker Use

495

Anne M. Gillis

This article summarizes recommendations for the clinical use of antiarrhythmic drugs for the treatment and prevention of atrial and ventricular arrhythmias based on current guideline and consensus documents. The choice of antiarrhythmic drug is based on the efficacy and safety profile and influenced by the presence or absence of structural heart disease. Because of its adverse side-effect profile, amiodarone is recommended for the management of atrial fibrillation only when other agents have failed or are contraindicated. For treatment of symptomatic ventricular arrhythmias in the setting of structural heart disease, amiodarone is generally the preferred agent.

CARDIAC ELECTROPHYSIOLOGY CLINICS

THE CLINICS ARE AVAILABLE ONLINE!
Access your subscription at:
www.theclinics.com

Foreword
The K$^+$ Channel: One Channel, Many Arrhythmias!

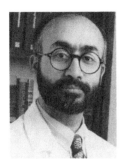
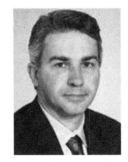

Ranjan K. Thakur, MD, MPH, MBA, FACC, FHRS   Andrea Natale, MD, FACC, FHRS

Consulting Editors

Potassium channels are potassium-selective pores that span the cell membrane; they are the most widely distributed type of ion channel and are found in virtually all living organisms. They control a variety of cellular processes, but in the cardiac muscle, these channels regulate repolarization of the cell membrane and thereby, the action potential duration. Potassium channels regulate the action potential by controlling a number of inward and outward ionic currents during various phases of the action potential to restore the transmembrane potential after depolarization. Malfunction of these channels may lead to life-threatening arrhythmias.

Structurally, the potassium channel consists of four subunits encoded by 80 distinct genes. Genetic mutations may lead to gain or loss of function in the potassium channels, resulting in a number of channelopathies: long QT syndrome, short QT syndrome, Brugada syndrome, and familial atrial fibrillation.

Over the past decade, numerous genotype–phenotype correlations and pathophysiologic mechanisms associated with potassium channel disorders have been elucidated. These crucial insights are paving the way to developing gene-specific and mutation-specific approaches to risk stratification and clinical management of individuals with these disorders.

Gene and molecular level understanding of these arrhythmias is proceeding at a breakneck pace, and most clinical electrophysiologists don't have a comprehensive understanding of these developments. This is due in large part to a lack of direct translation of molecular understanding into daily practice of clinical electrophysiology. But this is the next frontier.

We want to congratulate Drs Shenasa and Nattel for editing this issue of *Cardiac Electrophysiology Clinics* and assembling contributors leading this field to give us expert summaries of the important advances to date. This issue of *Cardiac Electrophysiology Clinics* is of interest to clinical electrophysiologists as well as experts in the field, who may need to catch up with advances outside of their own focused research interest.

Ranjan K. Thakur, MD, MPH, MBA, FACC, FHRS
Sparrow Thoracic and Cardiovascular Institute
Michigan State University
1200 East Michigan Avenue, Suite 580
Lansing, MI 48912, USA

Andrea Natale, MD, FACC, FHRS
Texas Cardiac Arrhythmia Institute
Center for Atrial Fibrillation at
St. David's Medical Center
1015 East 32nd Street, Suite 516
Austin, TX 78705, USA

E-mail addresses:
thakur@msu.edu (R.K. Thakur)
andrea.natale@stdavids.com (A. Natale)

http://dx.doi.org/10.1016/j.ccep.2016.03.002
1877-9182/16/$ – see front matter © 2016 Published by Elsevier Inc.

cardiacEP.theclinics.com

Preface

Cardiac Potassium Channel Disorders: From Basics to Clinics

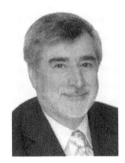 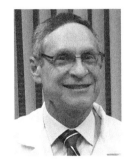

Mohammad Shenasa, MD   Stanley Nattel, MD

Editors

The last two decades have witnessed dramatic progress in our understanding of cardiac ion channels, and their structure, function, and regulation. We have learned about the role of various ion channels in cardiac physiology and their involvement in cardiac pathophysiology. We have also learned a great deal about the genetic control of channels, by both genes encoding the subunits that form channels and associated/regulatory subunits that are essential for normal ion channel properties. A great deal of information has been obtained by studying mutations in ion channel genes that cause cardiac disease. Sodium, potassium, and calcium ion channels are crucial for cardiac homeostasis and are implicated in physiologic regulation and pathologic conditions; potassium channels constitute the most diverse and complex cardiac ion channel family.

In December 2014, *Cardiac Electrophysiology Clinics* published an issue dedicated to cardiac sodium channel disorders.

We are delighted that the Consulting Editors invited us to be the Guest Editors of the current issue on "Cardiac Potassium Channel Disorders: From Basics to Clinics." Despite the presence of much material in the literature about cardiac

potassium channels, the editors felt, and we agree, that a comprehensive issue dedicated to potassium channel disorders from basics to clinics would be useful and timely.

We are also pleased that a group of leading experts from around the world have accepted our invitation to participate in this up-to-date, comprehensive, and unique issue on the subject and have provided a remarkable set of outstanding contributions.

This issue discusses cardiac potassium channel properties under both normal and abnormal conditions, including biophysical and structural (molecular) profiles, along with clinical relevance for the management of patients with potassium channel disorders. The concept of ion channel remodeling in different pathologic conditions, like left ventricular hypertrophy, myocardial infarction, and heart failure, is discussed. The properties of potassium channel blocking agents are reviewed, along with the factors that determine success as antiarrhythmic agents as well as their adverse consequences like torsadogenic effects.

We are confident that this issue will be equally informative and useful for basic and clinical

Card Electrophysiol Clin 8 (2016) xv–xvi
http://dx.doi.org/10.1016/j.ccep.2016.03.001
1877-9182/16/$ – see front matter © 2016 Elsevier Inc. All rights reserved.

electrophysiologists as well as for general cardiologists and fellows in training.

Mohammad Shenasa, MD
Heart and Rhythm Medical Group
105 North Bascom Avenue, Suite 204
San Jose, CA 95117, USA

Department of Cardiovascular Services
O'Connor Hospital
105 North Bascom Avenue, Suite 204
San Jose, CA 95128, USA

Stanley Nattel, MD
Department of Medicine
University of Montreal
Research Center
Montreal Heart Institute
5000 Belanger Street E.
Montreal, Quebec H1T1C8, Canada

E-mail addresses:
mohammad.shenasa@gmail.com (M. Shenasa)
stanley.nattel@icm-mhi.org (S. Nattel)

Molecular Basis of Functional Myocardial Potassium Channel Diversity

 CrossMark

Jeanne M. Nerbonne, PhD[a,b,*]

KEYWORDS

- Action potentials • Propagation • Repolarization • Dispersion • K^+ channels
- Pore-forming subunits • Accessory subunits • Macromolecular protein complexes

KEY POINTS

- Cellular electrophysiological studies have distinguished multiple types of voltage-gated inward and outward currents that contribute to action potential repolarization in mammalian cardiac cells.
  - Considerable progress has been made in identifying the pore-forming Kv and Kir α subunits contributing to the formation of most of the K^+ channels expressed in mammalian cardiac myocytes.
  - Biochemical studies have provided some insights into the molecular mechanisms underlying the observed heterogeneities in the expression of myocardial Kv and Kir currents.
- Considerable evidence suggests that native myocardial K^+ channels, like other ion channels, likely function in macromolecular protein complexes, comprising pore-forming α subunits and multiple cytosolic and transmembrane accessory/regulatory subunits.
- An important focus of future work will likely be on defining the physiologic roles of the many K^+ channel accessory subunits in the generation of native myocardial K^+ channels and on defining the molecular mechanisms controlling the properties and the cell surface expression of native cardiac K^+ channels.

INTRODUCTION

The normal mechanical functioning of the mammalian heart depends on proper electrical function, evident in the sequential generation of action potentials in cells in the "pacemaker" regions and the propagation of activity through the ventricles.[1–3] The waveforms of action potentials in individual cardiac cells (**Fig. 1**) reflect the coordinated activation and inactivation of inward (Na^+ and Ca^{2+}) and outward (K^+) current-carrying ion channels.[1] The propagation of electrical activity and the coordinated electromechanical

functioning of the heart also depend on electrical coupling between cells, mediated by gap junctions.[4] The rapid upstroke of action potentials in atrial and ventricular myocytes, attributed to inward currents through voltage-gated Na^+ (Nav) channels, is followed by slower repolarization and plateau phases (see **Fig. 1**), reflecting increased outward currents through multiple types of K^+ channels and inward currents through voltage-gated Ca^{2+} (Cav) channels. Cell-type–specific and regional differences in the waveforms of action potentials, which impact the normal spread of excitation in the myocardium and the

[a] Department of Internal Medicine, Washington University Medical School, 660 South Euclid Avenue, Box 8086, St Louis, MO 63110, USA; [b] Department of Developmental Biology, Washington University Medical School, St Louis, MO 63110, USA
* Corresponding address.
E-mail address: jnerbonne@wustl.edu

Card Electrophysiol Clin 8 (2016) 257–273
http://dx.doi.org/10.1016/j.ccep.2016.01.001
1877-9182/16/$ – see front matter © 2016 Elsevier Inc. All rights reserved.

cardiacEP.theclinics.com

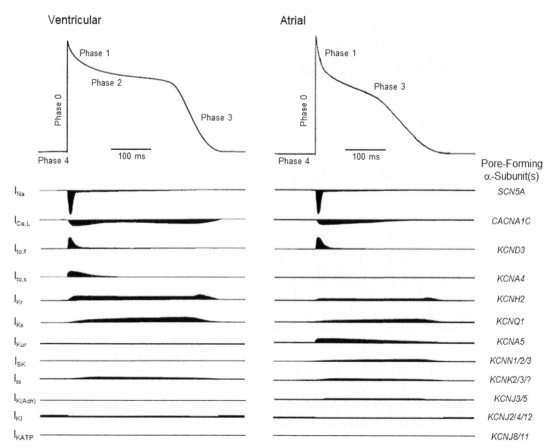

Fig. 1. Action potentials and underlying ionic currents in adult human ventricular and atrial myocytes. The major ionic currents shaping action potential waveforms in human atrial and ventricular myocytes are schematized. The names of the individual ionic currents are indicated to the left of the records, and the main pore-forming (α) subunits encoding the K$^+$ channel underlying these currents are indicated to the right of the records. There are differences in the relative expression levels of several of the repolarizing K$^+$ currents and/or in the relative contributions the various K$^+$ currents make to shaping action potential waveforms and controlling repolarization in ventricular and atrial myocytes.

dispersion of repolarization in the ventricles, reflect differences in the expression and/or the properties of inward Nav and Cav, as well as several outward K$^+$, channels.[1–3]

In contrast to the Nav and Cav channels, there are multiple types of cardiac K$^+$ channels, both voltage-gated K$^+$ (Kv) and non–voltage-gated, inwardly rectifying, K$^+$ (Kir) channels (**Table 1**)[5–7] encoded by Kv and Kir subunits (**Fig. 2**). As in other tissues and cell types, there are additional (non–voltage-gated) "leak" K$^+$ channels thought to be encoded by a novel class of K$^+$ channel (K2P) subunits with 2 pore domains (see **Fig. 2**), several of which are also expressed in the heart.[1] It is well-documented that changes in the densities, distributions, and properties of Kv and Kir channels are evident in a variety of myocardial diseases, and these changes alter repolarization, influence propagation, and decrease rhythmicity, effects

that can produce substrates for the generation of life-threatening arrhythmias.[1] Although less well studied, changes in K2P channel expression and/or function in inherited/acquired cardiac disease would also be expected to impact myocardial excitability and arrhythmia susceptibility.[1]

Considerable progress has been made in defining the biophysical properties, the functional roles, and the cell-type–specific differences in expression of the various myocardial K$^+$ currents (see **Table 1**). In addition, a large number of Kv, Kir, and K2P channel pore-forming (α) subunits[8] that encode the underlying K$^+$ current-carrying ion channels have been identified (see **Fig. 2**), and many of these are expressed in the heart.[1] Considerable progress also has been made in defining the relationships between expressed Kv and Kir α subunits and functional myocardial Kv and Kir channels, and studies completed to date

Table 1
Functional and molecular diversity of cardiac potassium currents

Channel Type	Current Name	Activation	Gating	Function	Pharmacology	Human α Subunit Gene	Chromosomal Location	α Subunit Protein	Auxiliary Subunits
Kv	$I_{to,f}$	Fast	Voltage	Plateau potential, repolarization	mM 4-AP, HaTX, HpTX, Ba^{2+}	KCND3	1p13.3	Kv4.3 or Kv4.2	KChIP2, DPP6/10, NCS-1 (minK, MiRP2/3 ?)
	$I_{to,s}$	Fast	Voltage	Plateau potential, repolarization	μM4-AP	KCNA4	11p14	Kv1.4	??
	I_{kr}	Fast	Voltage	Plateau potential, repolarization	E-4031, Dofetilide, NE-10064, NE-10133	KCNH2	7q36.1	Kv12.1 (hERG)	minK, MiRP1/2??
	I_{ks}	Slow	Voltage	Repolarization		KCNQ1	11p15.5	Kv7.1 (KvLQT1)	minK (MiRPs?)
	I_{kur} [$I_{K,slow2}$][a]	Fast	Voltage	Repolarization	μM 4-AP	KCNA5	12p13	Kv1.5	SAP97
		Slow	Voltage	Repolarization	mM TEA	[Kcnb1][b]	2H3	Kv2.1	Amigo?
K2P	[I_{ss}][a]	—	H⁺, fatty acids, anesthetics	Resting potential, repolarization, diastolic potential	mM TEA, A1899	[Kcnk2/3][b]	1q41, 2p23	K2p2 (TREK1)/k2p3 (TASK1)	??
	[I_{Kp}][c]	—	??	Resting potential, repolarization	Ba^{2+}	??	??	??	??
KCa	I_{SK}	Slow	Ca²⁺-Calmodulin	Repolarization	Apamin	KCNN1/2/3	19p13.1, 5q22.2,1q21.3	KCa2.1, KCa2.2, KCa2.3	??
KNa	I_{NaK}	Fast	Na	??[b]	Quinidine, Clofilium	KCNT1/2	9q34.3, 1q31.3	KNa1.1 (Slick), KNa1.2 (Slack)	??
Kir	I_{K1}	—	Spermines, Mg²⁺	Resting potential, diastolic potential	Ba^{2+}	KCNJ2/4/12	17q24.1, 17p11.2, 22q13.1	Kir2.1, Kir2.2, Kir2.3	??
	$I_{K(Ach)}$	—	Ach	Resting potential, diastolic potential	Tertiapin-Q	KCNJ3/5	2q24.1, 11q24	Kir3.1, Kir3.4	??
	$I_{K(ATP)}$	—	ATP, ADP	??[d]	SURs	KCNJ8/11	12p11.23, 11p15.1	Kir6.1, Kir6.2	SUR1/2

Abbreviations: 4-AP, 4-aminopyridine; HaTX, hanatoxin; HpTX, heteropodatoxin; SURs, sulfonylureas; TEA, tetraethylammonium.

[a] Current found in rodents, but has not, to date, been reported in human cardiac cells.
[b] Pore-forming subunit encoding K⁺ current in mouse heart.
[c] Current reported in guinea pig ventricular myocytes.
[d] Current has been suggested to function to hyperpolarize membrane potential under conditions of ischemia/metabolic stress.

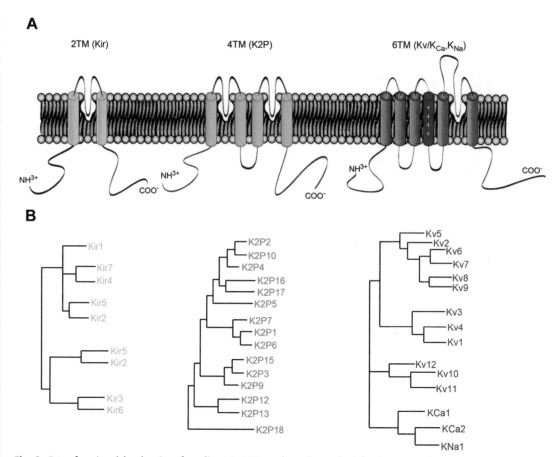

Fig. 2. Pore-forming (α) subunits of cardiac Kir, K2P, and Kv channels. (*A*) Schematics illustrating the transmembrane topologies of the α subunits encoding inwardly rectifying (Kir), 2-pore domain (K2P), and voltage-gated (Kv) K$^+$ channels. (*B*) Phylogenetic dendrograms of K$^+$ channel α subunits of the Kir, K2P, and Kv (including KCa and KNa) α subunit subfamilies.

have revealed that the various types of Kv and Kir channels distinguished electrophysiologically (see **Table 1**) are encoded by different α subunits.[1] To date, there have been many fewer studies focused on defining the functional correlates of expressed K2P subunits. A rather large number of K$^+$ channel, particularly Kv channel, accessory subunits also have been identified, and accumulating evidence suggests that myocardial K$^+$ channels,[9–12] like other types of ion channels,[13–16] likely function in macromolecular protein complexes comprising the pore-forming α subunits and one or more different types of (cytosolic or transmembrane) auxiliary proteins. Identification of the molecular components and the stoichiometric native myocardial Kv, Kir, and K2P channels is necessary for future studies focused on defining the mechanisms controlling regional differences in the expression of these channels in the normal myocardium, as well as the derangements in the expression/functioning of these channels associated with myocardial disease.

MYOCARDIAL Kv CHANNELS: TRANSIENT OUTWARD AND DELAYED RECTIFIER Kv CHANNELS

Voltage-gated K$^+$ (Kv) currents, activated on membrane depolarization, influence the amplitudes and durations of myocardial action potentials and, in most cardiac cell types, 2 broad classes of Kv currents have been distinguished: transient outward K$^+$ currents, I$_{to}$; and delayed, outwardly rectifying K$^+$ currents, I$_K$ (see **Table 1**). The transient currents (I$_{to}$) activate rapidly and underlie early (*phase 1*) repolarization, whereas the delayed rectifiers (I$_K$) determine the latter phase (*phase 3*) of membrane repolarization (see **Fig. 1**) back to the resting membrane potential.

These are broad classifications, however, and there are multiple functionally (and molecularly) distinct types of transient (I$_{to}$) and delayed rectifier (I$_K$) Kv currents (see **Table 1**) expressed in cardiac cells. Electrophysiologic and pharmacologic studies in mouse myocytes, for example, have revealed the presence of 2 types of rapidly activating and inactivating, "transient" outward K$^+$ currents, referred to as Ito,fast (I$_{to,f}$) and Ito,slow (I$_{to,s}$).[17] The rapidly activating and inactivating transient outward K$^+$ current, I$_{to,f}$, is also characterized by rapid recovery from inactivation, whereas I$_{to,s}$ recovers slowly.[17,18] In addition, I$_{to,f}$ is readily distinguished from other Kv currents, including I$_{to,s}$,[17,18] using the Heteropoda toxin-2 or toxin-3.[19]

Although originally identified in Purkinje fibers, I$_{to,f}$ is a prominent repolarizing Kv current in atrial and ventricular myocytes, as well as in nodal cells, in most species.[20–22] There are, however, marked regional differences in I$_{to,f}$ densities, with the highest densities typically in atrial myocytes.[21] In addition, I$_{to,f}$ and I$_{to,s}$ are differentially expressed in ventricular myocytes. In adult mouse ventricles, for example, I$_{to,f}$ density is higher in ventricular myocytes isolated from the right, compared with the left, ventricle and, within the left ventricle, I$_{to,f}$ densities are significantly higher in the apex than in the base.[17,18] In addition, all interventricular septum cells express I$_{to,s}$, and most ($\approx$80%) also express I$_{to,f}$.[17] When present, however, I$_{to,f}$ density is significantly (P<.001) lower in septum than in right or left ventricular, cells.[17,18] Also, I$_{to,s}$ is not detected in mouse heart cells other than septum cells.[17,18] I$_{to,f}$ and I$_{to,s}$ are also differentially expressed in ferret left ventricles, and I$_{to,s}$ is detected only in endocardial left ventricular cells.[23] In spite of heterogeneities in functional expression, the time-dependent and voltage-dependent properties of I$_{to,f}$ and I$_{to,s}$ in different cardiac cell types and species are remarkably similar, suggesting that the molecular determinants of the underlying (I$_{to,f}$ and I$_{to,s}$) channels are also similar.

Electrophysiologic and pharmacologic studies have also distinguished multiple types of cardiac delayed rectifier K$^+$ currents, I$_K$ (see **Table 1**). In atrial myocytes, for example, the dominant repolarizing K$^+$ current is a very rapidly activating (ultrarapid), noninactivating K$^+$ current, I$_{Kur}$ (IK,ultrarapid), which is not detected in ventricular or nodal cells.[1,5–7] In ventricular myocytes, in contrast, there are 2 prominent components of delayed rectification, I$_{Kr}$ (IK,rapid) and I$_{Ks}$ (IK,slow), that are distinct from I$_{Kur}$ in terms of time-dependent and voltage-dependent properties: I$_{Kr}$ activates and inactivates rapidly, and displays marked inward rectification, whereas I$_{Ks}$ activates slowly and is outwardly rectifying.[24] Similar to the transient outward K$^+$ currents, I$_{Ks}$ and I$_{Kr}$ are differentially expressed in the ventricular cells.[1,5] The density of I$_{Ks}$ in guinea pig left ventricular free wall is significantly higher in

subepicardial than in subendocardial or midmyocardial, cells.[25] At the base of the left ventricle, in contrast, I$_{Kr}$ and I$_{Ks}$ densities are lower in myocytes in the endocardium, compared with either midmyocardium or the epicardium.[25] Heterogeneities in I$_{Kr}$ and I$_{Ks}$ densities also contribute to the stereotypical differences in action potential waveforms recorded in different regions (eg, in atria and ventricles, right and left ventricles, apex and base of the ventricles) and through the thickness of the left and right ventricular free walls.[1,2]

In mouse ventricles, additional novel components of I$_K$, with properties distinct from I$_{Ks}$ and I$_{Kr}$, have also been identified (see **Table 1**) and referred to as IK,slow1, IK,slow2, and I$_{ss}$.[17,18,26,27] IK,slow1 is blocked by μM concentrations of 4-aminopyridine and appears to be indistinguishable from human atrial I$_{Kur}$, whereas IK,slow2 is blocked selectively by tetraethylammonium (see **Table 1**). In addition to being functionally distinct, IK,slow1 and IK,slow2 also reflect the expression of unique molecular entities.[28–31] An additional component of the total depolarization-activated outward K$^+$ current in mouse ventricular myocytes is noninactivating and has been referred to as Isteady-state or I$_{ss}$.[17,18] Similar currents are evident in voltage-clamp recordings from ventricular myocytes isolated from a number of other species, although, to date, these currents have not been extensively studied. In contrast to the differential distribution of I$_{to,f}$ and I$_{to,s}$, the densities of IK,slow1, IK,slow2, and I$_{ss}$ are similar in mouse atrial and ventricular myocytes.[17,18,27–32]

In addition to the Kv channels, it has recently been demonstrated that apamin-sensitive, small-conductance Ca^{2+}-dependent K$^+$ (I$_{SK}$) channels are also expressed in mammalian atrial myocytes.[33,34] Importantly, these channels have been shown to contribute to action potential repolarization in mouse atrial myocytes,[35] and dysregulation of I$_{SK}$ has been linked to atrial arrhythmias.[35,36] In addition, it has been reported that I$_{SK}$ is upregulated in ventricular myocytes in the failing heart, and it was suggested that this upregulation increases the susceptibility to ventricular arrhythmias.[37,38] A recent study has also suggested a role for large-conductance K$^+$ (BK) channels in mouse sino-atrial nodal cells,[39] although it is unclear whether there are BK channels in nodal cells in other species. In addition, Na$^+$-dependent K$^+$ channels have been described in (guinea pig) ventricular myocytes,[39] a channel that may be activated under conditions of elevated intracellular Na$^+$ and play a protective role.

INWARDLY RECTIFYING (Kir) MYOCARDIAL K⁺ CHANNELS

In addition to the Kv currents, inwardly rectifying K⁺ (Kir) currents, including I_{K1} and the ATP-dependent K⁺ current, I_{KATP} (see **Table 1**), are expressed in the mammalian myocardium.[33–35] Similar to the Kv currents, the densities of the Kir currents vary in different regions; that is, in atria, ventricles, and conducting tissue. In contrast to the Kv currents, however, myocardial Kir current densities are similar in myocytes in different regions of the ventricles.[1] In mammalian atrial and ventricular myocytes, I_{K1} is thought to play a role in establishing resting membrane potentials and plateau potentials, and to contribute to phase 3 repolarization (see **Fig. 1**). The fact that I_{K1} conductance is high at negative membrane potentials has been suggested to be important in the establishment of the relatively hyperpolarized resting membrane potentials of ventricular and atrial myocytes.[40] Although the properties of I_{K1} channels are such that conductance is low at potentials positive to −40 mV, these channels do contribute outward K⁺ currents during the action plateau potential, as well as during phase 3 repolarization,[40] potentials at which the driving force on K⁺ is high.

In contrast with I_{K1} channels, myocardial ATP-dependent K⁺ channels are weakly inwardly rectifying, and these channels are inhibited by intracellular ATP and activated by nucleotide diphosphates, suggesting a link between I_{KATP} channels and cell metabolism.[41] In ventricular myocytes, activation of I_{KATP} channels during periods of hypoxia/ischemia results in action potential shortening,[41–43] and the opening of I_{KATP} channels is thought to contribute to cardioprotection in ischemic preconditioning.[42–45] Interestingly, and in contrast with I_{K1} (and Kv) channels, however, I_{KATP} channels have high single channel conductance, such that activation of only a few I_{KATP} channels is expected to result in marked action potential shortening.[41] I_{KATP} channels appear to be distributed uniformly and at high density[41,43] in the right and left ventricles and through the thicknesses of the right and left ventricular walls.

Acetylcholine, which is released on stimulation of the vagus, has negative chronotropic and inotropic effects on the heart, mediated by activation of acetylcholine (Ach)-regulated K⁺ channels, I_{KAch}.[46] In atrial myocytes, application of Ach reveals large conductance inwardly rectifying K⁺ channels, a process that requires GTP[47] and is mediated by the βδ subunits of heterotrimeric GTP-binding proteins.[48] Interestingly, although the expression of I_{KAch} in atrial and nodal cells has long been appreciated, it is also clear that I_{KAch} channels are expressed in ventricular myocytes.[49] In addition, although somewhat less sensitive to Ach than atrial or nodal I_{KAch} channels, the properties of single ventricular I_{KAch} channels are similar to atrial/nodal I_{KAch},[49] suggesting that the molecular determinants of I_{KAch} channels in different cardiac cell types and in different species are the same. It is also of interest to note that accumulating evidence indicates that I_{KAch} channels can be open (ie, constitutively active) in the absence of Ach,[50] suggesting a role for these channels under baseline conditions.

PORE-FORMING (α) AND ACCESSORY/ AUXILIARY SUBUNITS OF MYOCARDIAL K⁺ CHANNELS

Multiple K⁺ channel pore-forming (α) subunits have been identified in the genome, and these have been organized into subfamilies based on sequence and structural similarities (see **Fig. 2**). Kv channel α subunits are 6 transmembrane spanning domain proteins (see **Fig. 2**) with a region between the fifth and sixth transmembrane domains that contributes to the K⁺- selective pore.[8] The positively charged fourth transmembrane domain in the Kv α subunits (see **Fig. 2**) is homologous to the corresponding regions in Nav and Cav channel α subunits, placing them in the "S4" superfamily of voltage-gated channels.[8] In contrast to Nav and Cav channels, in which only a single α subunit is required to form a channel, however, functional Kv channels comprise 4 α subunits. Similar to the diversity of functional myocardial Kv channels (see **Table 1**), multiple Kv α subunits in several distinct Kv α subunit subfamilies,[8] including Kv1.x, Kv2.x, Kv3.x, Kv4.x (see **Fig. 2**), have been identified. In addition, many of the individual Kv α subunits in several different subfamilies have been shown to be expressed in the mammalian heart.[1] Further functional Kv channel diversity could arise through alternative splicing of transcripts, as well as through the formation of heteromultimeric channels between 2 or more Kv α subunit proteins in the same Kv α subunit subfamily,[1,8] although the physiologic roles of alternative splicing and heteromeric assembly of Kv α subunits in the generation of native cardiac Kv channels remain to be determined.

Additional subfamilies of Kv α subunits were revealed with the cloning of the human eag-related (HERG) gene, KCNH2, which encodes the Kv11.1 α subunit and has been identified as the locus of mutations underlying familial long-QT syndrome type 2 (LQt2) and KCNQ1, which encodes Kv7.1, the locus of mutations in another inherited long-QT syndrome, LQT1.[51] Expression of Kv11.1 in heterologous cells reveals inwardly rectifying Kv currents[51] with properties similar to cardiac I$_{Kr}$ (see **Table 1**). Although expression of *KCNQ1* (Kv7.1) in heterologous cells reveals rapidly activating, non-inactivating Kv currents, the addition of the Kv channel accessory subunit, minK, results in the production of slowly activating Kv currents[43] that resemble the slow component of cardiac delayed rectification, I$_{Ks}$. Additional Kv α subunit gene subfamilies that underlie the generation of Ca^{2+} and Na$^+$ regulated K$^+$ channels also have been identified (see **Fig. 2**). Structurally much simpler than the Kv α subunits, the inwardly rectifying K$^+$ (Kir) α subunits have only 2 transmembrane domains flanking the pore region (see **Fig. 2**). Similar to the Kv family, however, there are multiple subfamilies of Kir α subunits. The Kir2.x subfamily members underlie I$_{K1}$, whereas the Kir6 and Kir3 subfamilies generate I$_{KATP}$ and I$_{KAch}$ channels, respectively. Another novel type of K$^+$ channel α subunit (K2P) with 4 transmembrane-spanning regions and 2 pore domains (see **Fig. 2**) was identified with the cloning of TWIK-1.[52] Both pore domains contribute to the formation of the K$^+$ selective pore, and TWIK-1 subunits assemble as dimers,[52] rather than as tetramers, like the Kir and Kv channels. Like the Kir and Kv subunits, however, a large number of 2 pore domain K$^+$ (K2P) channel α subunit genes also have been identified (see **Fig. 2**), and several of these are expressed in the mammalian myocardium.[53] Heterologous expression of K2P subunits reveals currents with distinct biophysical properties and sensitivities to several potential intracellular and extracellular modulators, including anesthetics, pH, and fatty acids.[53]

In addition to the Kv α subunits, a number of Kv channel accessory (Kv β) subunits also have been identified. The first of these was *KCNE1*, which encodes a small (130 amino acid) protein (minK) with a single transmembrane spanning domain.[54] It appears that minK coassembles with Kv7.1 (KvLQT1) to form functional cardiac I$_{Ks}$ channels.[51] Additional minK homologues, MiRP1 (*KCNE2*), MiRP2 (*KCNE3*), and MiRP3 (*KCNE4*) also have been identified, and it has been suggested that MiRP1 (*KCNE2*) functions as an accessory subunit coassembling with Kv11.1 to generate cardiac I$_{Kr}$.[55] It also has been reported that the MiRP subunits interact with multiple Kv α subunit subfamilies and modify channel properties.[54] MiRP2, for example, coassembles with Kv3.4 in mammalian skeletal muscle[56] and MiRP1 coassembles with Kv4.x α subunits when coexpressed in heterologous cells.[57] These observations suggest that the MiRP (*KCNE*)

accessory subunits can assemble with a variety of Kv α subunits and contribute to the formation of multiple types of myocardial Kv channels. Direct experimental support for this hypothesis, however, has not been provided to date, and the roles of the various *KCNE* subunits in the generation of functional cardiac Kv (or other) channels remain to be identified.

Several cytosolic accessory Kvβ subunits, Kvβ1, Kvβ2, and Kvβ3, first identified in brain[58] as well as alternatively spliced transcripts, are expressed in heart,[1] and biochemical studies suggest that Kvβ subunits interact with the intracellular domains of Kv1 α subunits and alter the time-dependent and voltage-dependent properties and the cell surface expression of Kv1 α subunit-encoded Kv currents.[58] Although Kvβ1 and Kvβ2 reportedly associate with Kv4 α subunits in the mouse myocardium and the targeted deletion of Kvβ1 results in the attenuation of Kv4-encoded I$_{to,f}$ in mouse ventricular myocytes,[59] the role(s) of Kvβ subunits in the generation of myocardial Kv channels in other species has not been explored.

There are 4 Kv Channel Interacting Proteins, KChIP1-4 in brain,[60] although only KChIP2 is expressed in heart.[60,61] KChIP2, like the other KChIPs, belongs to the recoverin family of neuronal Ca^{2+}-sensing (NCS) proteins,[62] containing 4 EF-hand domains.[60] There are multiple splice variants of KChIP2 in heart,[63–65] although the relative abundances of these variants, particularly in the human heart, and the functional significance of splicing are not known. When coexpressed with Kv4 α subunits, the KChIPs increase K$^+$ current densities, slow inactivation, speed recovery from inactivation, and shift the voltage-dependence of current activation.[60] Although KCHIP2 does not appear to affect non–Kv4-encoded K$^+$ channels, it has been reported that loss of KChIP2 affects myocardial Cav channels.[27,66] In addition, although KChIP binding to Kv4 α subunits does not appear to be Ca^{2+}-dependent, mutations in EF-hand domains 2, 3, and 4 eliminate the modulatory effects of KChIP1 on Kv4-encoded Kv currents,[60] suggesting a role for voltage-dependent Ca^{2+} entry and intracellular Ca^{2+} levels in the regulation of functional cardiac (Kv4-encoded) I$_{to,f}$ channels, as has been demonstrated for neuronal Kv4-encoded channels.[67]

The transmembrane diaminopeptidyl transferase-like proteins (DPP6 and DPP10) have also been suggested to be an accessory subunit of cardiac[68] and neuronal[69] Kv4-encoded channels. Coexpression with DPP6 increases the cell surface expression of Kv4 α subunits, shifts the voltage dependences of Kv4-encoded current activation and inactivation, and accelerates the rates of current activation, inactivation, and recovery.[68,69] Interestingly, heterologous coexpression of DPP6 with Kv4.3 and KChIP2, produces Kv currents that closely resemble native cardiac $I_{to,f}$.[68] DPP10, which has been demonstrated to associate with Kv4.2 and KChIP3 in brain and to have regulatory effects similar to DPP6 on heterologously expressed Kv4,[70,71] is expressed in human ventricles.[72] The expression levels of both DPP6 and DPP10, however, are quite low in the heart, raising some concern about the likely physiologic relevance of DPP6- (or DPP10-) mediated regulation of cardiac $I_{to,f}$ channels. Interestingly, however, it was recently suggested that the molecular compositions of $I_{to,f}$ channels in ventricular and Purkinje cells are distinct, and that DPP6 plays a unique role in the generation of Purkinje cell (but not ventricular) $I_{to,f}$ channels.[73] A selective role for Neuronal Calcium Sensor-1 (NCS-1), previously shown to associate with Kv4 α subunits in mouse ventricles,[74] was also suggested to play a role (with DPP6) in the generation of $I_{to,f}$ in canine (and human) Purkinje cells.[73]

MOLECULAR DETERMINANTS OF NATIVE MYOCARDIAL Kv CHANNELS

Critical insights into the roles of individual Kv α subunits or subunit subfamilies in the generation of native cardiac Kv channels were provided in studies of $I_{to,f}$ channels in rat and mouse ventricular myocytes. Using antisense oligodeoxynucleotides (AsODNs) targeted against Kv4.2 or Kv4.3, for example, it was shown that $I_{to,f}$ density is selectively reduced by approximately 50%.[75,76] Rat ventricular $I_{to,f}$ density was also reduced in cells exposed to an adenoviral construct encoding a truncated Kv4.2 subunit (Kv4.2ST) that functions as a dominant negative.[77] In addition, $I_{to,f}$ was eliminated in ventricular and atrial myocytes isolated from transgenic mice expressing a dominant negative Kv4.2 pore mutant, Kv4.2W362 F (Kv4.2DN).[78,79] Although biochemical and electrophysiologic studies suggested that Kv4.2 and Kv4.3 are associated in mouse ventricles and that functional mouse ventricular $I_{to,f}$ channels are heteromeric,[76] targeted deletion of Kv4.2 eliminates mouse ventricular $I_{to,f}$,[80] whereas elimination of Kv4.3 has no measureable effects.[81] In mouse ventricles, therefore, Kv4.2 is the critical α subunit required for the generation of functional $I_{to,f}$ channels.[80,81] Given the similarities in the time-dependent and voltage-dependent properties of the fast transient currents in other species, it seems reasonable to suggest that Kv 4 α

subunits also underlie $I_{to,f}$ in other species. In canine and in human myocardium, however, the candidate subunit is Kv4.3, rather than Kv4.2.[82] Although 2 splice variants of Kv4.3 have been identified,[83] the expression levels of the 2 predicted Kv4.3 proteins and the functional roles of these variants in the generation of functional cardiac $I_{to,f}$ channels have not been determined.

The Kv channel accessory subunit KChIP2 coimmunoprecipitates with Kv4 α subunits from adult mouse ventricles, consistent with a role in the generation of Kv4-encoded mouse ventricular $I_{to,f}$ channels.[76] In ferret heart, a gradient in KChIP2 message expression is observed through the thickness of the ventricular wall,[64] leading to suggestions that the differential expression of KChIP2 underlies the epicardial-endocardial differences in $I_{to,f}$ densities. The patterns of expression of the KChIP2 message, the KChIP2 protein and $I_{to,f}$ densities are similar in canine ventricles,[84] consistent with an important role for KChIP2 in determining functional canine, as well as human, ventricular $I_{to,f}$ densities. In contrast, in rat and mouse ventricles, there is little or no gradient in KChIP2[80,85] expression, and it appears that regional differences in Kv4.2 expression underlie the heterogeneities in $I_{to,f}$ densities in rodent ventricles.[85,86] Molecular insights into the regulation of regional variations in Kv4.2 (transcript) expression were provided with the demonstrations that expression of the transcription factors, Irx5 and NFAT, are positively and negatively (respectively) correlated with the differences in Kv4.2 expression and $I_{to,f}$ densities.[87,88] Interestingly, approximately 25 transcription factors have been shown to be differentially expressed in the ventricles.[89]

Functional analysis of the role of KChIP2 in the generation of $I_{to,f}$ revealed that the targeted deletion of KChIP2 results in the elimination of $I_{to,f}$[27,90] and, interestingly, the complete loss of the Kv4.2 protein.[27] Additional putative channel regulatory proteins, including the voltage-gated Nav channel accessory subunit 1, Navβ1,[91] and semaphorin 3A,[92] have been shown to associate with Kv4 α subunits and suggested to function in the generation of native Kv4-encoded channels. The functional roles of these and other putative Kv4 channel accessory subunits, including the *KCNE* and *DPPX* subunits, in the generation of native myocardial $I_{to,f}$ channels and/or in determining regional differences in myocardial $I_{to,f}$ densities remain to be defined. Although accumulating evidence suggests that cardiac $I_{to,f}$ channels function in macromolecular complexes, comprising Kv4 α subunits and multiple cytosolic and transmembrane accessory subunits (**Fig. 3**), the molecular composition(s) of native

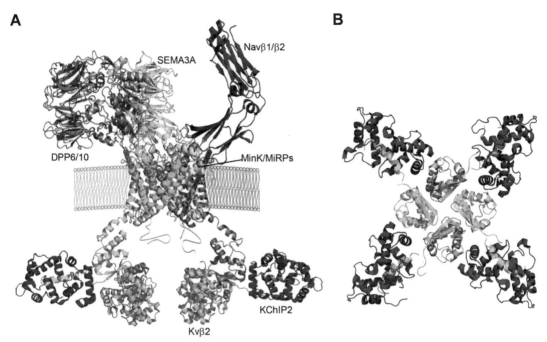

Fig. 3. Native Kv4.3-encoded, myocardial $I_{to,f}$ channels function in macromolecular protein complexes. (*A*) Cross section of a schematized cardiac $I_{to,f}$ channel complex in a membrane showing 2 Kv4.3 α subunits (blue), generated based on the structure of Kv1.2,[124] each interacting with a cytosolic KChIP2 (red) and a cytosolic Kvβ (green) accessory subunit (in a 1:1:1 stoichiometry) through distinct, nonoverlapping N-terminal domains. The transmembrane accessory subunits, DPP6/10[125] (brown), MinK/MiRPs (yellow), and Navβ1/Navβ2 (red), which also have been proposed to interact with Kv4.3 α subunits (each illustrated in a 2:1 stoichiometry) and to contribute to the formation of native Kv4-encoded channels, are also shown. (*B*) Structural analyses of Kv4.3N-KChIP1 complexes[126] revealed a 1:1 stoichiometry with each KChIP (red) bridging 2 adjacent Kv4.3 N termini (blue) and anchoring each hydrophobic Kv4.3 N terminus in a hydrophobic KChIP1 binding pocket. Protein structures illustrated were generated based on published structural data using PyMOL.

myocardial $I_{to,f}$ channels have not been determined directly.

The kinetic and pharmacologic properties of the slow transient outward K⁺ currents, $I_{to,s}$, in ventricular myocytes are quite different from $I_{to,f}$ (see **Table 1**), observations interpreted as suggesting that the molecular correlates of ventricular $I_{to,s}$ and $I_{to,f}$ channels are also distinct. Direct experimental support for this hypothesis was provided in electrophysiologic experiments on myocytes isolated from mice with a targeted deletion of the Kv1.4 gene, Kv1.4$^{-/-}$,[93] demonstrating that $I_{to,s}$ is undetectable in septum cells.[94] The properties and the densities of $I_{to,f}$, IK,slow1, IK,slow2, and I_{ss} in Kv1.4$^{-/-}$ left and right ventricular (and in atrial) myocytes, however, are indistinguishable from those in wild-type cells.[94] Interestingly, upregulation of $I_{to,s}$ is evident in the ventricles of Kv4.2DN-expressing mice in which $I_{to,f}$ is eliminated,[78] and this upregulation (of $I_{to,s}$) is eliminated on crossing Kv4.2DN with Kv1.4$^{-/-}$ mice.[95] Given the similarities in the time-dependent and voltage-dependent properties of the slow transient

outward K⁺ currents in other species with mouse $I_{to,s}$,[1] it seems reasonable to suggest that Kv1.4 likely also encodes $I_{to,s}$ in ferret, rabbit, and perhaps human, ventricular myocytes.

Heterologous expression of ERG1 reveals voltage-gated, inwardly rectifying K⁺-selective channels that are similar to cardiac I_{Kr}.[51] Alternatively processed forms of ERG1, with unique N-termini and C-termini, also have been identified in mouse and human heart and suggested to play roles in the generation of native cardiac I_{Kr} channels.[96–98] It also has been suggested that functional cardiac I_{Kr} channels are multimeric, comprising ERG1 and minK, and biochemical studies have demonstrated coimmunoprecipitation of ERG1 and minK from equine ventricles.[99] It is presently not clear, however, if ERG1 and minK or other members of the KCNE family are also found in association in other species.

Although heterologous expression of *KCNQ1*, the locus of mutations in LQT1, reveals rapidly activating, noninactivating Kv currents, coexpression with minK produces slowly activating Kv currents similar to cardiac I_{Ks}.[51] These observations, together with biochemical data demonstrating that heterologously expressed KvLQT1 and minK associate, were interpreted as suggesting that minK coassembles with KvLQT1 to form functional cardiac I_{Ks} channels.[51] Biochemical evidence for the in situ coassembly of KvLQT1 and minK in equine ventricles has been reported,[99] although similar data for human ventricular I_{Ks} has yet to be provided. Unexpectedly, however, it has been reported that KvLQT1 modulates the distribution and properties of ERG1-encoded channels, an observation interpreted as suggesting that cardiac I_{Ks} and I_{Kr} channels are regulated through direct Kv α subunit–Kv α subunit interactions.[100] The mechanisms controlling the cell surface expression of functional I_{Ks} channels, the regional differences in I_{Ks} densities, and the interaction(s) between I_{Ks} and I_{Kr} remain to be determined.

Similar to the transient outward Kv currents, molecular methods, in combination with biochemistry and electrophysiology, have provided insights into the molecular basis of functional delayed rectifier Kv channel diversity in the mouse myocardium. A role for Kv1 α subunits in the generation of mouse ventricular IK,slow1, for example, was suggested by the observation that IK,slow is selectively attenuated in ventricular myocytes isolated from transgenic mice expressing a truncated, dominant negative Kv1 α subunit, Kv1.1DN.[101] It was subsequently shown, however, that IK,slow is also reduced in ventricular myocytes expressing a dominant negative Kv 2.1 mutant, Kv2.1DN,[28] revealing that there are 2, molecularly distinct components of mouse ventricular IK,slow: IK,slow1, which is sensitive to μM concentrations of 4-aminopyridine and encoded by Kv1 α subunits and IK,slow2, which is sensitive to TEA and encoded by Kv2 α subunits.[28] Subsequent studies revealed that IK,slow1 is eliminated in ventricular myocytes isolated from mice harboring the targeted disruption of the KCNA5 (Kv1.5) locus, revealing that Kv1.5 encodes IK,slow1.[29] These findings, together with the previous studies completed on cells from Kv1.4$^{-/-}$ animals,[93] in which $I_{to,s}$ is eliminated,[94] reveal that, in contrast to the Kv 4 α subunits, Kv4.2 and Kv4.3,[76] the Kv 1 α subunits, Kv1.4 and Kv1.5, do not associate in adult mouse ventricles in situ. Rather, functional Kv1 α subunit-encoded Kv channels in mouse ventricular myocytes are homomeric, composed of Kv1.4 α subunits ($I_{to,s}$)[93] or Kv1.5 α subunits (IK,slow1).[29] The role(s) of Kv accessory subunits in the generation of native $I_{to,s}$, IK,slow1, and IK,slow2 channels and the mechanisms controlling the expression of these channels remain to be determined.

MOLECULAR DETERMINANTS OF NATIVE MYOCARDIAL Kir AND K2P CHANNELS

Inwardly rectifying K$^+$ channels in cardiac and other cells are encoded by a large and diverse subfamily of inward rectifier K$^+$ (Kir) channel pore-forming α subunit genes,[8] each of which encodes a protein with 2 transmembrane domains (see **Fig. 2**) that assemble as tetramers to form K$^+$ selective pores. Based on the properties of the currents produced in heterologous expression systems, Kir2 α subunits were long thought to encode the strongly inwardly rectifying cardiac I_{K1} channels,[102] and several members of the Kir 2 subfamily are expressed in the myocardium.[1] Direct insights into the role(s) of Kir 2 α subunits in the generation of cardiac I_{K1} channels was provided in studies completed on myocytes isolated from mice lacking KCNJ2 (Kir2.1$^{-/-}$) or KCNJ12 (Kir2.2$^{-/-}$).[103] Although Kir2.1$^{-/-}$ mice have cleft palate and die shortly after birth, precluding electrophysiologic studies on adult myocytes, voltage-clamp recordings from newborn Kir2.1$^{-/-}$ ventricular myocytes revealed that I_{K1} is absent, whereas I_{K1} was reduced (but not eliminated) in adult Kir2.2$^{-/-}$ ventricular myocytes,[103] suggesting that both Kir2.1 and Kir2.2 contribute to (mouse) ventricular I_{K1} and that functional cardiac I_{K1} channels are heteromeric. The quantitative differences between the effects of the deletion of KCNJ2 and KCNJ12 further suggest that Kv2.1 (KCNJ2) is the critical subunit underlying native (mouse) I_{K1} channels.[103]

Mutations in KCNJ2 have been linked to congenital long QT (Andersen-Tawil syndrome or LQT7), as well as short QT, syndromes,[104,105] and increasing expression of Kir2.1 in the mouse heart, which results in the upregulation of I_{K1}, is proarrhythmic.[106,107] Previous studies have identified regional differences in myocardial I_{K1} expression and properties in adult mouse heart[108,109] and it has been suggested that these differences reflect the variable subunit composition(s) of the channels, as well as differences in polyamine concentrations.[110] Studies focused on testing these hypotheses directly and on defining the mechanisms controlling regional differences in the expression and functioning of native I_{K1} channels in species other than mice are also clearly warranted.

In the heart, I_{KATP} channels appear not to contribute to action potential repolarization, but rather are thought to be important in myocardial ischemia and preconditioning.[41,42] In heterologous cells, I$_{KATP}$ channels can be reconstituted by coexpression of Kir6.x subunits with the accessory ATP-binding cassette sulfonylurea receptors, SURx, proteins.[111] Cardiac sarcolemmal I$_{KATP}$ channels are encoded by Kir6.2 and SUR2A, and the essential role of Kir6.2 was demonstrated directly in experiments on ventricular myocytes from Kir6.2$^{-/-}$ animals.[112]

In addition, cardiac I$_{KATP}$ channel activity is reduced in SUR2$^{-/-}$ myocytes[113] and unaffected in SUR1$^{-/-}$ myocytes,[114] suggesting an important role for SUR2. Interestingly, the properties of the residual I$_{KATP}$ channels in SUR2$^{-/-}$ myocytes are similar to those produced in heterologous cells on coexpression of Kir6.2 and SUR1,[113] suggesting that SUR1 may also contribute to the generation of cardiac I$_{KATP}$ channels by coassembling with Kir6.2 α subunits alone or in combination with SUR2A.

Although action potential waveforms in Kir6.2$^{-/-}$ and wild-type ventricular myocytes are indistinguishable, the action potential shortening observed in wild-type cells during ischemia is not observed in Kir6.2$^{-/-}$ myocytes.[112] Action potential durations are also largely unaffected in transgenic animals expressing mutant I$_{KATP}$ channels with markedly (40-fold) reduced ATP sensitivity, suggesting that there are also additional inhibitory mechanisms that regulate cardiac I$_{KATP}$ channel activity in vivo.[115] Similar to myocardial I$_{K1}$ channels, further studies focused on defining the mechanisms controlling the regional differences in the expression and properties of myocardial I$_{KATP}$ channels will be of interest.

The multiplicity of K2P α subunits, the widespread distribution of expressed subunits, and the finding(s) that the properties of the channels encoded by K2P subunits are regulated by a variety of physiologically (and pathophysiologically) relevant stimuli[52,53] suggest that K2P channels likely subserve a variety of important functions. As in other cell types, the physiologic roles of these subunits/channels in the myocardium are just beginning to be explored. The transcripts encoding TREK-1 and TASK-1 are detected in heart, and heterologous expression of either of these subunits gives rise to instantaneous, noninactivating K$^+$ currents that display little or no voltage dependence.[116,117] These properties suggest that K2P subunits likely contribute to "background" or "leak" K$^+$ channels; that is, channels with properties similar to the "steady-state" noninactivating K$^+$ current (I$_{ss}$) characterized in adult mouse and rat ventricular myocytes.[17,18,116–119] Clearly, experiments focused on testing these hypotheses directly are needed to provide clear insights into the molecular basis of I$_{ss}$ and to allow further studies focused on defining the mechanisms controlling the physiologic and the pathophysiologic regulation of these (I$_{ss}$) channels.

MECHANISMS CONTRIBUTING TO THE MOLECULAR REGULATION OF MYOCARDIAL K$^+$ CHANNELS

Considerable evidence suggests that multiple mechanisms contribute to the regulation of myocardial K$^+$ channel expression and functioning.[120] These include transcriptional mechanisms to control the temporal and spatial expression of K$^+$ channel pore-forming and accessory subunits and regulatory proteins during normal development and in response to myocardial damage or disease. Interestingly, signaling pathways, such as signaling mediated by phosphoinositide 3-kinase, also have been linked to transcriptional regulation of multiple cardiac K$^+$ channels.[121] Similarly, posttranscriptional/translational mechanisms, including pre-mRNA processing, RNA editing, microRNAs, and, perhaps other noncoding RNAs, also have been linked to the regulation of functional myocardial K$^+$ channel expression.[120] The various K$^+$ channel subunit proteins also are potential targets for posttranslational modifications, such as phosphorylation, sumoylation, glycosylation, and palmitoylation, and/or associations with membrane lipids, each of which has been implicated in the regulation of myocardial K$^+$ channel stability, trafficking, and functioning.[120] In addition, considerable evidence suggests that K$^+$ channel subunit expression levels are regulated epigenetically; that is, by modifications, such as methylation, through mechanisms that involve changes in DNA structure (and resulting transcription), but not changes in DNA sequences.[120] Future studies focused on defining the roles of each of these mechanisms in the generation and regulation of myocardial K$^+$ (and other) channels will be of considerable interest and import.

SUMMARY, OPEN QUESTIONS, AND FUTURE CHALLENGES

Cellular electrophysiologic studies have distinguished multiple types of voltage-gated inward and outward currents that contribute to action potential repolarization in mammalian cardiac cells (see **Table 1**). The outward (K$^+$) currents are more numerous and more diverse than the inward (Na$^+$, Ca^{2+}) currents, and most cardiac cells express a repertoire of voltage-gated and non–voltage-gated K$^+$ channels (see **Table 1**). In addition, some of these K$^+$ channels are expressed differentially in the heart, contributing to regional and cell-type–specific differences in action potential waveforms. Multiple voltage-gated (Kv), non–voltage-gated, inwardly rectifying (Kir) and weakly rectifying, noninactivating (K2P) K^+ channel pore-forming α subunits and a number of channel accessory (β) subunits have been identified and suggested to play roles in the generation of the native K^+ channels (see **Table 1**). Indeed, considerable progress has been made in identifying the pore-forming Kv and Kir α subunits (see **Fig. 2**) contributing to the formation of most of the K^+ channels expressed in mammalian cardiac myocytes. In addition, biochemical studies have provided some insights into the molecular mechanisms underlying the observed heterogeneities in the expression of myocardial Kv and Kir currents. For cardiac $I_{to,f}$, for example, regional differences in current densities are correlated with differences in Kv4.2 protein expression in rodents,[86] whereas variable expression of the $I_{to,f}$ channel accessory protein, KChIP2, has been suggested to underlie the transmural gradient in $I_{to,f}$ densities in canine and human ventricles.[61,84] For cardiac I_{K1} channels, in contrast, recent studies suggest that differences in Kir channel α subunit composition and/or differences in the concentrations of intracellular polyamines play roles in regulating the functional diversity of these channels.[40]

Considerable evidence suggests that native myocardial K^+ channels, like other ion channels,[13–16] likely function in macromolecular protein complexes (see **Fig. 3**), comprising pore-forming α subunits and multiple cytosolic and transmembrane accessory/regulatory subunits, although the molecular composition(s) of native myocardial K^+ channels have not been determined directly to date. In addition, and in contrast to the progress made in defining the α subunits encoding native myocardial K^+ channels/currents, very little is known about the functional roles of most of the K^+ channel auxiliary subunits that have been identified. An important focus of future work will likely be on defining the physiologic roles of the many K^+ channel accessory subunits in the generation of native myocardial K^+ channels and on defining the molecular mechanisms controlling the properties and the cell surface expression of native cardiac K^+ channels. In addition, as numerous studies have documented changes in functional K^+ channel expression in a variety of myocardial disease states, changes that could reflect modifications in channel properties, as well as alterations in the molecular compositions of the channels and/or in the (posttranslational) processing of the underlying channel subunits, it seems clear that a major focus of future research will be on defining

these mechanisms in detail. As discussed previously, there are a number of possible mechanisms, including transcriptional, posttranscriptional, translational, posttranslational, and epigenetic, that may play roles in regulating the functional expression and the biophysical properties of myocardial K^+ channels in the normal, as well as in the damaged or diseased, myocardium. Efforts to explore these mechanisms in depth will likely be enhanced by the increased availability and application of induced pluripotent stem cell–derived cardiac myocytes.[122,123] In addition to providing new insights into the molecular determinants of native cardiac K^+ channel functioning, studies focused on defining these mechanisms will facilitate efforts to develop novel therapeutic strategies to prevent or reverse K^+ channel remodeling associated with systemic or myocardial disease.

REFERENCES

1. Nerbonne JM, Kass RS. Molecular physiology of cardiac repolarization. Physiol Rev 2005;85: 1205–53.
2. Rudy Y. Modelling the molecular basis of cardiac repolarization. Europace 2007;9:vi17–9.
3. Amin AS, Tan HL, Wilde AA. Cardiac ion channels in health and disease. Heart Rhythm 2010; 7:117–26.
4. Magyar J, Banyas T, Szentandrassy N, et al. Role of gap junction channel in the development of beat-to-beat action potential repolarization variability and arrhythmias. Curr Pharm Des 2015;21: 1042–52.
5. Anumonwo JMB, Freeman LC, Kwok WM, et al. Potassium channels in the heart: electrophysiology and pharmacological regulation. Cardiovasc Drug Rev 1991;9:299–316.
6. Mitcheson JS, Sanguinetti MC. Biophysical properties and molecular basis of cardiac rapid and delayed rectifier potassium channels. Cell Physiol Biochem 1999;9:201–16.
7. Snyders DJ. Structure and function of cardiac potassium channels. Cardiovasc Res 1999;42: 377–90.
8. Coetzee WA, Amarillo Y, Chiu J, et al. Molecular diversity of K^+ channels. Ann N Y Acad Sci 1999; 868:233–85.
9. Marx SO, Kurokawa J, Reiken S, et al. Requirement of a macromolecular signaling complex for β adrenergic receptor modulation of the KCNQ1-KCNE1 potassium channel. Science 2002;295: 496–9.
10. Abbott GW, Xu X, Roepke TK. Impact of ancillary subunits on ventricular repolarization. J Electrocardiol 2007;40:S42–6.

11. Oudit GY, Kassiri Z, Sah R, et al. The molecular physiology of the cardiac transient outward potassium current (I_{to}) in normal and diseased myocardium. J Mol Cell Cardiol 2001;33:851–72.

12. Niwa N, Nerbonne JM. Molecular determinants of cardiac transient outward K$^+$ current (I_{to}) expression and regulation. J Mol Cell Cardiol 2010;48: 12–25.

13. Abriel H, Kass RS. Regulation of the voltage-gated cardiac sodium channel Nav1.5 by interacting proteins. Trends Cardiovasc Med 2005;15:35–40.

14. Abriel H. Cardiac sodium channel Na$_v$1.5 and interacting proteins: physiology and pathophysiology. J Mol Cell Cardiol 2010;48:2–11.

15. Dai S, Hall DD, Hell JW. Supramolecular assemblies and localized regulation of voltage- gated ion channels. Physiol Rev 2009;89:411–52.

16. Hund TJ, Mohler PJ. Na$_v$ channel complex heterogeneity: new targets for the treatment of arrhythmias? Circulation 2014;130:132–4.

17. Xu H, Guo W, Nerbonne JM. Four kinetically distinct depolarization-activated K+ currents in adult mouse ventricular myocytes. J Gen Physiol 1999; 113:661–78.

18. Brunet S, Aimond F, Li H, et al. Heterogeneous expression of repolarizing voltage-gated K$^+$ currents in adult mouse ventricles. J Physiol 2004; 559:103–20.

19. Sanguinetti MC, Johnson JH, Hammerland LG, et al. Heteropodatoxins: peptides isolated from spider venom that block Kv4.2 potassium channels. Mol Pharmacol 1997;51:491–8.

20. Campbell DL, Rasmusson RL, Comer MB, et al. The cardiac calcium independent transient outward potassium current: kinetics, molecular properties, and role in ventricular repolarization. In: Zipes DP, Jalife J, editors. Cardiac electrophysiology: from cell to bedside. 2nd edition. Philadelphia: W.B. Saunders Co; 1995. p. 83–96.

21. Giles WR, Clark RB, Braun AP. Ca^{2+}-independent transient outward current in mammalian heart. In: Morad M, Kurachi Y, Noma A, et al, editors. Molecular physiology and pharmacology of cardiac ion channels and transporters. Amsterdam: Klewer Press Ltd; 1996. p. 141–68.

22. Patel SP, Campbell DL. Transient outward potassium current, "I_{to}", phenotypes in the left ventricle: underlying molecular, cellular and biophysical mechanisms. J Physiol 2005;569:7–39.

23. Brahmajothi MV, Campbell DL, Rasmussen RL, et al. Distinct transient outward potassium current (Ito) phenotypes and distribution of fast-inactivating potassium channel alpha subunits in ferret left ventricular myocytes. J Gen Physiol 1999;113:581–600.

24. Jurkiewicz NK, Sanguinetti MC. Rate-dependent prolongation of cardiac action potentials by a methanesulfonanilide class III antiarrhythmic agent. Specific block of rapidly activating delayed rectifier K$^+$ current by dofetilide. Circ Res 1993;72: 75–83.

25. Bryant SM, Wan X, Shipsey SJ, et al. Regional differences in the delayed rectifier current (I_{Kr} and I_{Ks}) contribute to the differences in action potential duration in basal left ventricular myocytes in guinea-pig. Cardiovasc Res 1998;40:322–31.

26. Liu J, Kim K-H, London B, et al. Dissection of the voltage-activated potassium outward currents in adult mouse ventricular myocytes: I(to,f), I(to,s), I(K,slow1), I(K,slow2), and I(ss). Basic Res Cardiol 2011;106:189–204.

27. Foeger NC, Wang W, Mellor RL, et al. Stabilization of Kv4 protein by the accessory K$^+$ channel interacting protein 2 (KChIP2) subunit is required for the generation of native myocardial fast transient outward K$^+$ currents. J Physiol 2013;591(17): 4149–66.

28. Xu H, Barry DM, Li H, et al. Attenuation of the slow component of delayed rectification, action potential prolongation, and triggered activity in mice expressing a dominant-negative Kv2 alpha subunit. Circ Res 1999;85:623–33.

29. London B, Guo W, Pan XH, et al. Targeted replacement of Kv1.5 in the mouse leads to loss of the 4-aminopyridine-sensitive component of I(K,slow) and resistance to drug-induced QT prolongation. Circ Res 2001;88:940–6.

30. Zhou J, Kodirov S, Murata M, et al. Regional upregulation of Kv2.1-encoded current, IK,slow2, in Kv1DN mice is abolished by crossbreeding with Kv2DN mice. Am J Physiol Heart Circ Physiol 2003;284:H491–500.

31. Li H, Guo W, Yamada KA, et al. Selective elimination of I(K,slow1) in mouse ventricular myocytes expressing a dominant negative Kv1.5alpha subunit. Am J Physiol Heart Circ Physiol 2004;286: H319–28.

32. Bou-Abboud E, Li H, Nerbonne JM. Molecular diversity of the repolarizing voltage-gated K$^+$ currents in mouse atrial cells. J Physiol 2000;529: 345–58.

33. Tuteja D, Xu D, Timofeyev V, et al. Differential expression of small-conductance Ca^{2+}-activated K$^+$ channels SK1, SK2, and SK3 in mouse atrial and ventricular myocytes. Am J Physiol Heart Circ Physiol 2005;289:H2714–23.

34. Zhang XD, Timofeyev V, Li N, et al. Critical roles of a small conductance Ca^{2+}- activated K$^+$ channel (SK3) in the repolarization process of atrial myocytes. Cardiovasc Res 2014;101:317–25.

35. Li N, Timofeyev V, Tuteja D, et al. Ablation of a Ca^{2+}-activated K$^+$ channel (SK2 channel) results in action potential prolongation in atrial myocytes and atrial fibrillation. J Physiol 2009;587:1087–100.

36. Zhang XD, Lieu DK, Chiamvimonvat N. Small-conductance Ca^{2+}-activated K^+ channels and cardiac arrhythmias. Heart Rhythm 2015;12:1845–51.

37. Chang PC, Chen PS. SK channels and ventricular arrhythmias in heart failure. Trends Cardiovasc Med 2015;25:508–14.

38. Lai MH, Wu Y, Gao Z, et al. BK channels regulate sinoatrial node firing rate and cardiac pacing in vivo. Am J Physiol Heart Circ Physiol 2014;307:H1327–38.

39. Lawrence C, Rodrigo GG. A Na^+-activated K^+ current ($I_{K,Na}$) is present in guinea pig but not rat ventricular myocytes. Pflugers Arch 1999;437:831–8.

40. Lopatin AN, Nichols CG. Inward rectifiers in the heart: an update on I(K1). J Mol Cell Cardiol 2001;33:625–38.

41. Flagg TP, Nichols CG. Sarcolemmal K(ATP) channels: what do we really know? J Mol Cell Cardiol 2005;39:61–70.

42. Grover GJ, Garlid KD. ATP-sensitive potassium channels: a review of their cardioprotective pharmacology. J Mol Cell Cardiol 2000;32:677–95.

43. Flagg TP, Enkvetchakul D, Koster JC, et al. Muscle KATP channels: recent insights to energy sensing and myoprotection. Physiol Rev 2010;90:799–829.

44. Kefaloyianni E, Bao L, Rindler MJ, et al. Measuring and evaluating the role of ATP-sensitive K^+ channels in cardiac muscle. J Mol Cell Cardiol 2012;52:596–607.

45. Nakaya H. Role of ATP-sensitive K^+ channels in cardiac arrhythmias. J Cardiovasc Pharmacol Ther 2014;19:237–43.

46. Kurachi Y, Nakajima T, Sugimoto T. Acetylcholine activation of K^+ channels in cell-free membrane patches of atrial cells. Am J Physiol 1986;251:H681–4.

47. Breetweiser GE, Szabo G. Uncoupling of cardiac muscarinic and β-adrenergic receptors from ion channels by a quinine nucleotide analogue. Nature 1985;317:538–40.

48. Logothetis DE, Kurachi Y, Galper J, et al. The βδ subunits of GTP-binding proteins activate the muscarinic K^+ channel in heart. Nature 1987;325:321–6.

49. Kuomi S-I, Wasserstrom JA. Acetylcholine sensitive muscarinic K^+ channels in mammalian ventricular myocytes. Am J Physiol 1994;266:H1812–21.

50. Voigt N, Abu-Taha I, Heijman J, et al. Constitutive activity of the acetylcholine-activated potassium current IK,ACh in cardiomyocytes. Adv Pharmacol 2014;70:393–409.

51. Keating MT, Sanguinetti MC. Molecular and cellular mechanisms of cardiac arrhythmias. Cell 2001;104:569–80.

52. Lesage F, Lazdunski M. Molecular and functional properties of two-pore-domain potassium channels. Am J Physiol Renal Physiol 2000;279:F793–801.

53. Goldstein SA, Bockenhauer D, O'Kelly I, et al. Potassium leak channels and the KCNK family of two-P-domain subunits. Nat Rev Neurosci 2001;2:175–84.

54. Abbott GW, Goldstein SA. A superfamily of small potassium channel subunits: form and function of the MinK-related peptides (MiRPs). Q Rev Biophys 1998;31:357–98.

55. Abbott GW, Sesti F, Splawski I, et al. MiRP1 forms I_{Kr} potassium channels with HERG and is associated with cardiac arrhythmia. Cell 1999;97:175–87.

56. Abbott GW, Butler MH, Bendahhou S, et al. MiRP2 forms potassium channels in skeletal muscle with Kv3.4 and is associated with periodic paralysis. Cell 2001;104:217–31.

57. Zhang M, Jiang M, Tseng GN. minK-related peptide 1 associates with Kv4.2 and modulates its gating function: potential role as beta subunit of cardiac transient outward channel? Circ Res 2001;88:1012–9.

58. Pongs O, Leicher T, Berger M, et al. Functional and molecular aspects of voltage-gated K^+ channel β subunits. Ann N Y Acad Sci 1999;868:344–55.

59. Aimond F, Kwak SP, Rhodes KJ, et al. Accessory Kvbeta1 subunits differentially modulate the functional expression of voltage-gated K^+ channels in mouse ventricular myocytes. Circ Res 2005;96:451–8.

60. An WF, Bowlby MR, Betty M, et al. Modulation of A-type potassium channels by a family of calcium sensors. Nature 2000;403:553–6.

61. Rosati B, Pan Z, Lypen S, et al. Regulation of KChIP2 potassium channel beta subunit gene expression underlies the gradient of transient outward current in canine and human ventricle. J Physiol 2001;533:119–25.

62. Burgoyne RD, Weiss JL. The neuronal calcium sensor family of Ca^{2+}-binding proteins. Biochem J 2001;353:1–12.

63. Deschenes I, DiSilvestre D, Juang GJ, et al. Regulation of Kv4.3 current by KChIP2 splice variants: a component of native cardiac $I_{(to)}$? Circulation 2002;106:423–9.

64. Patel S, Campbell DL, Morales MJ, et al. Heterogenous expression of KChIP2 isoforms in the ferret heart. J Physiol 2002;539:649–56.

65. Decher N, Barth AS, Gonzalez T, et al. Novel KChIP2 isoforms increase functional diversity of transient outward potassium currents. J Physiol 2004;557:761–72.

66. Thomsen MB, Wang C, Ozgen N, et al. Accessory subunit KChIP2 modulates the cardiac L-type calcium current. Circ Res 2009;104:1382–9.

67. Anderson D, Mehaffey WH, Iftinca M, et al. Regulation of neuronal activity by Cav3-Kv4

channel signaling complexes. Nat Neurosci 2010;13:333–7.

68. Radicke S, Cotella D, Graf EM, et al. Expression and function of dipeptidyl-aminopeptidase-like protein 6 as a putative β-subunit of human cardiac transient outward current encoded by Kv4.3. J Physiol 2005;565:751–6.

69. Nadal MS, Ozaita A, Amarillo Y, et al. The CD26-related dipeptidyl aminopeptidase-like protein DPPX is a critical component of neuronal A-type K+ channels. Neuron 2003;37:449–61.

70. Jerng HH, Qian Y, Pfaffinger PJ. Modulation of Kv4.2 channel expression and gating by dipeptidyl peptidase 10 (DPP10). Biophys J 2004;87:2380–96.

71. Ren X, Hayashi Y, Yoshimura N, et al. Transmembrane interaction mediates complex formation between peptidase homologues and Kv4 channels. Mol Cell Neurosci 2005;29:320–32.

72. Turnow K, Metzner K, Cotella D, et al. Interaction of DPP10a with Kv4.3 channel complex results in a sustained current component of human transient outward current Ito. Basic Res Cardiol 2015;110:5.

73. Xiao L, Koopmann TT, Ördög B, et al. Unique cardiac Purkinje fiber transient outward current β-subunit composition: a potential molecular link to idiopathic ventricular fibrillation. Circ Res 2013;112:1310–22.

74. Guo W, Malin SA, Johns DC, et al. Modulation of Kv4-encoded K+ currents in the mammalian myocardium by neuronal calcium sensor-1. J Biol Chem 2002;277:26436–43.

75. Fiset C, Clark RB, Shimoni Y, et al. Shal-type channels contribute to the Ca2+- independent transient outward K+ current in rat ventricle. J Physiol 1997;500:51–64.

76. Guo W, Li H, Aimond F, et al. Role of heteromultimers in the generation of myocardial transient outward K+ currents. Circ Res 2002;90:586–93.

77. Johns DC, Nuss HB, Marban E. Suppression of neuronal and cardiac transient outward currents by viral gene transfer of dominant-negative Kv4.2 constructs. J Biol Chem 1997;272:31598–603.

78. Barry DM, Xu H, Schuessler RB, et al. Functional knockout of the transient outward current, long-QT syndrome, and cardiac modeling in mice expressing a dominant-negative Kv4 alpha subunit. Circ Res 1998;83:560–7.

79. Xu H, Li H, Nerbonne JM. Elimination of the transient outward current and action potential prolongation in mouse atrial myocytes expressing a dominant negative Kv4 alpha subunit. J Physiol 1999;519:11–21.

80. Guo W, Jung WE, Marionneau C, et al. Targeted deletion of Kv4.2 eliminates I(to,f) and results in electrical and molecular remodeling, with no evidence of ventricular hypertrophy or myocardial dysfunction. Circ Res 2005;97:1342–50.

81. Niwa N, Wang W, Sha Q, et al. Kv4.3 is not required for the generation of functional I(to,f) channels in adult mouse ventricles. J Mol Cell Cardiol 2008;44:95–104.

82. Dixon JE, Shi W, Wang HS, et al. Role of the Kv4.3 K+ channel in ventricular muscle. A molecular correlate for the transient outward current. Circ Res 1996;79:659–68.

83. Kong W, Po S, Yamagishi T, et al. Isolation and characterization of the human gene encoding Ito: further diversity by alternative mRNA splicing. Am J Physiol 1998;275:H1963–70.

84. Rosati B, Grau F, Rodriguez S, et al. Concordant expression of KChIP2 mRNA, protein and transient outward current throughout the canine ventricle. J Physiol 2003;548:815–22.

85. Teutsch C, Kondo RP, Dederko DA, et al. Spatial distributions of Kv4 channels and KChIP2 isoforms in the murine heart based on laser capture microdissection. Cardiovasc Res 2007;73:739–49.

86. Dixon JE, McKinnon D. Quantitative analysis of potassium channel mRNA expression in atrial and ventricular muscle of rats. Circ Res 1994;75:252–60.

87. Costantini DL, Arruda EP, Agarwal P, et al. The homeodomain transcription factor Irx5 establishes the mouse cardiac ventricular repolarization gradient. Cell 2005;123:347–58.

88. Rossow CF, Dilly KW, Santana LF. Differential calcineurin/NFATc3 activity contributes to the Ito transmural gradient in the mouse heart. Circ Res 2006;98:1306–13.

89. Rosati B, Grau F, McKinnon D. Regional variation in mRNA transcript abundance within the ventricular wall. J Mol Cell Cardiol 2006;40:295–302.

90. Kuo HC, Cheng CF, Clark RB, et al. A defect in the Kv channel interacting protein 2 (KChIP2) gene leads to a complete loss of Ito and confers susceptibility to ventricular arrhythmias. Cell 2001;107:801–13.

91. Marionneau C, Carrasquillo Y, Norris AJ, et al. The sodium channel accessory subunit Navβ1 regulates neuronal excitability through modulation of repolarizing voltage-gated K+ channels. J Neurosci 2012;32:5716–27.

92. Boczek NJ, Ye D, Johnson EK, et al. Characterization of SEMA3A-encoded semaphorin as a naturally occurring Kv4.3 protein inhibitor and its contribution to Brugada syndrome. Circ Res 2014;115:460–9.

93. London B, Wang DW, Hill JA, et al. The transient outward current in mice lacking the potassium channel gene Kv1.4. J Physiol 1998;509:171–82.

94. Guo W, Xu H, London B, et al. Molecular basis of transient outward K+ current diversity in

mouse ventricular myocytes. J Physiol 1999;521: 587–99.

95. Guo W, Li H, London B, et al. Functional consequences of elimination of I(to,f) and I(to,s): early afterdepolarizations, atrioventricular block, and ventricular arrhythmias in mice lacking Kv1.4 and expressing a dominant-negative Kv4 alpha subunit. Circ Res 2000;87:73–9.

96. Jones EM, Roti Roti EC, Wang J, et al. Cardiac IKr channels minimally comprise hERG 1a and 1b subunits. J Biol Chem 2004;279:44690–4.

97. Phartiyal P, Jones EM, Robertson GA. Heteromeric assembly of human ether-a-go-go- related gene (hERG) 1a/1b channels occurs cotranslationally via N-terminal interactions. J Biol Chem 2007;282: 9874–82.

98. Jones DK, Liu F, Vaidyanathan R, et al. hERG 1b is critical for human cardiac repolarization. Proc Natl Acad Sci U S A 2014;111:18073–7.

99. Finley MR, Li Y, Hua F, et al. Expression and coassociation of ERG1, KCNQ1, and KCNE1 potassium channel proteins in horse heart. Am J Physiol 2002; 283:H126–38.

100. Ehrlich JR, Pourrier M, Weerapura M, et al. KvLQT1 modulates the distribution and biophysical properties of HERG. A novel alpha-subunit interaction between delayed rectifier currents. J Biol Chem 2004; 279:1233–41.

101. London B, Jeron A, Zhou J, et al. Long QT and ventricular arrhythmias in transgenic mice expressing the N terminus and first transmembrane segment of a voltage-gated potassium channel. Proc Natl Acad Sci U S A 1998;95:2926–31.

102. Liu GX, Derst C, Schlichthorl G, et al. Comparison of cloned Kir2 channels with native inward rectifier K+ channels from guinea-pig cardiomyocytes. J Physiol 2001;532:115–26.

103. Zaritsky JJ, Redell JB, Tempel BL, et al. The consequences of disrupting cardiac inwardly rectifying K+ current (IK1) as revealed by the targeted deletion of the murine Kir2.1 and Kir2.2 genes. J Physiol 2001;533:697–710.

104. Tristani-Firouzi M, Jensen JL, Donaldson MR, et al. Functional and clinical characterization of KCNJ2 mutations associated with LQT7 (Andersen Syndrome). J Clin Invest 2002;110:381–8.

105. Priori SG, Pandit SV, Rivolta I, et al. A novel form of short QT syndrome (SQT3) is caused by a mutation in the KCNJ2 gene. Circ Res 2005;96:800–7.

106. Noujaim SF, Pandit SV, Berenfeld O, et al. Up-regulation of the inward rectifier K+ current (IK1) in the mouse heart accelerates and stabilizes rotors. J Physiol 2007;578:315–26.

107. Piao L, Li J, McLerie M, et al. Transgenic upregulation of IK1 in the mouse heart is proarrhythmic. Basic Res Cardiol 2007;102:416–28.

108. Dhamoon AS, Pandit SV, Sarmast F, et al. Unique Kir2.x properties determine regional and species differences in the cardiac inward rectifier K+ current. Circ Res 2004;94:1332–9.

109. Panama BK, McLerie M, Lopatin AN. Heterogeneity of IK1 in the mouse heart. Am J Physiol Heart Circ Physiol 2007;293:H3558–67.

110. Panama BK, Lopatin AN. Differential polyamine sensitivity in inwardly rectifying Kir2 potassium channels. J Physiol 2006;571:287–302.

111. Babenko AP, Aguilar-Bryan L, Bryan J. A view of sur/KIR6.X, KATP channels. Annu Rev Physiol 1998;60:667–87.

112. Suzuki M, Li RA, Miki T, et al. Functional roles of cardiac and vascular ATP-sensitive potassium channels clarified by Kir6.2-knockout mice. Circ Res 2001;88:570–7.

113. Pu J, Wada T, Valdivia C, et al. Evidence of KATP channels in native cardiac cells without SUR. Biophys J 2001;80:625–6.

114. Seghers V, Nakazaki M, DeMayo F, et al. SUR1 knockout mice. A model for K(ATP) channel-independent regulation of insulin secretion. J Biol Chem 2000;275:9270–7.

115. Koster JC, Knopp A, Flagg TP, et al. Tolerance for ATP-insensitive K(ATP) channels in transgenic mice. Circ Res 2001;89:1022–9.

116. Terrenoire C, Lauritzen I, Lesage F, et al. A TREK-1-like potassium channel in atrial cells inhibited by beta-adrenergic stimulation and activated by volatile anesthetics. Circ Res 2001;89:336–42.

117. Barbuti A, Ishii S, Shimizu T, et al. Block of the background K+ channel TASK-1 contributes to arrhythmogenic effects of platelet-activating factor. Am J Physiol Heart Circ Physiol 2002;282: H2024–30.

118. Besana A, Barbuti A, Tateyama MA, et al. Activation of protein kinase C epsilon inhibits the two-pore domain K+ channel, TASK-1, inducing repolarization abnormalities in cardiac ventricular myocytes. J Biol Chem 2004;279:33154–60.

119. Putzke C, Wemhoner K, Sachse FB, et al. The acid-sensitive potassium channel TASK-1 in rat cardiac muscle. Cardiovasc Res 2007;75:59–68.

120. Yang KC, Nerbonne JM. Mechanisms contributing to myocardial potassium channel diversity, regulation and remodeling. Trends Cardiovasc Med 2015. [Epub ahead of print].

121. Ballou LM, Lin RZ, Cohen IS. Control of cardiac repolarization by phosphoinositide 3- kinase signaling to ion channels. Circ Res 2015;116: 127–37.

122. Karakikes I, Ameen M, Termglinchan V, et al. Human induced pluripotent stem cell-derived cardiomyocytes: insights into molecular, cellular, and functional phenotypes. Circ Res 2015;117:80–8.

123. Sallam K, Li Y, Sager PT, et al. Finding the rhythm of sudden cardiac death: new opportunities using induced pluripotent stem cell-derived cardiomyocytes. Circ Res 2015;116:1989–2004.

124. Long SB, Tao X, Campbell EB, et al. Atomic structure of a voltage-dependent K+ channel in a lipid membrane-like environment. Nature 2009;450: 376–82.

125. Strop P, Bankovich AJ, Hansen KC, et al. Structure of a human A-type potassium channel interacting protein DPPX, a member of the dipeptidyl aminopeptidase family. J Mol Biol 2004;343:1055–65.

126. Pioletti M, Findeisen F, Hura GL, et al. Three-dimensional structure of the KChIP1-Kv4.3 T1 complex reveals a cross-shaped octamer. Nat Struct Mol Biol 2006;13:987–95.

Molecular Basis of Cardiac Delayed Rectifier Potassium Channel Function and Pharmacology

Wei Wu, PhD, Michael C. Sanguinetti, PhD*

KEYWORDS

- Gating • hERG • KCNA5 • KCNE1 • KCNQ1 • Pharmacology • Potassium channel

KEY POINTS

- Although the structures of cardiac delayed rectifier potassium ion (K^+) channels, including Kv1.5, Kv7.1 (KCNQ1), and Kv11.1 (human *ether-a-go-go*–related gene [hERG1]), have not been determined, the molecular basis of their function can be inferred from biophysical studies and known structural features of other K^+ channels.
- The molecular basis of action for several blockers and activators of cardiac delayed rectifier K^+ channels have been determined primarily by functional analysis of mutant channels that alter drug affinity.
- Most blockers inhibit K^+ conductance by binding to the central cavity of the channel. In contrast, hERG1 and KCNQ1 activators bind outside the cavity to 4 symmetric sites and alter one or more gating properties.

INTRODUCTION

In cardiomyocytes, multiple types of outward delayed rectifier potassium ion current (I_K) mediate the late repolarization phase of action potentials.[1] In human cardiomyocytes, 3 distinct types of I_K are recognized. A rapidly activating current (I_{Kr}) is conducted by channels formed by coassembly of human *ether-a-go-go*-related gene (hERG1) (Kv11.1; gene: *KCNH2*) subunits, both full-length hERG1a α-subunits,[2,3] and alternatively spliced hERG1b α-subunits.[4] A slowly activating current (I_{Ks}) is conducted by channels formed by coassembly of KCNQ1 (Kv7.1; gene: *KCNQ1*) α-subunits and auxiliary KCNE1 β-subunits.[5,6] In human atrial, but not ventricular, myocytes, an ultrarapid activating current (I_{Kur}) is also present and conducted by channels formed by Kv1.5 (gene: *KCN5A*) α-subunits.[7,8] Identification of the molecular basis of I_{Kur}, I_{Kr}, and I_{Ks} combined with patch clamp studies of heterologously expressed channels spawned copious biophysical studies designed to probe the molecular mechanisms of channel gating and enabled the screening of small molecule libraries to discover novel compounds that either inhibit or activate these channels. Detailed descriptions of the molecular basis of Kv1.5, hERG1, and KCNQ1 channel gating are reviewed elsewhere.[9–12] Here the authors provide a general overview of the structural basis of channel gating and feature recent findings regarding modulation of the cardiac delayed rectifier K^+ channel by low-molecular-weight compounds and peptides.

Disclosure: The authors have nothing to disclose.
Department of Medicine, Nora Eccles Harrison Cardiovascular Research and Training Institute, University of Utah, 95 South 2000 East, Salt Lake City, UT 84112, USA
* Corresponding author.
E-mail address: m.sanguinetti@utah.edu

Card Electrophysiol Clin 8 (2016) 275–284
http://dx.doi.org/10.1016/j.ccep.2016.01.002
1877-9182/16/$ – see front matter © 2016 Elsevier Inc. All rights reserved.

STRUCTURAL BASIS OF VOLTAGE-DEPENDENT POTASSIUM CHANNEL GATING

Insights into the molecular mechanisms of K^+ channel gating have been provided by early biophysical studies of *Drosophila* Shaker and other voltage-gated K^+ (Kv) channels combined with structural biology studies of several bacterial channels (KcsA, MthK, KvAP) and vertebrate Kv1.2 channels. Similar to other Kv channel subunits, hERG1, KCNQ1, and Kv1.5 subunits each contain 6 transmembrane α-helical segments (S1–S6), and functional channels are formed by coassembly of 4 identical or highly similar α-subunits into a tetrameric complex (**Fig. 1A**). In each subunit, segments S1 to S4 form a voltage-sensing domain (VSD); segments S5 and S6 contribute to the central pore-forming domain. The S6 segments line the central cavity of the channel, and the cytoplasmic ends of each segment crisscross one another (the S6 bundle crossing) to form a narrow aperture (the activation gate) when the channel is in a closed state. The S4 segment contains multiple basic (positively charged) amino acids and, thus, serves as the primary voltage sensing structure. In response to membrane depolarization, the S4 segments move in an outward direction and the attached cytoplasmic S4-S5 linker acts as an electromechanical coupler to link the S4 movement to the opening of the activation gate (ie, an outward splaying of the S6 bundle crossing).[13] When the activation gate is in an open configuration, hydrated K^+ ions within the cytoplasm diffuse into the central cavity in response to the outwardly directed electrochemical driving force. As K^+ ions enter the selectivity filter (**Fig. 1B**), they are stripped of their surrounding water molecules and move stepwise from one high-affinity binding site to another until they reach the extracellular vestibule where they are again rehydrated. The selectivity filter of K^+-selective channels is a narrow lumen that is lined by 5 amino acid residues (ThrValGlyTyrGly) contributed by each of the 4 subunits. The hydroxyl group from the Thr residue and the backbone carbonyl oxygen atoms of 4 following amino acids together form an oxygen network (**Fig. 1C**) that coordinate dehydrated K^+ ions in a manner that closely resembles the oxygen atoms from 8 water molecules that form the hydration shell surrounding the ion in solution.[14]

ACTIVATION GATING

The amino acid sequence of the Kv1.5 channel is highly homologous to Kv1.2, and so it is reasonable to assume the structural basis of gating described for Kv1.2 also applies to cardiac Kv1.5 channels. Some of the details differ for hERG1 and KCNQ1/KCNE1 channels. Recently it was

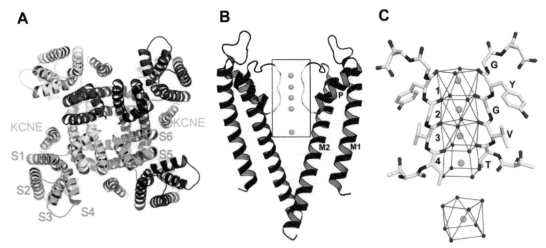

Fig. 1. Structural features of voltage-gated K^+ channels. (*A*) Functional channels are composed of 4 identical or highly related α-subunits. The S1 to S4 transmembrane segments form the voltage-sensing domain. The S5 and S6 segments form the pore domain. In I_{Ks} channels, 4 KCNQ1 α-subunits are joined by 2 (or more) KCNE1 β-subunits that are positioned in the cleft as indicated. (*B*) Side view of the pore domain of the KcsA bacterial K^+ channel in a closed state. Only 2 of the 4 subunits are shown; selectivity filter is boxed. (*C*) The selectivity filter of a K^+ channel (KcsA) is a narrow lumen where dehydrated K^+ ions (*green sphere*) transiently bind to sites (1–4) formed by oxygen atoms contributed by TYGYG residues that form the structure. Bottom panel shows a single K^+ ion surrounded by 8 water molecules. (*From* [*A*] Nakajo K, Kubo Y. KCNQ1 channel modulation by KCNE proteins via the voltage-sensing domain. J Physiol 2015;593:2618; and [*B, C*] Alam A, Youxing J. Structural studies of ion selectivity in tetrameric cation channels. J Gen Physiol 2011;137(5):398; with permission.)

reported that physical continuity between the S4 segment and pore domain is not required for normal voltage dependent activation (and inactivation) gating in hERG1 channels. Channels could still gate relatively normally when subunits were split into 2 pieces at the S4-S5 linker, a finding inconsistent with the simple idea of electromechanical coupling.[15] For hERG1 channels, specific interactions between Asp540 in the S4-S5 linker and Leu666 in the S6 segment are a key component of activation gating.[16,17] Presumably these interactions can still occur in a split channel. In the heart, the biophysical properties of KCNQ1 channels are modified by KCNE1 β-subunits. Channels formed by coassembly of KCNE1 subunits (1 - 4 per channel) to KCNQ1 homotetramers exhibit an increased single-channel conductance, open at more positive potentials, and have a slower rate of activation. Voltage sensor movement associated with KCNQ1 channel activation is divided into 2 steps with distinct voltage dependences and kinetics,[18] corresponding to an intermediate-open or a high permeation activated–open state.[19] KCNE1 subunits inhibit the intermediate-open state and facilitate the activated-open states by altering the interactions between the VSDs and the pore domain.[19] The binding of intracellular phosphatidylinositol 4,5-bisphosphate (PIP2) or ATP promotes coupling between voltage sensing at S4 segments and the pore domain in KCNQ1/KCNE1 channels.[20,21]

INACTIVATION GATING

Kv1.5 channels exhibit a very slow and time-independent C-type inactivation at depolarized potentials, a process that involves cooperative subunit interactions in related Kv1 channels.[22,23] Auxiliary Kvβ1.2 and Kvβ1.3 subunits interact with the C-terminal domain of Kv1.5[24] to induce rapid inactivation.[25] It is unclear to what extent Kvβ subunits alter Kv1.5 channel gating in human atrial myocytes. KCNQ1 channels inactivate slightly at positive potentials, but KCNQ1/KCNE1 channels do not inactivate.[26] In hERG1, C-type inactivation is extremely fast and voltage dependent[27,28] and occurs in sequential steps that culminate in a subtle change in the conformation of the selectivity filter.[29] The authors used concatenated tetramers to demonstrate that the extent of subunit cooperativity depended on the location of the mutations used to probe inactivation and that the final step in the gating process was mediated by a concerted, all-or-none cooperative interaction between subunits.[30]

DEACTIVATION GATING

Return of the transmembrane potential to a negative level (as occurs during repolarization of an action potential) induces channel transition from an open to a closed state, a process called deactivation. The slow rate of deactivation of hERG1 channels depends on multiple interactions between the cytoplasmic N-terminus of one subunit with the cytoplasmic C-terminus of an adjacent subunit.[31–33] Slow deactivation is a fully cooperative process (ie, all or none), requiring the N-C interaction between all 4 subunits. Disruption of a single N-C interaction is sufficient to greatly accelerate deactivation.[34] These interactions have physiologic significance, as hERG1 channels can be formed by coassembly of hERG1a subunits that contain a full-length N-terminus and hERG1b subunits that have a truncated N-terminus[4,35] that cannot interact with the C-terminus to slow deactivation.

MOLECULAR PHARMACOLOGY OF CARDIAC DELAYED RECTIFIER POTASSIUM ION CHANNELS
Inhibitors

Most Kv1.5 inhibitors are pore blockers. Several potent open channel blockers of Kv1.5, including AVE0118, S0100176, vernakalant, DPO-1, MK-0448, anandamide, and acacetin, were developed to selectively block I_{Kur} in atria as a potential therapy for atrial fibrillation (AF).[36–42] These Kv1.5 blockers share an overlapping binding site, including 5 critical residues that face toward the lumen of the central cavity: Thr479, Thr480, Val505, Ile508, and Val512.[39,43–46] More recently, Marzian and colleagues[47] identified Psora-4 as a unique Kv1.5 inhibitor that is both a pore blocker and an allosteric gating modifier. Besides direct pore blockage, Psora-4 also binds to 4 symmetric side pockets distant from the central cavity (Fig. 2A). The amino acids that form the pore of Kv1 channels are highly conserved, challenging efforts to develop specific Kv1.5 blockers. Allosteric gating inhibitors, such as Psora-4, offer an alternative approach to the design of channel-specific drugs.

The primary motivation driving the discovery of Kv1.5 blockers has been its predicted usefulness for pharmacologic cardioversion of recent-onset AF or prevention of AF episodes by a mechanism that would not affect the electrophysiologic properties of the ventricles. Specifically, because Kv1.5 is highly expressed in human atria but not in the ventricles, the block of these channels would

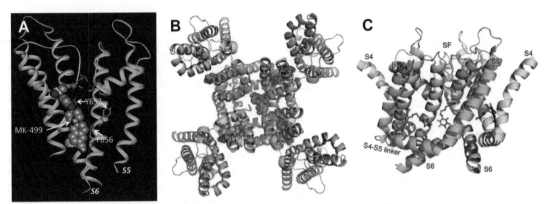

Fig. 2. K$^+$ channel inhibitors. (*A*) Model of the hERG1 channel pore domain showing block of the central cavity by MK-499, a class III antiarrhythmic agent. The S5 and S6 segments for 2 of the 4 subunits are shown. The key binding residues in the S6 segment (Y652 and F656) are indicated. (*B, C*) Psora-4 (*orange*) binds to multiple sites on the Kv1.5 channel viewed from the extracellular space (*B*) or from the side (*C*). (*From [A]* Mitcheson JS, Chen J, Lin M, et al. A structural basis for drug-induced long QT syndrome. Proc Natl Acad Sci U S A 2000;97:12332; and [*B, C*] Marzian S, Stansfeld PJ, Rapedius M, et al. Side pockets provide the basis for a new mechanism of Kv channel-specific inhibition. Nat Chem Biol 2013;9:509; with permission.)

be expected to specifically prolong the APD of atrial myocytes (and atrial effective refractory period [AERP]) without risk of inducing QT prolongation. The clinical experience to date has not been encouraging for this mechanism. Although MK-0448 was shown in preclinical studies to prolong AERP without effects on the ventricle, the compound was without effect on AERP in healthy human subjects. This finding was predicted by previous mathematical modeling of human atrial action potentials. Simulated inhibition of I_{Kur} was shown to increase plateau height, leading to additional activation of I_{Kr} and no net change in APD.[48] Moreover, as noted by Ravens and colleagues,[49] MK-0448 was evaluated by electrophysiologic testing over a frequency range lower than what is typically observed during AF. It remains to be demonstrated that Kv1.5 channel inhibition will provide protection against AF in relevant patient populations.

hERG1 channels are blocked by a wide spectrum of compounds, including quinidine, d-sotalol, and many other class III antiarrhythmic agents, such as the highly potent methanesulfonanilides dofetilide and ibutilide. All of these compounds block hERG1 channels by preferentially plugging the central cavity of the channel (**Fig. 2**B, C). In addition to these antiarrhythmic drugs, several other commonly used medications with diverse chemical structures (eg, cisapride, terfenadine, astemizole, moxifloxacin, and tamoxifen) are high-affinity blockers of hERG1 channels and, hence, prolong the QT interval.[50] Many hERG1 blockers have an unacceptable risk of inducing arrhythmia. Unintended drug-induced QT prolongation increases

the risk of ventricular tachyarrhythmia (most commonly, torsade de pointes) in patients and, hence, has prompted the withdrawal or restriction of these marketed drugs. The structural basis for high-affinity binding of hERG1 channel blockers was revealed using a site-directed mutagenesis approach. Two aromatic residues (ie, Tyr652 and Phe656) located in all 4 S6 segments that line the central cavity of the channel are the most critical determinants for drug interaction.[51,52] Inactivation-deficient hERG1 mutant channels (eg, S620T, S631A, G628C/S631C) are much less sensitive to block by these compounds,[53–56] so it was commonly assumed that drugs can only bind with high affinity to the inactivated state of the channel. However, a detailed analysis of concatenated hERG1 tetramers containing a variable number of S620T, G628C/S631C, or S631A mutation subunits indicate instead that these mutant subunits allosterically interrupt drug block in a manner that is independent of their ability to disrupt inactivation gating.[57] Peptide toxins isolated from scorpion venoms, such as ErgTx1 and BeKm-1, bind to the external region of the pore to block channels with nanomolar potency.[58,59] Other peptide toxins act as allosteric modifiers of activation gating, including APETx1 from sea anemone and several tarantula toxins. These peptides directly interact with the VSD of hERG1 and reduce current magnitude by shifting the voltage dependence of activation to more positive potentials.[60,61]

Chromanol 293B is a relatively selective I_{Ks} blocker that was initially developed as a class III antiarrhythmic drug to prolong action potential duration.[62,63] The benzodiazepine L-7 is a more potent blocker that binds to specific residues in the S6 segments of KCNQ1 channels.[64,65] Other compounds, such as indapamide, propofol, and thiopentone, exert lower affinity block of KCNQ1 channels.[66,67] KCNE1 subunits increase the affinity of chromanol 293B binding to KCNQ1 channels by up to 100-fold.[68]

The amino acids in the S6 segments that line the central cavity of K$^+$ channels are often highly conserved among members of closely related channels (eg, Kv1.1, 1.2, 1.3, 1.4, and 1.5). This conservation has been a major impediment to the discovery of pore blockers that are highly channel specific. Another approach to inhibiting K$^+$ flux is to modulate channel gating processes (eg, shift the voltage dependence of activation to more positive potentials) with compounds that bind to structural elements (eg, voltage-sensor domain) that are not as highly conserved as the residues in the S6 segment that form the channel pore. The authors anticipate that this approach will be greatly facilitated as more K$^+$ channel structures are elucidated.

Activators

Congenital LQTS is a disorder of cardiac repolarization that predisposes affected individuals to an increased risk of cardiac arrhythmia and sudden cardiac death. The most common cause of LQTSs are loss of function mutations in either hERG1 or KCNQ1 channels, resulting in a reduction of I_{Kr} and I_{Ks}, and a prolongation of ventricular repolarization that is easily quantified as a longer QTc interval.[69–71] Thus, compounds that activate hERG1 or KCNQ1 channels are an obvious potential approach to restoring normal repolarization for most patients with congenital LQTS.

In the past 10 years, routine safety screening of compounds for undesirable hERG1 activity led to the serendipitous discovery of several hERG1 activators that act by different mechanisms to allosterically modify channel gating. These agents can slow deactivation, attenuate C-type inactivation, enhance single channel open probability, induce a hyperpolarizing shift in the voltage dependence of activation, or exert a combination of 2 or more of these actions.[72] RPR-260243 was the first reported synthetic hERG1 activator. This compound markedly slows the rate of hERG1 channel deactivation and causes a mild attenuation of inactivation with no effect on the voltage dependence of activation.[73,74] Ginsenoside Rg3, a natural product isolated from ginseng root, also dramatically slows hERG1 deactivation rate; but it also causes a modest negative shift in the voltage dependence of activation.[75] ICA-105574,[76,77] ML-T531,[78] and

AZSMO-23[79] profoundly enhance outward hERG1 current by greatly attenuating C-type inactivation and modestly slow deactivation without affecting the voltage dependence of channel activation. PD-118057 enhances hERG1 current by increasing channel open probability and causing a positive shift in the voltage dependence of inactivation.[80] The putative binding sites for RPR-260243, ICA-105574, and PD-118057 were revealed by the combined approach of alanine-scanning mutagenesis and molecular modeling. Although the specific residues of hERG1 that interact with these agonists vary, all 3 compounds interact with the channel via a hydrophobic pocket located between 2 adjacent subunits of the pore domain (**Fig. 3**).[74,77,80] Thus, each homotetrameric hERG1 channel contains 4 identical binding sites. Analysis of concatenated hERG1 tetramers revealed that all 4 binding sites and cooperative subunit interactions are required to achieve maximal effects by ICA-105574 or PD-118057.[81] Maximal slowing of deactivation by RPR-260243 requires all 4 hERG1 subunits, whereas only 2 or more subunits were sufficient to achieve a maximal effect on inactivation.[82] In addition to ginsenoside Rg3,[75] mallotoxin[83] and KB130015[84] also shift the voltage dependence of hERG1 activation to more negative potentials; however, the binding site for these agents has not yet been defined. NS1643 shifts the voltage dependence of activation to more negative potentials and inactivation to more positive potentials, but effects vary depending on the heterologous expression system used.[85–87] The binding site for NS1643 has eluded definitive identification; but based on detailed molecular modeling and analysis of L529I hERG1 mutant channels, it is likely that NS1643 interacts indirectly with the VSD to facilitate opening of hERG1 channels.[88]

R-L3 was the first I_{Ks} activator to be described[89,90] and was shown to slow the rate of deactivation and cause a hyperpolarizing shift in the voltage dependence of channel activation. Overexpression of KCNE1 subunits with KCNQ1 channels abolished the action of R-L3, suggesting that the single transmembrane domain KCNE1 subunit either competes directly or allosterically with R-L3 for binding to KCNQ1 channel subunits. The putative binding site for R-L3, located between S5 and S6 segments[90] strongly suggests that it too will bind with 4-fold symmetry as described for the hERG1 activators. Zinc pyrithione (ZnPy) is a potent activator of KCNQ2 and KCNQ3 channels but also activates KCNQ1.[91,92] ZnPy attenuates inactivation and slows the rate of activation and deactivation of KCNQ1 channels; like R-L3, its actions are abolished by

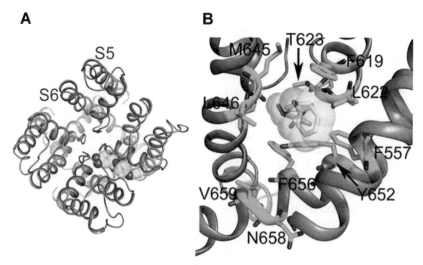

Fig. 3. Binding site for ICA-105574, a hERG1 channel activator. (*A*) Open-state pore domain of the channel as viewed from the extracellular space. ICA is shown in space fill–occupying one of the 4 symmetric sites available. VSDs are not shown. (*B*) Side view of the hydrophobic binding pocket with important binding site residues indicated in single letter code. (*From* Garg V, Stary-Weinzinger A, Sachse F, et al. Molecular determinants for activation of human *ether-a-go-go*-related gene 1 potassium channels by 3-nitro-n-(4-phenoxyphenyl) benzamide. Mol Pharmacol 2011;80:635; with permission.)

overexpression of KCNE1 subunits.[91] Most recently, high-throughput screening identified the compound ML277 as a potent KCNQ1 agonist[93,94] whose efficacy is also reduced by KCNE1.[95] A combined approach of electrophysiology and molecular dynamics simulation indicated that ML277 binds to the side pockets between adjacent KCNQ1 subunits to allosterically modify channel gating.[94] Nonspecific compounds, such as the chloride channel blockers mefenamic acid and DIDS, and the antibacterial hexachlorophene can also activate I_{Ks}; but these compounds exert stronger potentiation on KCNQ1/KCNE1 channels than on homomeric KCNQ1 channels.[96,97] Unlike other KCNQ1 channel activators, the negative shift of voltage dependence of channel activation produced by phenylboronic acid is independent of KCNE1 subunits.[98] Polyunsaturated fatty acids (PUFAs) are the most recently identified KCNQ1 agonists.[99] Electrostatic interactions between the negatively charged head group of PUFAs, such as docosahexaenoic acid, and the basic residues in the S4 segment of KCNQ1 shift the voltage dependence of channel activation to more negative potentials (maximal shift of -15 mV) at concentrations similar to total circulating plasma levels of PUFAs. Interestingly, KCNE1 subunits abolish the agonist effect by promoting PUFA protonation, indicating that natural PUFAs do not affect I_{Ks} channels in the heart.[99] If excessive shortening of QT_c can be avoided, hERG1 or KCNQ1/KCNE1 activators may be useful for the

prevention of arrhythmia associated with prolonged ventricular repolarization in patients with LQTS. They might be particularly useful for patients with particularly aggressive arrhythmia syndromes who enter periods of arrhythmic storm refractory to conventional management with repeated defibrillation shocks and increased mortality risk.

SUMMARY

Fueled by the molecular cloning of genes encoding the many channels that conduct the wide diversity of known ionic currents, the last 2 decades have witnessed a great leap forward in our understanding of the structural and mechanistic basis of potassium channel function. Because of their well-recognized importance in cardiac repolarization and the severe medical consequence of inherited gene mutations, the pharmacology of cardiac delayed rectifier K$^+$ channels has been explored extensively. In the past few decades, high-throughput drug screening efforts have focused on the discovery of compounds to treat AF (Kv1.5 channel blockers) or ventricular arrhythmia (hERG1 and KCNQ1/ KCNE1 blockers). More recently, hERG1 and KCNQ1 channel activators were discovered that may prove useful for the treatment of ventricular arrhythmia associated with prolonged QT_c intervals. It is anticipated that future antiarrhythmic drug discovery efforts will rely less on screening of large compound libraries and instead capitalize on our increasingly sophisticated understanding of channel structure and gating mechanisms to enable a rational, knowledge-based drug design approach.

REFERENCES

1. Noble D, Tsien RW. Outward membrane currents activated in the plateau range of potentials in cardiac Purkinje fibres. J Physiol 1969;200:205–31.
2. Sanguinetti MC, Jiang C, Curran ME, et al. A mechanistic link between an inherited and an acquired cardiac arrhythmia: HERG encodes the I_{Kr} potassium channel. Cell 1995;81:299–307.
3. Trudeau MC, Warmke JW, Ganetzky B, et al. HERG, a human inward rectifier in the voltage-gated potassium channel family. Science 1995;269:92–5.
4. Jones EM, Roti Roti EC, Wang J, et al. Cardiac I_{Kr} channels minimally comprise hERG 1a and 1b subunits. J Biol Chem 2004;279:44690–4.
5. Sanguinetti MC, Curran ME, Zou A, et al. Coassembly of K_VLQT1 and minK (IsK) proteins to form cardiac I_{Ks} potassium channel. Nature 1996;384:80–3.
6. Barhanin J, Lesage F, Guillemare E, et al. K_VLQT1 and IsK (minK) proteins associate to form the I_{Ks} cardiac potassium current. Nature 1996;384:78–80.
7. Li GR, Feng J, Wang Z, et al. Adrenergic modulation of ultrarapid delayed rectifier K+ current in human atrial myocytes. Circ Res 1996;78:903–15.
8. Wang Z, Fermini B, Nattel S. Sustained depolarization-induced outward current in human atrial myocytes. Evidence for a novel delayed rectifier K+ current similar to Kv1.5 cloned channel currents. Circ Res 1993;73:1061–76.
9. Vandenberg JI, Perry MD, Perrin MJ, et al. hERG K+ channels: structure, function, and clinical significance. Physiol Rev 2012;92:1393–478.
10. Nakajo K, Kubo Y. KCNQ1 channel modulation by KCNE proteins via the voltage-sensing domain. J Physiol 2015;593:2617–25.
11. Liin SI, Barro-Soria R, Larsson HP. The KCNQ1 channel - remarkable flexibility in gating allows for functional versatility. J Physiol 2015;593:2605–15.
12. Schmitt N, Grunnet M, Olesen SP. Cardiac potassium channel subtypes: new roles in repolarization and arrhythmia. Physiol Rev 2014;94:609–53.
13. Long SB, Campbell EB, Mackinnon R. Voltage sensor of Kv1.2: structural basis of electromechanical coupling. Science 2005;309:903–8.
14. Zhou Y, Morais-Cabral JH, Kaufman A, et al. Chemistry of ion coordination and hydration revealed by a K+ channel-Fab complex at 2.0 A resolution. Nature 2001;414:43–8.
15. Lorinczi E, Gomez-Posada JC, de la Pena P, et al. Voltage-dependent gating of KCNH potassium channels lacking a covalent link between voltage-sensing and pore domains. Nat Commun 2015;6:6672.
16. Ferrer T, Rupp J, Piper DR, et al. The S4-S5 linker directly couples voltage sensor movement to the activation gate in the human *ether-a'-go-go*-related gene (hERG) K+ channel. J Biol Chem 2006;281:12858–64.
17. Tristani-Firouzi M, Chen J, Sanguinetti MC. Interactions between S4-S5 linker and S6 transmembrane domain modulate gating of HERG K+ channels. J Biol Chem 2002;277:18994–9000.
18. Barro-Soria R, Rebolledo S, Liin SI, et al. KCNE1 divides the voltage sensor movement in KCNQ1/KCNE1 channels into two steps. Nat Commun 2014;5:3750.
19. Zaydman MA, Kasimova MA, McFarland K, et al. Domain-domain interactions determine the gating, permeation, pharmacology, and subunit modulation of the I_{Ks} ion channel. Elife 2014;3:e03606.
20. Zaydman MA, Silva JR, Delaloye K, et al. Kv7.1 ion channels require a lipid to couple voltage sensing to pore opening. Proc Natl Acad Sci U S A 2013;110:13180–5.
21. Li Y, Gao J, Lu Z, et al. Intracellular ATP binding is required to activate the slowly activating K+ channel I_{Ks}. Proc Natl Acad Sci U S A 2013;110:18922–7.
22. Ogielska EM, Zagotta WN, Hoshi T, et al. Cooperative subunit interactions in C-type inactivation of K channels. Biophys J 1995;69:2449–57.
23. Panyi G, Sheng Z, Deutsch C. C-type inactivation of a voltage-gated K+ channel occurs by a cooperative mechanism. Biophys J 1995;69:896–903.
24. Tipparaju SM, Li XP, Kilfoil PJ, et al. Interactions between the C-terminus of Kv1.5 and Kvbeta regulate pyridine nucleotide-dependent changes in channel gating. Pflugers Arch 2012;463:799–818.
25. Heinemann SH, Rettig J, Graack HR, et al. Functional characterization of Kv channel beta-subunits from rat brain. J Physiol 1996;493:625–33.
26. Tristani-Firouzi M, Sanguinetti MC. Voltage-dependent inactivation of the human K+ channel KvLQT1 is eliminated by association with minimal K+ channel (minK) subunits. J Physiol 1998;510:37–45.
27. Spector PS, Curran ME, Zou A, et al. Fast inactivation causes rectification of the I_{Kr} channel. J Gen Physiol 1996;107:611–9.
28. Smith PL, Baukrowitz T, Yellen G. The inward rectification mechanism of the HERG cardiac potassium channel. Nature 1996;379:833–6.
29. Wang DT, Hill AP, Mann SA, et al. Mapping the sequence of conformational changes underlying selectivity filter gating in the K_V11.1 potassium channel. Nat Struct Mol Biol 2011;18:35–41.
30. Wu W, Gardner A, Sanguinetti MC. Cooperative subunit interactions mediate fast C-type inactivation of hERG1 K+ channels. J Physiol 2014;592:4465–80.

31. Ng CA, Phan K, Hill AP, et al. Multiple interactions between cytoplasmic domains regulate slow deactivation of Kv11.1 channels. J Biol Chem 2014;289: 25822–32.

32. Gianulis EC, Liu Q, Trudeau MC. Direct interaction of eag domains and cyclic nucleotide-binding homology domains regulate deactivation gating in hERG channels. J Gen Physiol 2013;142:351–66.

33. Gustina AS, Trudeau MC. hERG potassium channel gating is mediated by N- and C-terminal region interactions. J Gen Physiol 2011;137:315–25.

34. Thomson SJ, Hansen A, Sanguinetti MC. Concerted all-or-none subunit interactions mediate slow deactivation of human *ether-a-go-go*-related gene K$^+$ channels. J Biol Chem 2014;289:23428–36.

35. Jones DK, Liu F, Vaidyanathan R, et al. hERG 1b is critical for human cardiac repolarization. Proc Natl Acad Sci U S A 2014;111:18073–7.

36. Friederich P, Pfizenmayer H. The novel Kv1.5 channel blocker vernakalant for successful treatment of new-onset atrial fibrillation in a critically ill abdominal surgical patient. Br J Anaesth 2011;107: 644–5.

37. Li GR, Wang HB, Qin GW, et al. Acacetin, a natural flavone, selectively inhibits human atrial repolarization potassium currents and prevents atrial fibrillation in dogs. Circulation 2008;117:2449–57.

38. Knobloch K, Brendel J, Rosenstein B, et al. Atrial-selective antiarrhythmic actions of novel I$_{Kur}$ vs. I$_{Kr}$, I$_{Ks}$, and I$_{KAch}$ class Ic drugs and beta blockers in pigs. Med Sci Monit 2004;10:BR221–228.

39. Decher N, Pirard B, Bundis F, et al. Molecular basis for Kv1.5 channel block: conservation of drug binding sites among voltage-gated K$^+$ channels. J Biol Chem 2004;279:394–400.

40. Blaauw Y, Gogelein H, Tieleman RG, et al. "Early" class III drugs for the treatment of atrial fibrillation: efficacy and atrial selectivity of AVE0118 in remodeled atria of the goat. Circulation 2004;110: 1717–24.

41. Lagrutta A, Wang J, Fermini B, et al. Novel, potent inhibitors of human Kv1.5 K$^+$ channels and ultrarapidly activating delayed rectifier potassium current. J Pharmacol Exp Ther 2006;317:1054–63.

42. Barana A, Amoros I, Caballero R, et al. Endocannabinoids and cannabinoid analogues block cardiac hKv1.5 channels in a cannabinoid receptor-independent manner. Cardiovasc Res 2010;85: 56–67.

43. Eldstrom J, Wang Z, Xu H, et al. The molecular basis of high-affinity binding of the antiarrhythmic compound vernakalant (RSD1235) to Kv1.5 channels. Mol Pharmacol 2007;72:1522–34.

44. Decher N, Kumar P, Gonzalez T, et al. Binding site of a novel Kv1.5 blocker: a "foot in the door" against atrial fibrillation. Mol Pharmacol 2006;70:1204–11.

45. Wu HJ, Wu W, Sun HY, et al. Acacetin causes a frequency- and use-dependent blockade of hKv1.5 channels by binding to the S6 domain. J Mol Cell Cardiol 2011;51:966–73.

46. Du YM, Zhang XX, Tu DN, et al. Molecular determinants of Kv1.5 channel block by diphenyl phosphine oxide-1. J Mol Cell Cardiol 2010;48:1111–20.

47. Marzian S, Stansfeld PJ, Rapedius M, et al. Side pockets provide the basis for a new mechanism of Kv channel-specific inhibition. Nat Chem Biol 2013;9:507–13.

48. Courtemanche M, Ramirez RJ, Nattel S. Ionic targets for drug therapy and atrial fibrillation-induced electrical remodeling: insights from a mathematical model. Cardiovasc Res 1999;42:477–89.

49. Ravens U, Poulet C, Wettwer E, et al. Atrial selectivity of antiarrhythmic drugs. J Physiol 2013;591:4087–97.

50. Drici MD, Barhanin J. Cardiac K$^+$ channels and drug-acquired long QT syndrome. Therapie 2000; 55:185–93.

51. Mitcheson JS, Chen J, Lin M, et al. A structural basis for drug-induced long QT syndrome. Proc Natl Acad Sci U S A 2000;97:12329–33.

52. Fernandez D, Ghanta A, Kauffman GW, et al. Physicochemical features of the HERG channel drug binding site. J Biol Chem 2004;279:10120–7.

53. Ficker E, Jarolimek W, Kiehn J, et al. Molecular determinants of dofetilide block of HERG K$^+$ channels. Circ Res 1998;82:386–95.

54. Numaguchi H, Mullins FM, Johnson JP Jr, et al. Probing the interaction between inactivation gating and Dd-sotalol block of HERG. Circ Res 2000;87: 1012–8.

55. Perrin MJ, Kuchel PW, Campbell TJ, et al. Drug binding to the inactivated state is necessary but not sufficient for high-affinity binding to human *ether-a-go-go*-related gene channels. Mol Pharmacol 2008;74:1443–52.

56. Suessbrich H, Schonherr R, Heinemann SH, et al. Specific block of cloned Herg channels by clofilium and its tertiary analog LY97241. FEBS Lett 1997;414: 435–8.

57. Wu W, Gardner A, Sanguinetti MC. The link between inactivation and high-affinity block of hERG1 channels. Mol Pharmacol 2015;87:1042–50.

58. Gurrola GB, Rosati B, Rocchetti M, et al. A toxin to nervous, cardiac, and endocrine ERG K$^+$ channels isolated from *Centruroides noxius* scorpion venom. FASEB J 1999;13:953–62.

59. Korolkova YV, Kozlov SA, Lipkin AV, et al. An ERG channel inhibitor from the scorpion Buthus eupeus. J Biol Chem 2001;276:9868–76.

60. Diochot S, Loret E, Bruhn T, et al. APETx1, a new toxin from the sea anemone Anthopleura elegantissima, blocks voltage-gated human *ether-a-go-go*-related gene potassium channels. Mol Pharmacol 2003;64:59–69.

61. Redaelli E, Cassulini RR, Silva DF, et al. Target promiscuity and heterogeneous effects of tarantula venom peptides affecting Na⁺ and K⁺ ion channels. J Biol Chem 2010;285:4130–42.

62. Varro A, Balati B, Iost N, et al. The role of the delayed rectifier component I_{Ks} in dog ventricular muscle and Purkinje fibre repolarization. J Physiol 2000; 523:67–81.

63. Bosch RF, Gaspo R, Busch AE, et al. Effects of the chromanol 293B, a selective blocker of the slow, component of the delayed rectifier K⁺ current, on repolarization in human and guinea pig ventricular myocytes. Cardiovasc Res 1998;38:441–50.

64. Seebohm G, Chen J, Strutz N, et al. Molecular determinants of KCNQ1 channel block by a benzodiazepine. Mol Pharmacol 2003;64:70–7.

65. Lengyel C, Iost N, Virag L, et al. Pharmacological block of the slow component of the outward delayed rectifier current (I_{Ks}) fails to lengthen rabbit ventricular muscle QT_c and action potential duration. Br J Pharmacol 2001;132:101–10.

66. Turgeon J, Daleau P, Bennett PB, et al. Block of I_{Ks}, the slow component of the delayed rectifier K⁺ current, by the diuretic agent indapamide in guinea pig myocytes. Circ Res 1994;75:879–86.

67. Heath BM, Terrar DA. Separation of the components of the delayed rectifier potassium current using selective blockers of I_{Kr} and I_{Ks} in guinea-pig isolated ventricular myocytes. Exp Physiol 1996;81: 587–603.

68. Busch AE, Busch GL, Ford E, et al. The role of the IsK protein in the specific pharmacological properties of the I_{Ks} channel complex. Br J Pharmacol 1997;122:187–9.

69. Sanguinetti MC, Tristani-Firouzi M. hERG potassium channels and cardiac arrhythmia. Nature 2006;440: 463–9.

70. Hedley PL, Jorgensen P, Schlamowitz S, et al. The genetic basis of long QT and short QT syndromes: a mutation update. Hum Mutat 2009;30:1486–511.

71. Brunner M, Peng X, Liu GX, et al. Mechanisms of cardiac arrhythmias and sudden death in transgenic rabbits with long QT syndrome. J Clin Invest 2008; 118:2246–59.

72. Sanguinetti MC. HERG1 channel agonists and cardiac arrhythmia. Curr Opin Pharmacol 2014; 15:22–7.

73. Kang J, Chen XL, Wang H, et al. Discovery of a small molecule activator of the human *ether-a-go-go*-related gene (HERG) cardiac K⁺ channel. Mol Pharmacol 2005;67:827–36.

74. Perry M, Sachse FB, Sanguinetti MC. Structural basis of action for a human *ether-a-go-go*-related gene 1 potassium channel activator. Proc Natl Acad Sci U S A 2007;104:13827–32.

75. Choi SH, Shin TJ, Hwang SH, et al. Ginsenoside Rg₃ decelerates hERG K⁺ channel deactivation through Ser631 residue interaction. Eur J Pharmacol 2011; 663:59–67.

76. Gerlach AC, Stoehr SJ, Castle NA. Pharmacological removal of human *ether-a-go-go*-related gene potassium channel inactivation by 3-nitro-N-(4-phenoxyphenyl) benzamide (ICA-105574). Mol Pharmacol 2010;77:58–68.

77. Garg V, Stary-Weinzinger A, Sachse F, et al. Molecular determinants for activation of human *ether-a-go-go*-related gene 1 potassium channels by 3-nitro-n-(4-phenoxyphenyl) benzamide. Mol Pharmacol 2011;80:630–7.

78. Zhang H, Zou B, Yu H, et al. Modulation of hERG potassium channel gating normalizes action potential duration prolonged by dysfunctional KCNQ1 potassium channel. Proc Natl Acad Sci U S A 2012;109:11866–71.

79. Mannikko R, Bridgland-Taylor MH, Pye H, et al. Pharmacological and electrophysiological characterization of AZSMO-23, an activator of the hERG K⁺ channel. Br J Pharmacol 2015;172: 3112–25.

80. Perry M, Sachse FB, Abbruzzese J, et al. PD-118057 contacts the pore helix of hERG1 channels to attenuate inactivation and enhance K⁺ conductance. Proc Natl Acad Sci U S A 2009;106:20075–80.

81. Wu W, Sachse FB, Gardner A, et al. Stoichiometry of altered hERG1 channel gating by small molecule activators. J Gen Physiol 2014;143:499–512.

82. Wu W, Gardner A, Sanguinetti MC. Concatenated hERG1 tetramers reveal stoichiometry of altered channel gating by RPR-260243. Mol Pharmacol 2015;87:401–9.

83. Zeng H, Lozinskaya IM, Lin Z, et al. Mallotoxin is a novel human *ether-a-go-go*-related gene (hERG) potassium channel activator. J Pharmacol Exp Ther 2006;319:957–62.

84. Gessner G, Macianskiene R, Starkus JG, et al. The amiodarone derivative KB130015 activates hERG1 potassium channels via a novel mechanism. Eur J Pharmacol 2010;632:52–9.

85. Hansen RS, Diness TG, Christ T, et al. Activation of human *ether-a-go-go*-related gene potassium channels by the diphenylurea 1,3-bis-(2-hydroxy-5-trifluoromethyl-phenyl)-urea (NS1643). Mol Pharmacol 2006;69:266–77.

86. Casis O, Olesen SP, Sanguinetti MC. Mechanism of action of a novel human *ether-a-go-go*-related gene channel activator. Mol Pharmacol 2006;69: 658–65.

87. Guo J, Cheng YM, Lees-Miller JP, et al. NS1643 interacts around L529 of hERG to alter voltage sensor movement on the path to activation. Biophys J 2015; 108:1400–13.

88. Perissinotti LL, Guo J, De Biase PM, et al. Kinetic model for NS1643 drug activation of WT and L529I

variants of Kv11.1 (hERG1) potassium channel. Biophys J 2015;108:1414–24.

89. Salata JJ, Jurkiewicz NK, Wang J, et al. A novel benzodiazepine that activates cardiac slow delayed rectifier K^+ currents. Mol Pharmacol 1998; 54:220–30.

90. Seebohm G, Pusch M, Chen J, et al. Pharmacological activation of normal and arrhythmia-associated mutant KCNQ1 potassium channels. Circ Res 2003;93:941–7.

91. Gao Z, Xiong Q, Sun H, et al. Desensitization of chemical activation by auxiliary subunits: convergence of molecular determinants critical for augmenting KCNQ1 potassium channels. J Biol Chem 2008;283:22649–58.

92. Xiong Q, Sun H, Li M. Zinc pyrithione-mediated activation of voltage-gated KCNQ potassium channels rescues epileptogenic mutants. Nat Chem Biol 2007;3:287–96.

93. Mattmann ME, Yu H, Lin Z, et al. Identification of (R)-N-(4-(4-methoxyphenyl)thiazol-2-yl)-1-tosylpiperidine-2-carboxamide, ML277, as a novel, potent and selective $K_V7.1$ (KCNQ1) potassium channel activator. Bioorg Med Chem Lett 2012;22:5936–41.

94. Xu Y, Wang Y, Zhang M, et al. Probing binding sites and mechanisms of action of an I_{Ks} activator by computations and experiments. Biophys J 2015; 108:62–75.

95. Yu H, Lin Z, Mattmann ME, et al. Dynamic subunit stoichiometry confers a progressive continuum of pharmacological sensitivity by KCNQ potassium channels. Proc Natl Acad Sci U S A 2013;110: 8732–7.

96. Abitbol I, Peretz A, Lerche C, et al. Stilbenes and fenamates rescue the loss of I_{Ks} channel function induced by an LQT5 mutation and other IsK mutants. EMBO J 1999;18:4137–48.

97. Zheng Y, Zhu X, Zhou P, et al. Hexachlorophene is a potent KCNQ1/KCNE1 potassium channel activator which rescues LQTs mutants. PLoS One 2012;7: e51820.

98. Mruk K, Kobertz WR. Discovery of a novel activator of KCNQ1-KCNE1 K channel complexes. PLoS One 2009;4:e4236.

99. Liin SI, Silvera Ejneby M, Barro-Soria R, et al. Polyunsaturated fatty acid analogs act antiarrhythmically on the cardiac I_{Ks} channel. Proc Natl Acad Sci U S A 2015;112:5714–9.

Genetic Control of Potassium Channels

Ahmad S. Amin, MD, PhD[a], Arthur A.M. Wilde, MD, PhD[a,b],*

KEYWORDS

- Cardiac potassium channel • Gene • Long QT syndrome • Short QT syndrome
- Brugada syndrome • Atrial fibrillation • Ventricular fibrillation

KEY POINTS

- Approximately 80 genes in the human genome code for pore-forming subunits of potassium (K^+) channels.
- Rare variants (mutations) in K^+ channel–encoding genes may cause heritable arrhythmia syndromes.
- Not all rare variants in K^+ channel–encoding genes are necessarily disease-causing mutations.
- Common variants in K^+ channel–encoding genes are increasingly recognized as modifiers of phenotype in heritable arrhythmia syndromes and in the general population.
- Although difficult, distinguishing pathogenic variants from benign variants is of utmost importance to avoid false designations of genetic variants as disease-causing mutations.

INTRODUCTION

Cardiac K^+ channels play a pivotal role in the electrical activity of atrial and ventricular myocytes by controlling the shape and duration of the repolarization during phases 1, 2, and 3 of the action potential and by stabilizing the negative resting membrane potential during phase 4 of the action potential. In addition, K^+ channels contribute to the regulation of the heart rate by influencing the pacemaker activity in sinoatrial node (SAN) and atrioventricular node (AVN) cells. Understanding of the molecular identity of K^+ channels started in the late 1980s, when the first gene encoding a K^+ channel was identified in *Drosophila*.[1] Flies with a shaker phenotype, which involves leg shaking on exposure to ether, were found to miss a K^+ current in their leg and flight muscles. Isolation of the gene responsible for this defective K^+ current resulted in the cloning of the first K^+ channel. Next, by using the molecular cloning technique and the *shaker* gene as a homology probe, other *Drosophila* K^+ channel genes and their mammalian homologues were isolated. In addition, by using the cDNA expression method and heterologous expression systems (eg, *Xenopus* oocytes or mammalian cell lines), the products of these cloned K^+ genes were characterized and correlated with endogenous K^+ currents.[2] In this manner, numerous human K^+ channel–encoding genes have been identified. Knowledge of the genetic control of cardiac K^+ channels has greatly expanded from the early 1990s, when genetic

This article was supported by the Netherlands CardioVascular Research Initiative, the Dutch Heart Foundation, Dutch Federation of University Medical Centers, the Netherlands Organisation for Health Research and Development, the Royal Netherlands Academy of Sciences (PREDICT; AAMW), and the Netherlands Heart Foundation (td/dekk/2388 2013T042; ASA).
Conflicts of Interest: None.
[a] Department of Clinical and Experimental Cardiology, Heart Centre, Academic Medical Center, University of Amsterdam, Meibergdreef 9, Amsterdam 1105 AZ, The Netherlands; [b] King Abdulaziz University, Princess Al-Jawhara Al-Brahim Centre of Excellence in Research of Hereditary Disorders, PO Box 80200, Jeddah 21589, Kingdom of Saudi Arabia
* Corresponding author.
E-mail address: a.a.wilde@amc.uva.nl

cardiacEP.theclinics.com

linkage studies started to link rare variants (mutations) in genes encoding for cardiac K^+ channels to heritable arrhythmia syndromes.[3,4] To do this, genetic linkage studies used both positional cloning technique and candidate gene approach. The positional cloning technique links a gene to a phenotype by its approximate location on the chromosome without earlier information on the molecular basis of the disease. The candidate gene approach uses mechanistic hypotheses based on pathophysiology to associate some genes of interest to a certain phenotype. Currently, mutations in cardiac K^+ channel genes have been implicated in the etiology of various heritable arrhythmia syndromes, including long QT syndrome (LQTS), short QT syndrome (SQTS), and Brugada syndrome (BrS).[5] Experimental studies have provided further mechanistic insights into the role of these mutations by exploring their effects on expression and function of cardiac K^+ channels. Last but not least, the past decade faced trying to unravel the results of increasing numbers of large-scale genome-wide association studies (GWAS) and candidate gene studies that have discovered significant associations between common variants in cardiac K^+ channel genes and risk of sudden cardiac death and/or ECG indices of conduction and repolarization in the general population and risk of atrial fibrillation (AF).[6] This article is part of the *Cardiac Electrophysiology Clinics* issue, "Cardiac Potassium Channel Disorders." Current knowledge on the genetic control of cardiac K^+ channels in health and disease is reviewed. The molecular biology, structure, and function of K^+ channels and the clinical features of diseases linked to K^+ channel dysfunction are described in detail elsewhere in this issue (see Wu W, Sanguinetti MC: Molecular Basis of Cardiac Delayed Rectifier K+ Channel Function and Pharmacology, in this issue).

CARDIAC K^+ CHANNEL GENES IN HEALTH

A gene is a DNA fragment coding for a functional RNA or protein product. It consists of several regions of nucleotide sequences, including (1) 1 or more promoter regions that bind transcription factors and RNA polymerase to initiate transcription, (2) regulatory regions (enhancers or silencers) upstream (5'end) or downstream (3'end) of the open reading frame that can bind activator or repressor proteins to control transcription, (3) untranslated regions immediately flanking the open reading frame, which can influence mRNA translation, and (4) the open reading frame, which is the region from the start codon to the stop codon and has the potential to encode a protein (encompassing protein-coding exons and untranslated introns). Introns are removed from mRNA before translation through splicing, a process that is dictated by specific splice sites (ie, nucleotide sequences at both ends of introns). Through alternative splicing, genes are able to generate multiple mRNA variants from the same gene, thereby giving rise to diversity of the final product. This may explain why the diversity of K^+ currents in cardiac myocytes exceeds the number of K^+ channels genes identified. K^+ channel genes encode a diverse family of membrane-spanning proteins, all containing a homologous pore that selectively allows K^+ ions to flow across the cell membrane.[2] The superfamily of K^+ channels is usually classified based on the amino acid sequence of their pore-forming α-subunit. This results in 3 main families: (1) channels with 2 membrane-spanning (transmembrane) segments and a single pore, (2) channels with 6 transmembrane segments and a single pore, and (3) channels with 4 transmembrane segments and 2 pores, also called 2-pore K^+ (K_{2P}) channels.

K^+ Channels with Two Transmembrane Segments and a Single Pore

K^+ channels with 2 transmembrane segments and a single pore are also known as inwardly rectifying K^+ (K_{ir}) channels. Inward rectification refers to the functional properties of K_{ir} channel current, which involve preferential conduction of K^+ into the cell (inward) rather than out of the cell (outward). Each K_{ir} channel α-subunit contains a pore loop between its 2 transmembrane segments, a cytosolic N-terminus and a cytosolic C-terminus. **Fig. 1** shows a topological model of the α-subunit of the K_{ir} channel and the phylogenic tree of the 15 human K_{ir} channels based on the amino acid sequence of their α-subunits.[7] Subfamilies of the K_{ir} channel family in the heart include $K_{ir}2.x$, $K_{ir}3.x$, and $K_{ir}6.x$, which are responsible for the inward rectifier K^+ current (I_{K1}), the acetylcholine-activated G-protein-gated K^+ current ($I_{K,Ach}$), and the adenosine-5'-triphosphate-sensitive K^+ current ($I_{K,ATP}$), respectively (**Table 1**).[8]

Four $K_{ir}2.1$ α-subunits, encoded by *KCNJ2*, coassemble to form 1 homotetrameric I_{K1} channel.[9] Other $K_{ir}2.x$ members, including $K_{ir}2.2$, $K_{ir}2.3$, and $K_{ir}2.4$, are also expressed in the heart and may coassemble with $K_{ir}2.1$ to form heterotetrameric channels. I_{K1} conducts an inward K^+ current at membrane potentials negative to the K^+ equilibrium potential (approximately -90 mV) and a smaller but substantial outward K^+ current at potentials between -40 mV and -90 mV. These properties enable I_{K1} to maintain a negative

A

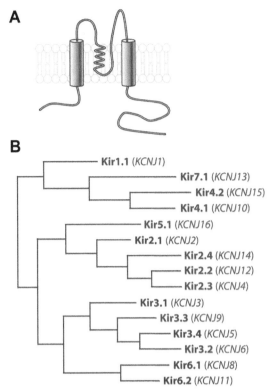

B

Kir1.1 (*KCNJ1*)
Kir7.1 (*KCNJ13*)
Kir4.2 (*KCNJ15*)
Kir4.1 (*KCNJ10*)
Kir5.1 (*KCNJ16*)
Kir2.1 (*KCNJ2*)
Kir2.4 (*KCNJ14*)
Kir2.2 (*KCNJ12*)
Kir2.3 (*KCNJ4*)
Kir3.1 (*KCNJ3*)
Kir3.3 (*KCNJ9*)
Kir3.4 (*KCNJ5*)
Kir3.2 (*KCNJ6*)
Kir6.1 (*KCNJ8*)
Kir6.2 (*KCNJ11*)

Fig. 1. K_{ir} channels. (*A*) Topological model of the pore-forming α-subunit of the K_{ir} channel. Each K_{ir} α-subunit contains 2 transmembrane segments, a pore-forming loop, and cytosolic N-terminus and C-terminus. (*B*) Phylogenic tree of the α-subunits of human K_{ir} channels based on the amino acid sequence alignments. In red are channels that play an important role in cardiac electricity. Gene names are shown between parenthesis.

membrane potential during phase 4 of atrial and ventricular action potentials and to contribute to the terminal portion of repolarization during phase 3.[8] I_{K1} is almost absent in SAN and AVN cells.

Four $K_{ir}3.1$ and $K_{ir}3.4$ α-subunits coassemble to form 1 heterotetrameric $I_{K,Ach}$ channel. *KCNJ3* and *KCNJ5* code for $K_{ir}3.1$ and Kir3.4, respectively.[10,11] $I_{K,Ach}$ is mainly expressed in SAN, atrial, and AVN cells. Binding of acetylcholine to muscarinic M_2 receptors leads to opening of $I_{K,Ach}$ channels via the βγ subunits of membrane G protein.[12] The resulting outward $I_{K,Ach}$ hyperpolarizes the membrane potential and slows the speed of spontaneous depolarization during phase 4 in pacemaker cells of SAN and AVN. This results in a lower heart rate and delayed AV conduction during parasympathetic activity. In addition, $I_{K,Ach}$ accelerates atrial repolarization and shortens atrial refractoriness.

The K^+ channel responsible for $I_{K,ATP}$ is a hetero-octameric protein complex formed by the coassembly of 4 $K_{ir}6.1$ α-subunits or 4 $K_{ir}6.2$ α-subunits and 4 sulfonylurea receptor (SUR) subunits (SUR1 or SUR2). *KCNJ8*, encoding $K_{ir}6.1$ (424 amino acids), is approximately 10.6 kilobases (kb) in length and has 3 exons.[13] *KCNJ11*, encoding Kir6.2 (390 amino acids), is a smaller gene (approximately 4.1 kb) with only 1 exon.[14] Compared with K_{ir} proteins, SUR subunits are much larger, with more than 1,500 amino acids and 3 transmembrane domains, each containing 5, 5, and 6 transmembrane segments. The genes coding for SUR1 and SUR2 are *ABCC8* and *ABCC9*, respectively (**Table 2**).[14,15] Alternative splicing of mRNA products give rise to multiple SUR variants (eg, SUR2A and SUR2B), which confer distinct functional and pharmacologic properties on $I_{K,ATP}$ channels. Both *KCNJ8* and *ABCC9* are located on chromosome 12p, whereas *KCNJ11* and *ABCC8* are located on chromosome 11p (at a distance of only approximately 4.5 kb from each other), suggesting their coregulation at gene level and that *KCNJ8/ABCC9* and *KCNJ11/ABCC8* may evolutionarily have been 1 gene. In healthy conditions, $I_{K,ATP}$ channels are closed due to the inhibitory effects of ATP at their cytoplasmic surface. Hypoxic conditions lead to lower intracellular ATP levels and thereby opening of $I_{K,ATP}$ channels. This results in an outward K^+ current, which leads to earlier repolarization and less influx of Ca^{2+} ions and, thereby, reduced contractile force and cellular energy consumption.[8] Thus, $I_{K,ATP}$ channels act as metabolic sensors by coupling membrane excitability to the energy demand of myocytes.[16] Current evidence suggests that $I_{K,ATP}$ channels in ventricular myocytes are composed primarily of Kir6.2 and SUR2A subunits whereas $I_{K,ATP}$ channels in atrial myocytes are composed primarily of Kir6.2 and SUR1 subunits. Kir6.1 subunits may contribute to the formation of $I_{K,ATP}$ channels in SAN, AVN, and Purkinje fiber cells.[15]

K^+ Channels with Six Transmembrane Segments and a Single Pore

K^+ channels with 6 transmembrane segments and a single pore include voltage-gated K^+ (K_v) channels and calcium-activated K^+ (K_{Ca}) channels.[2,5,17] The α-subunits contain a pore loop between the 5th and 6th transmembrane segments, a cytosolic N-terminus, and a cytosolic C-terminus (**Figs. 2A and 3A**). The phylogenic tree of human K_v and K_{Ca} channels based on the amino acid sequence of their α-subunit is shown in **Figs. 2B and 3B**.[7]

Table 1
Cardiac K^+ channel pore-forming α-subunits

Current	Tissue	α-Subunit	Topology	Protein Size (Amino Acids)	Chromosome	Gene	Gene Size (Bases)	Exons (Coding)
Inwardly activating channels								
I_{K1}	Atria, ventricles	Kir2.1	2 TM tetramer	427	17q24.3	KCNJ2	11,376	2 (1)
I_{KAch}	SAN, atria, AVN	Kir3.1	2 TM tetramer	501	2q24.1	KCNJ3	160,054	3 (3)
		Kir3.4		419	11q24.3	KCNJ5	29,810	3 (2)
I_{KATP}	Atria, ventricles	Kir6.1	2 TM tetramer	424	12p12.1	KCNJ8	10,627	3 (2)
		Kir6.2		390	11p15.1	KCNJ11	4,095	1 (1)
Voltage-gated channels								
$I_{to,slow}$	Atria, ventricles	K_v1.4	6 TM tetramer	653	11p14.1	KCNA4	7,290	2 (1)
$I_{to,fast}$	Atria, ventricles	K_v4.2	6 TM tetramer	630	7q31.31	KCND2	476,699	6 (6)
		K_v4.3		655	1p13.2	KCND3	218,869	8 (7)
I_{Kur}	Atria	K_v1.5	6 TM tetramer	613	12p13.32	KCNA5	2,870	1 (1)
I_{Ks}	Atria, ventricles	K_v7.1	6 TM tetramer	676	11p15.5	KCNQ1	404,427	16 (16)
I_{Kr}	Atria, ventricles	K_v11.1	6 TM tetramer	1159	7q36.1	KCNH2	33,374	15 (15)
Calcium-activated channels								
I_{KCa}	Atria	K_{Ca}2.1	6 TM tetramer	543	19p13.11	KCNN1	48,788	11 (9)
		K_{Ca}2.2	6 TM tetramer	579	5q22.3	KCNN2	135,696	9 (8)
		K_{Ca}2.3	6 TM tetramer	731	1q21.3	KCNN3	172,826	8 (8)
Two-pore channels								
I_{TWIK-1}	Atria, ventricles	K_{2p}1.1	4 TM dimer	336	1q42.2	KCNK1	58,509	3 (3)
I_{TASK-1}	Atria, AVN	K_{2p}3.1	4 TM dimer	394	2p23.3	KCNK3	40,731	2 (2)
I_{TALK-2}	Purkinje cells	K_{2p}17.1	4 TM dimer	332	6p21.2	KCNK17	15,553	5 (5)

Abbreviation: TM, transmembrane segments.

Table 2
Cardiac K$^+$ channel obligatory[a] and modulatory subunits

Subunit	Current	Protein Size (Amino Acids)	Chromosome	Gene	Gene Size (Bases)	Exons (Coding)
AKAP5	I_{K1}	427	14q23.3	AKAP5	9,005	2 (1)
Cav3	I_{K1} I_{Kr}	151	3p25.3	CAV3	198,009	3 (2)
DPP6	$I_{to,fast}$	865	7q36.2	DPP6	1,146,097	26 (26)
K$_v$β1	$I_{to,slow}$ I_{Kur}	419	3q25.31	KCNAB1	501,438	14 (14)
K$_v$β2	$I_{to,slow}$ I_{Kur}	367	1p36.31	KCNAB2	109,728	16 (15)
K$_v$β3	$I_{to,slow}$ I_{Kur}	404	17p13.1	KCNAB3	8,004	14 (14)
KChIP2	$I_{to,fast}$[a]	270	10q24.32	KCNIP2	17,947	10 (10)
Mink	I_{Ks}[a] I_{Kr}	129	21q22.12	KCNE1	65,588	2 (1)
MiRP1	I_{Ks} I_{Kr}[a]	123	21q22.11	KCNE2	7,366	2 (1)
MiRP2	I_{Ks} I_{Kr}	103	11q13.4	KCNE3	12,889	3 (1)
MiRP3	I_{Ks}	221	2q36.1	KCNE4	146,586	2 (2)
MiRP4	I_{Ks}	142	Xq23	KCNE5	1,473	1 (1)
SAP97	I_{K1} I_{Kur}	904	3q29	DLG1	256,741	26 (25)
SUR1	I_{KATP}[a]	1581	11p15.1	ABCC8	83,961	39 (39)
SUR2	I_{KATP}[a]	1549	12p12.1	ABCC9	144,475	38 (38)
Yotiao	I_{Ks}	3911	7q21.2	AKAP9	169,807	50 (50)

[a] Subunit is obligatory for the current.

Voltage-gated K$^+$ channels

K$_v$ channels are responsible for K$^+$ currents essential for repolarization during phases 1 to 3 of the atrial and ventricular action potential. These currents are the rapidly activating and inactivating transient outward current (I_{to}) and the ultrarapidly activating (I_{Kur}), the rapidly activating (I_{Kr}), and the slowly activating (I_{Ks}) delayed rectifier outward currents. In contrast to K$_{ir}$ channels, channels carrying outward rectifying currents preferentially conduct K$^+$ out of the cell (outward) than into the cell (inward).

I_{to} has 2 components. Its slow component, $I_{to,slow}$, recovers slowly from inactivation and is mainly present in the endocardium and Purkinje fiber cells. Its fast component, $I_{to,fast}$, recovers rapidly from inactivation and is mainly expressed in the epicardium. In the endocardium, 4 K$_v$1.4 α-subunits, encoded by KCNA4, coassemble to form the channel responsible for $I_{to,slow}$.[18] Channels responsible for $I_{to,slow}$ in Purkinje cells may require the composition of 4 K$_v$4.3 α-subunits, encoded by KCND3, and the regulatory subunits dipeptidyl-aminopeptidase-like protein-6 (DPP6) and frequenin (neuronal calcium sensor 1).[19] In the epicardium, the closely related K$_v$4.2 (KCND2) and K$_v$4.3 (KCND3) α-subunits can coassemble to form the tetrameric $I_{to,fast}$ channel.[20] In the human heart, however, K$_v$4.2 is minimally expressed and $I_{to,fast}$ channels are predominantly formed by K$_v$4.3 subunits.[21] Heterologous expression of KCND2 and KCND3 cDNA does not fully recapitulate native $I_{to,fast}$, unless coexpressed with the modulatory subunit KChIP2 (ie, K$^+$ channel interacting protein 2).[22] In the ventricles, KChIP2 mRNA displays 25-fold higher expression levels in the epicardium than in the endocardium, and this corresponds to the expression levels of $I_{to,fast}$.[23] It is, therefore, believed that transcriptional regulation of KCNIP2, the gene encoding KChIP2,

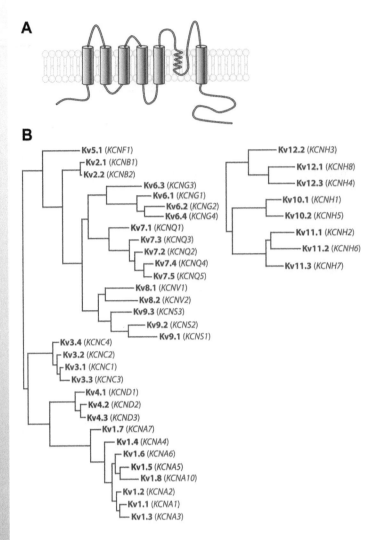

Fig. 2. K$_v$ channels. (*A*) Topological model of the pore-forming α-subunit of the K$_v$ channel. Each K$_v$ α-subunit contains 6 transmembrane segments, a pore-forming loop, intracellular and extracellular linkers, and cytosolic N-terminus and C-terminus. (*B*) Phylogenic tree of the α-subunits of human K$_v$ channels based on the amino acid sequence alignments. In red are channels that play an important role in cardiac electricity. Gene names are shown between parenthesis.

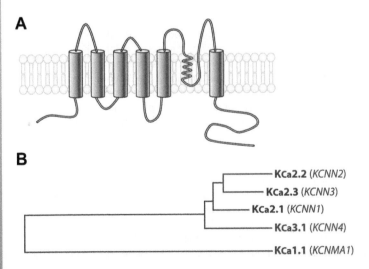

Fig. 3. K$_{Ca}$ channels. (*A*) Topological model of the pore-forming α-subunit of the K$_{Ca}$ channel. Each K$_{Ca}$ α-subunit contains 6 transmembrane segments, a pore-forming loop, intracellular and extracellular linkers, and cytosolic N-terminus and C-terminus. (*B*) Phylogenic trees of the α-subunits of human K$_{Ca}$ channels based on the amino acid sequence alignments. In red are channels that may play an important role in cardiac electricity. Gene names are shown between parenthesis.

primarily determines the transmural gradient of $I_{to,fast}$ expression across the ventricular wall.

I_{Kur} is carried by a channel composed of 4 $K_v1.5$ α-subunits. *KCNA5*, which encodes $K_v1.5$, is a small intron-less gene.[24] I_{Kur} is mainly expressed in the atria and plays a role in atrial repolarization.

I_{Kr} is one of the most, if not the most, important current for human cardiac repolarization. The α-subunit of the homotetrameric channel conducting I_{Kr} ($K_v11.1$) is encoded by *KCNH2*, a gene traditionally called the Human Ether-a-go-go Related Gene *(HERG)* due to its homology to the *Drosophila ether-a-go-go gene (eag)*.[3] Interaction of $K_v11.1$ with MinK-related peptide 1 (MiRP1), a β-subunit encoded by *KCNE2*, is thought to be required to recapitulate native I_{Kr}.[25] The role of MiRP1 in I_{Kr} modulation remains, however, controversial, especially because its expression is very low in the ventricles and only significantly high in Purkinje fiber cells.[26] *KCNH2* has 15 exons. Alternative splicing of KCNH2 transcripts leads to production of several $K_v11.1$ isoforms with different N-termini or C-termini.[27] The HERG1a transcript translates into the full-length $K_v11.1a$ protein. The HERG1b transcript translates into Kv11.1 b, which lacks the first 376 amino acids of $K_v11.1a$ and has an alternate 36–amino acids N-terminus. The Kv11.1-USO transcript codes for a protein in which the last 359 amino acids of $K_v11.1a$ or $K_v11.1$ b are replaced by an alternate 88–amino acids C-terminus. Kv11.1 b cDNA, but not Kv11.1-USO cDNA, can form functional channels in heterologous systems. Coassembly of $K_v11.1a$ with Kv11.1b results in higher expression levels of channels with different functional properties and drug sensitivity, whereas coassembly of $K_v11.1a$ with Kv11.1-USO results in lower expression levels of $K_v11.1a$.

I_{Ks} plays also an important role in human repolarization, particularly during increased sympathetic activity. The I_{Ks} channel consists of 4 $K_v7.1$ α-subunits.[4] *KCNQ1*, encoding $K_v7.1$, is initially imprinted during early embryogenesis (ie, expressed only from the maternal allele) but the expression becomes biallelic during fetal cardiac development.[28] For *KCNQ1*-encoded channels to conduct a current resembling I_{Ks}, the presence of the β-subunit MinK (encoded by *KCNE1*) is required. In addition, MinK is believed to enable phosphorylation of $K_v7.1$ channels by protein kinase C on β-adrenergic stimulation, a process that significantly augments I_{Ks} and underlies the physiologic response (abbreviation) of repolarization to fast heart rates during sympathetic activity.

Calcium-activated K^+ channels

K_{Ca} channels have recently been implicated in the human cardiac electricity—for a long time they were thought to be absent in cardiac myocytes.[5,17] K_{Ca} channels are categorized into 3 subfamilies according to their single-channel conductance properties: big-conductance ($K_{Ca}1.1$), intermediate-conductance ($K_{Ca}3.1$), and small-conductance ($K_{Ca}2.1$, $K_{Ca}2.2$, and $K_{Ca}2.3$) channels. To date, only small-conductance channels have been identified as functional in the cell membranes of cardiac myocytes. $K_{Ca}1.1$ channels may be expressed in mitochondrial membranes. Genes encoding $K_{Ca}2.1$, $K_{Ca}2.2$, and $K_{Ca}2.3$ are *KCNN1*, *KCNN2*, and *KCNN3*, respectively (see **Table 1**).[29–31] Four $K_{Ca}2.1$, $K_{Ca}2.2$, and/or $K_{Ca}2.3$ α-subunits coassemble to form homotetrameric or heterotetrameric channels, which are activated by low concentrations of cytoplasmic Ca^{2+}. Ca^{2+} does not directly bind to the channels but through constitutively binding of calmodulin to the C-terminus of $K_{Ca}2.x$. Current evidence suggests that $K_{Ca}2.x$ channels are atrial specific and play a role in the pathophysiology of AF.[17]

K^+ Channels with Four Transmembrane Segments and Two Pores

K_{2P} channels are recently added as members to the K^+ channel superfamily. The α-subunits of K_{2P} channels have both unique structural and functional features. Structurally, they are composed of 2 pore loops, 4 transmembrane segments, a cytosolic N-terminus, and a cytosolic C-terminus (**Fig. 4A**). The presence of 2 pores enables them to form homodimers or heterodimers instead of tetramers like other K^+ channels. Functionally, they are distinguished by their lack of voltage sensitivity, their open state at all membrane potentials, and their regulation by numerous chemical and physical stimuli, including lipids, pH, temperature, oxygen, membrane stretch, neurotransmitters, and second messengers.[32] As a result, K_{2P} channels can conduct a background (leak) K^+ current through all phases of the cardiac action potential, thereby stabilizing the resting potential near the equilibrium potential of K^+ during phase 4, ensuring the availability of Na^+ channels during phase 0 and facilitating repolarization during phase 1 to 3 of the action potential. So far, 15 K_{2P} channels are discovered and divided into subfamilies based on the amino acid sequence of their α-subunit (**Fig. 4B**).[7] Based on their functional properties, K_{2P} channels are classified into 6 different subfamilies: 2-pore domain in a weakly K_{ir} channel (TWIK); TWIK-related K^+ channel

A

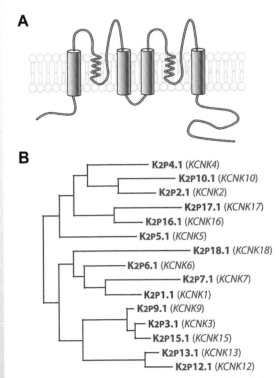

B

Fig. 4. K_{2P} channels. (A) Topological model of the pore-forming α-subunit of the K_{2P} channel. Each K_{2P} α-subunit contains 4 transmembrane segments, 2 pore-forming loops, an intracellular linker, and cytosolic N-terminus and C-terminus. (B) Phylogenic trees of the α-subunits of human K_{2P} channels based on the amino acid sequence alignments. In red are channels that may play an important role in cardiac electricity. Gene names are shown between parenthesis.

(TREK); TWIK-related acid-sensitive K^+ channel (TASK); TWIK-related alkaline-sensitive K^+ channel (TALK); tandem pore domain halothane-inhibited K^+ channel (THIK); and TRESK TWIK-related spinal cord K^+ channel (TRESK).[32] Cardiac expression in humans has been shown at mRNA level for $K_{2P}1.1$ (coded by *KCNK1*), $K_{2P}3.1$ (coded by *KCNK3*), $K_{2P}4.1$ (coded by *KCNK4*), $K_{2P}5.1$ (coded by *KCNK5*), $K_{2P}15.1$ (coded by *KCNK15*), and $K_{2P}17.1$ (coded by *KCNK17*). Further studies are needed to understand the importance of each of these channels for cardiac rhythm. So far, available data suggest a role for $K_{2P}3.1$ in atrial repolarization and for $K_{2P}17.1$ in AVN conduction.[33–35]

MODULATORY SUBUNITS OF CARDIAC K^+ CHANNEL GENES

The α-subunits of cardiac K^+ channels are usually able to form functional channels in heterologous expression systems (in vitro). The resulting currents, however, often display different functional properties compared with their correlated native K^+ currents. This may be partially due to different post-translational modification processes and heterologous coassembly of α-subunits within the same subfamily with each other in vivo. In addition, expression levels and functional properties of K^+ channels are well known to be modulated by the interaction of their α-subunits with multiple regulatory proteins and β-subunits.[36] It is beyond the scope of this review to discuss the regulatory proteins of cardiac K^+ channels in detail. A list of the most well-known proteins is provided in **Table 2**. Expression of some of these proteins, however, and thereby their modulatory effects on K^+ channels may be tissue specific. For example, expression level of DPP6, a regulatory subunit of I_{to}, is low in the ventricles and only significantly high in Purkinje fibers, whereas KChIP2, another regulatory subunit I_{to}, is relatively more expressed in the ventricles than in Purkinje fibers.[19]

CARDIAC K^+ CHANNEL GENES IN HERITABLE CARDIAC DISEASES

In the mid-1990s, *KCNH2* (coding for $K_v11.1$) and *KCNQ1* (coding for $K_v7.1$) were among the first genes linked to a heritable cardiac phenotype, that is, the LQTS, a repolarization disease characterized by prolonged heart rate–corrected QT interval (QTc), syncope, and sudden death due to torsades de pointes ventricular tachycardia and ventricular fibrillation.[3,4] These discoveries created great enthusiasm among geneticists around the world to search for mutations in families or in single individuals with a heritable cardiac phenotype using the positional cloning technique and more often the candidate gene approach. Through these efforts, large numbers of mutations in several genes of cardiac K^+ channels or other cardiac ion channels were associated with distinct heritable cardiac phenotypes (so-called ion channelopathies), including LQTS, SQTS, BrS, and familial AF (**Table 3**).[5] Most of these associations, however, do not fulfill to a combination of criteria required to draw definite conclusions regarding the causative link between a rare variant (mutation) and a phenotype. These criteria include detailed knowledge about the frequency of the variant in the general population, verification of the association in independent populations, evaluation of cosegregation in families, and experimental evidence for a mechanistic pathway between the variant and the phenotype. Fulfilling these criteria has become of great importance because increasing availability and analysis of human genomic data have revealed that many variants

Table 3
Cardiac K$^+$ channels associated with a heritable arrhythmic phenotype

Current	Gene	Subunit	Effect of Mutation	Phenotype	Reference
I$_{K1}$	KCNJ2	Kir2.1	Loss of function	LQT7[a]	41
			Gain of function	SQT3[a]	42
			Gain of function	AF[a]	43
I$_{KAch}$	KCNJ5	Kir3.4	Loss of function	LQTS type	44
			Loss of function	AF	45
I$_{KATP}$	KCNJ8	Kir6.1	Gain of function	BrS	46
	ABCC9	SUR2	Gain of function	ERS	47
			Loss of function	BrS	48
			Loss of function	AF	49
I$_{to,fast}$	KCND2	K$_v$4.2	Gain of function	ERS	50
	KCND3	K$_v$4.3	Gain of function	BrS	51
	KCND3	K$_v$4.3	Gain of function	AF	52
	KCNE3	MiRP2	Gain of function	BrS	53
	KCNE3	MiRP2	Gain of function	AF	54
	KCNE5	MiRP4	Gain of function	BrS	55
I$_{Kur}$	KCNA5	K$_v$1.5	Loss of function	AF	56
I$_{Ks}$	KCNQ1	K$_v$7.1	Loss of function	LQT1[a]	4
			Loss of function	JLNS[a]	57
			Gain of function	SQT2[a]	58
			Gain of function	AF[a]	59
	KCNE1	minK	Loss of function	LQT5[a]	60
			Loss of function	JLNS[a]	61
			Gain of function	AF	62
	KCNE2	MiRP1	Gain of function	AF	63
	KCNE3	MiRP2	Loss of function	LQTS	64
	KCNE5	MiRP4	Gain of function	AF	65
	AKAP9	Yotiao	Loss of function	LQTS type	66
I$_{Kr}$	KCNH2	K$_v$11.1	Loss of function	LQT2[a]	3
			Gain of function	SQT1[a]	67
			Gain of function	BrS	68
	KCNE2	MiRP1	Loss of function	LQT6[a]	25
	KCNE3		Gain of function	AF	54
I$_{TASK-1}$	KCNK3	K$_{2p}$3.1	Loss of function	AF	69
I$_{TALK-2}$	KCNK17	K$_{2p}$17.1	Gain of function	Cardiac conduction defect[b]	33

[a] Diseases with a strong (causal) association with mutations in the corresponding gene.
[b] Effect only in the copresence of a splice-site mutation in SCN5A.
  Data from Refs.[3,4,25,33,41–51,53–69]

previously linked to cardiac diseases are not rare but actually common variants and that a significant number of rare variants in genes encoding cardiac ion channels are present in individuals with no history of cardiac diseases.[37–39] Obtaining experimental evidence for a mechanistic relation between a variant and a phenotype is, however, difficult and time consuming, and evaluation of cosegregation in families is greatly hampered by small family sizes (often single affected individuals), low penetrance, and variable expressivity of a potential disease-causing mutation.[40] Low penetrance means that not all mutation carriers within a family develop a phenotype, whereas variable expressivity refers to the variable degree in which carriers of an identical mutation manifest a certain phenotype. Thus, although the ascription of ion channelopathies to an increasing number of cases is currently being challenged by the growing knowledge on human genome, extreme caution is needed in the interpretation of data from genetic studies to avoid false designations of variants as pathogenic mutations.

Long QT Syndrome

The autosomal dominant form of LQTS, traditionally called Romano-Ward syndrome, is classified into different subtypes based on the chronologic order in which they are reported. Based on the available evidence, mutations in 5 different K+ channel genes can be regarded as causative in the etiology of LQTS, including *KCNQ1* (LQT1), *KCNH2* (LQT2), and *KCNJ2* (LQT7; also known as Andersen syndrome) encoding pore-forming α-subunits,[3,4,41] and *KCNE1* (LQT5) and *KCNE2* (LQT6) encoding modulatory β-subunits.[25,60] The autosomal recessive form of LQTS is called Jervell and Lange-Nielsen syndrome (JLNS) and is caused by homozygous mutations in *KCNQ1* or *KCNE1*.[57,61]

LQTS-related mutations are often single-nucleotide substitutions. When located in exons, single-nucleotide substitutions alter a codon and result in the replacement of one amino acid by a different one (missense mutations) or create a premature stop codon, leading to the generation of a truncated protein (nonsense mutations). Single-nucleotide substitutions may also affect the splicing when located at specific splice sites at intron/exon (acceptor site) and exon/intron (donor site) boundaries. Mutations within these highly conserved sites may result in deletion of entire exons (or exon parts) or inclusion of entire introns (or intron parts) in the mature mRNA. This often changes the open reading frame of translation and leads to addition of an altered sequence of amino acids to the protein (ie, frameshift). Mutations also involve insertion or deletion of 1 or more nucleotides, which may lead to a shift in the open reading frame or (when a multiple of 3 nucleotides is inserted or deleted) to addition or removal of 1 or more amino acids in the protein, without changing the reading frame.[70] Whatever the type, all LQTS-linked mutations cause loss of function, meaning that they lead to a reduction of the corresponding outward K+ currents (I_{Ks} in cases of LQT1, LQT5, and JLNS; I_{Kr} in cases of LQT2 and LQT6; and I_{K1} in the case of LQT7).[71] Loss of function is achieved through a decrease in the number of functional channels in the cell membrane (reduced expression) or defective channel opening/closing (unfavorable gating) (**Fig. 5**). When mutated α-subunits still possess the ability to interact with normal α-subunits, both expression and gating may be adversely affected (dominant-negative effect). Loss of ability to participate in tetramer assembly often leads to premature degradation of the mutated subunits, which results in lower expression levels, whereas gating of the channels composed of normal subunits remains unaltered (haploinsufficiency). Dominant-negative mutations are associated with worse clinical outcomes than mutations that cause haploinsufficiency.[72,73]

I_{Ks}-related long QT syndrome: long QT1, long QT5, and Jervell and Lange-Nielsen syndrome

LQT1 accounts for approximately 40% of all LQTS cases, and to date, more than 300 mutations have been linked to LQT1. It remains unknown, however, how many of these *KCNQ1* mutations are really pathogenic. LQT1 mutations are missense (approximately 70%), frameshift (approximately 10%), splice-site (approximately 10%), nonsense (approximately 5%), in-frame deletions or insertions (approximately 5%), or large genomic rearrangements (copy number variants) with complete deletion of 1 or more exons. LQT1 mutations are located in the transmembrane segments (approximately 60%), C-terminus (approximately 30%), and N-terminus (approximately 10%) of $K_v7.1$.[74,75] Different, but not mutually exclusive, mechanisms underlie I_{Ks} loss of function, including defective $K_v7.1$ synthesis, deficient trafficking of mutated $K_v7.1$ to the cell membrane, loss of ability to coassemble into tetramers, altered gating, disrupted interaction with modulatory subunits, abnormal phosphorylation, and defective endosomal recycling (see **Fig. 5**). Type and location of a mutation may predict the clinical outcome and whether it is pathogenic or an innocuous variant. Mutations with dominant-negative effects and mutations located in the transmembrane segments and cytoplasmic loops between the segments are associated with higher rates of cardiac events.[71,72] Nonmissense mutations have an estimated predictive value of greater than 99% to be pathogenic. Missense mutations have a high predictive value to be pathogenic only if located in the transmembrane segments, pore loop, and C-terminus of $K_v7.1$ proteins.[76]

LQT5-related mutations in *KCNE1* are responsible for approximately 3% of all LQTS cases.[74] LQT5 mutations are mainly missense mutations, but in-frame deletions, nonsense, and frameshift mutations have also been reported. Most mutations impair the ability of MinK to modulate I_{Ks} gating. Other mechanisms include defective trafficking of mutated MinK (and thereby $K_v7.1$) to cell membrane, impaired tetramer assembly, and abnormal interaction of MinK with phosphatidylinositol-4, 5-bisphosphate (PIP2), which mediates I_{Ks} channel phosphorylation.[71]

JLNS is the rare autosomal recessive form of LQTS with concomitant congenital bilateral sensory neural deafness. JLNS is caused by homozygous or compound heterozygous mutations in *KCNQ1* or *KCNE1*.[57,61] Hearing loss is due to I_{Ks} channel loss of function in the inner ear, where it act as a K$^+$ charge carrier for sensory transduction and generation of endocochlear potential in the endolymph. *KCNQ1* mutations account for approximately 90% of all JLNS cases. Most JLNS-linked mutations are nonsense, frameshift, and splice-site mutations and cause haploinsufficiency. This is probably why heterozygous parents of JLNS patients have a much less severe phenotype compared with LQT1 patients.[77]

I_{Kr}-related long QT syndrome: long QT2 and long QT6

LQT2 accounts for approximately 30% of all LQTS cases. LQT2-linked *KCNH2* mutations involve missense (approximately 60%), frameshift (approximately 25%), nonsense (approximately 10%), splice-site mutations and in-frame deletions or insertions (approximately 5%), and large genomic rearrangements. LQT2 mutations are located in the C-terminus (approximately 40%), transmembrane segments (approximately 30%), and N-terminus (approximately 30%) of K$_v$11.1.[74] Missense mutations in transmembrane segments, the linkers, and the pore loop have a predictive value of 100% to be pathogenic and are associated with a worse phenotype.[73,76] I_{Kr} reduction is most often caused by impaired intracellular trafficking of mutated subunits.[78] Other less prevalent mechanisms include defective K$_v$11.1 synthesis, nonsense-mediated decay (NMD), altered gating, abnormal channel phosphorylation, and reduced K$^+$ permeation (see **Fig. 5**).[71,78,79] NMD is an RNA surveillance mechanism that selectively degrades mRNA transcripts with a premature stop codon due to the presence of a nonsense or frameshift mutation. In this way, NMD prevents the generation of mutated subunits with a potential dominant-negative effect on normal K$_v$11.1 subunits.[79] Mutations in *KCNE2* may be responsible for less than 1% of all LQTS cases.[74] LQT5-related mutations in MiRP2 lead to I_{Kr} loss of function through adverse modulatory effects on K$_v$11.1. channel expression and gating.[71]

I_{K1}-related long QT syndrome: long QT7 (Andersen syndrome)

Andersen syndrome is characterized by K$^+$-sensitive periodic paralysis, dysmorphic features (eg, short stature, scoliosis, clinodactyly, and hypertelorism), and ventricular arrhythmias. Although this rare disease is often considered a subtype of LQTS (LQT7), this may be argued because of the presence of the noncardiac manifestations, prominent U waves, and no or only mild QT prolongation.[41] Mutations in *KCNJ2* account for approximately 60% of all cases with Andersen syndrome. Virtually all these mutations lead to the formation of proteins, which are still able to coassemble with normal K$_{ir}$2.1 subunits, thereby exerting dominant-negative effects on their gating and altering their sensitivity to PIP2, an essential activator of the I_{K1} channel.[80]

Other K$^+$ channel genes associated with long QT syndrome

AKAP9, *KCNE3*, and *KCNJ5* are 3 K$^+$ channel genes that are yet anecdotally linked to LQTS. AKAP9 and KCNE3 code for modulatory subunits of the I_{Ks} channel. AKAP9 interacts with I_{Ks} channel proteins to mediate their phosphorylation on β-adrenergic stimulation. The only *AKAP9* missense mutation described so far was found in a patient with LQTS. The mutation was shown to disrupt the interaction of AKAP9 with K$_v$7.1, leading to reduced K$_v$7.1 phosphorylation after β-adrenergic stimulation.[66] This could theoretically impair I_{Ks} increase during sympathetic activity. The 2 mutations in *KCNE3*, encoding MiRP2, were found in 3 of 485 patients with LQTS and were shown to lead to I_{Ks} loss of function in vitro.[64] Finally, a loss-of-function mutation in *KCNJ5*, encoding the α-subunit (K$_{ir}$3.4) of I_{K-ACh} channel, was found in the affected members of a large Chinese family with LQTS.[44] Because I_{K-Ach} is mainly present in SAN, atria, and AVN, the precise effect of this mutation on ventricular repolarization is yet unclear.

Short QT Syndrome

SQTS is a rare disease characterized by persistent shorter-than-normal QT intervals, syncope, and sudden death due to ventricular fibrillation. SQTS patients may also suffer from AF.[81] After its first description in 2000, genetic studies using candidate gene approach in unrelated families with SQTS soon linked SQTS to mutations in 3 K$^+$ channel genes: *KCNH2* (SQTS type 1; SQT1), *KCNQ1* (SQTS type 2; SQT2), and *KCNJ2* (SQTS type 3; SQT3).[42,58,67,82,83] Only a small number of mutations have been described so far, all of them being missense mutations and causing gain of function by altering gating properties (see **Fig. 5**). The anticipated increase in I_{Kr} (SQT1), I_{Ks} (SQT2) or the outward component of I_{K1} (SQT3) is expected to speed up repolarization and thereby shorten the QTc. Based on these studies and the extensive data available for LQTS, it is reasonable to assume that gain-of-function mutations may mirror the effects of loss-of-function mutations in *KCNH2*, *KCNQ1*, and *KCNJ2* and thus be causally related to SQTS. It is important to emphasize, however, that in the absence of detailed information about

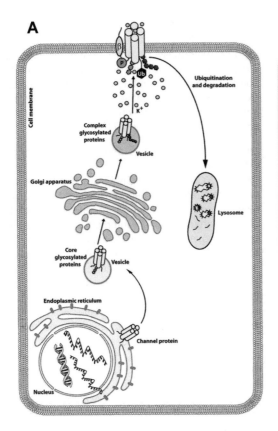

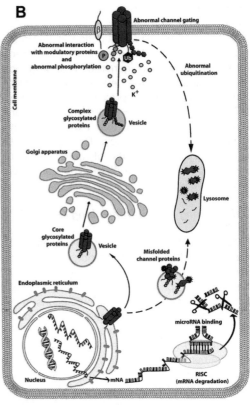

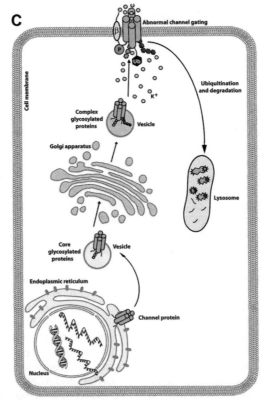

their frequency in the general population, not all variants found in patients with SQTS can be regarded as mutations and thus disease-causing.

Brugada Syndrome and Early Repolarization Syndrome

BrS is associated with characteristic coved-type ST segment (or J-point) elevation in the right precordial ECG leads V_1–V_3, often prolonged conduction intervals (PR and QRS), and increased risk for ventricular tachycardia and fibrillation. Early repolarization syndrome (ERS) is characterized by J-point elevation with either terminal QRS slurring or notching in at least 2 contiguous leads.[84] Although early repolarization is a prevalent ECG sign in the general population, it is more frequently observed in patients with who have experienced a syncope or out-of-hospital cardiac arrest due to idiopathic ventricular fibrillation. BrS is traditionally considered an Na^+ channelopathy because of its association with loss-of-function mutations in SCN5A, the gene encoding the α-subunit of the cardiac Na^+ channel. BrS-linked mutations in SCN5A lead to decreased I_{Na} during phase 0 of the cardiac action potential. This is speculated to give I_{to} more repolarizing power during action potential phases 0–1, leading to loss of action potential plateau because the membrane potential is not able anymore to reach voltages required for L-type Ca^{2+} channels to activate. Because I_{to} is more present in epicardium than endocardium, loss of action potential plateau may aggravate transmural voltage gradients and provide a substrate for electrical reentry.[85] Driven by this theory and the fact that SCN5A mutations are found in only approximately 20% of all BrS cases, scientists started to search for mutations in genes encoding cardiac K^+ channels that are active during phases 0–1 of the action potential. These efforts have resulted in the identification of several rare variants in genes coding for different subunits of I_{to} (ie, KCND2, KCND3, KCNE3, and KCNE5)[50,51,53,55] and $I_{K\text{-}ATP}$ (ie, KCNJ8 and ABCC9)[46–48] in individuals with BrS or ERS. As expected, all these variants caused I_{to} or $I_{K\text{-}ATP}$ gain of function in vitro. Missense variants in KCNH2 with putative gain-of-function effects have also been found in unrelated BrS patients.[68] A recent study, however, searched for the presence of rare coding variants in 45 arrhythmia-susceptibility genes (including KCND3, KCNE3, KCNE5, KCNJ8, and ABCC9) in 167 BrS cases and an equal number of healthy controls with no history of cardiac arrhythmia and found an association only between BrS and variants in SCN5A.[38] In this study, rare coding variants in most other BrS-susceptibility genes were observed in a similar extent among BrS cases and controls. In addition, another study identified a rare variant in KCNJ8, previously linked to both BrS and ERS, as a common variant in Ashkenazi Jews,[86] suggesting that this variant may be benign. Therefore, extreme caution should be taken in designating rare variants in genes other than SCN5A as causal mutations in BrS or ERS.

Atrial Fibrillation

The pathophysiologic mechanisms underlying the development AF are complex, probably involving both environmental and acquired triggers as well as genetic factors.[87] The latter may play a more

---

Fig. 5. Common molecular mechanisms for mutations to cause loss of function or gain of function of the cardiac K^+ channels in heritable K^+ channel diseases. (A) Displays post-transcriptional and post-translational processes of K^+ channel proteins in the healthy condition. After transcription in the nucleus, mRNA is processed in the nucleus (eg, splicing) and translated into protein in the ER. Next, channels proteins are folded, core-glycosylated, and coassembled into tetramers in the ER and transported via vesicles to the Golgi apparatus, where they undergo complex glycosylation. From the Golgi apparatus, channel proteins travel to the cell membrane where they interact with modulatory proteins (eg, β-subunits) and undergo further post-translational modification (eg, phosphorylation [P] and ubiquitination [Ub]). Ubiquitination leads to endocytosis and degradation of the channels in the lysosome or proteasome. The expression of modulatory proteins of cardiac K^+ channel (eg, β-subunits) proteins involves a similar molecular pathway from the nucleus to the cell membrane (not shown). (B) Displays post-transcriptional and post-translational processes for mutations with loss-of-function effects. Mutated mRNA transcripts may be degraded through NMD (not shown) or miRNA-mediated repression of translation. Variations in the 3'UTR may increase the binding affinity of the 3'UTR to target miRNAs, leading to the degradation of the mRNA by the RNA-induced silencing complex (RISC). Misfolded mutated proteins are transported to the lysosome where they undergo proteolysis. If not misfolded, channel proteins may travel through the Golgi apparatus to the cell membrane. Loss-of-function effects at the cell membrane include defective interaction of channel proteins with their modulatory proteins, abnormal phosphorylation, and abnormal ubiquitination. Finally, defective channel opening and closing (gating) may cause loss of function. (C) Displays posttranscriptional and posttranslational processes for mutations that cause gain of function. Gain-of-function effects are primarily mediated by changes in channel gating.

important role in the case of familial AF. Several mutations in K^+ channel genes have been found in families or individuals with AF, including gain-of-function mutations in *KCNJ2* (I_{K1}),[43] *KCND3* (I_{to}),[52] *KCNE3* $(I_{to}$ and $I_{Kr})$,[54] *KCNQ1* (I_{Ks}),[59] *KCNE1* (I_{Ks}),[62] *KCNE2* (I_{Ks}),[63] and *KCNE5* (I_{Ks}),[65] and loss-of-function mutations in *KCNJ5* (I_{K-Ach}),[45] *ABCC9* (I_{K-ATP}),[49] *KCNA5* (I_{Kur}),[56] and *KCNK3* encoding the newly discovered $K_{2P}3.1$ channel responsible for $I_{TASK,}$ a background K^+ current in the atria.[69] Although these mutations are speculated to shorten or prolong atrial repolarization and thereby facilitate reentry, their precise contribution to the multifactorial etiologic pathway of AF remains unresolved. A similar association bias, however, as observed in BrS and ERS, may be imperative in the association of rare variants in K^+ channel genes and AF.

CARDIAC K^+ CHANNEL GENES AS MODIFIERS OF PHENOTYPE

Major challenges in the concept of monogenetic arrhythmia syndromes are the low penetrance and variable expressivity of a putative disease-causing mutation. There are several examples of pedigrees with a heritable phenotype, in particular LQTS, in which members with an identical mutation display large differences in disease severity, ranging from lifelong asymptomatic to sudden cardiac death at young age.[88,89] Although some demographic and environmental factors, such as age, gender, exercise, auditory stimuli, circadian rhythm, and drugs, and some physiologic changes, such as fever and electrolyte changes, have been recognized as modifiers of phenotype in LQTS or BrS, these factors only partially explain the incomplete penetrance and variable expressivity in these monogenetic syndromes.[40] Recently, coinheritance of additional common genetic variants has been proposed as an explanation for the differences in phenotype among carriers of an identical mutation. Common variants are naturally occurring DNA sequence variations with a minor allele frequency (MAF) between 1% and 5% in the general population, which are expected to exert an intermediate effect on a certain phenotype. These common variants contrast with rare variants with less than 1% MAFs that are assumed to be pathogenic, such as mutations found in patients with LQTS, SQTS, or BrS, and very common variants with greater than 5% MAFs that are expected to have a minor effect on the phenotype. Common variants include (1) mutations with low penetrance, such as those identified in LQTS patients with a relatively benign phenotype; (2) variants associated with a phenotype only in the copresence of another disease-modifying factor, such as those found in subjects with drug-induced LQTS; and (3) variants associated with a certain phenotype in the general population by GWAS, for example single-nucleotide polymorphisms (SNPs) associated with the QTc duration or conduction intervals.[40]

Cardiac K^+ Channel Genes as Modifiers of Phenotype in Heritable Arrhythmia Syndromes

The discovery of common variants as modifiers of phenotype in heritable arrhythmia syndromes has moved the concept of these diseases from monogenic diseases to oligogenic or even polygenic diseases. This concept is based on the assumption that coinheritance of a second (or even more) genetic variant that modifies a certain phenotype may determine the final clinical outcome of a disease-causing mutation in a particular carrier (the so-called double-hit theory). Double hits include 2 mutations in the same gene (compound heterozygosity), 2 mutations in different genes (digenic heterozygosity), or a mutation and a common variant in the same gene or different genes (oligogenic inheritance). Compound heterozygosity and digenic heterozygosity are not uncommon in LQTS (prevalence between 5% and 10%) and are associated with a more severe outcome.[90] Common variants (SNPs) in several K^+ channel–encoding genes are proposed as genetic modifiers in LQTS, including coding variants in *KCNE1* (D85 N)[91] and *KCNH2* (K897 T),[92] an intronic variant in *KCNQ1*,[93] and noncoding variants in the 3′ untranslated region (3′UTR) of *KCNQ1* (**Table 4**).[94] The minor allele of D85 N is associated with a more severe phenotype in LQT1 and LQT2 and with loss of function of channels responsible for I_{Ks} and I_{Kr}.[91] The minor allele of K897 T is associated with more severe phenotype in LQT2 patients who carry the variant on their nonmutated *KCNH2* allele and is expected to cause I_{Kr} loss of function.[92] The minor allele of the intronic variant in *KCNQ1* (rs2074238) is associated with lower risk of symptoms and shorter QTc in LQT1 and LQT2.[93] The underlying mechanism, however, is as yet unclear. The role of variants in the 3′UTR of *KCNQ1* in LQTS is discussed later.

Case-control studies also have associated common variants in 3 K^+ channel–related genes with the risk of AF, including (1) a coding variant in the β-subunit of membrane G protein, which is associated with increased opening of the I_{K-Ach} channel (lower risk for AF)[97]; (2) a coding variant in

Table 4
Common variants in cardiac K+ channel genes associated with an arrhythmic phenotype

Current	Gene	Single-nucleotide Polymorphism	Location	Effect	Method	Cohort	Reference
I_{K1}	KCNJ2	rs17779747	Intergenic	QTc	Genome-wide	General population	95
		rs7219669	Intergenic	TPE	Genome-wide	General population	96
I_{KAch}	GNB3	rs5443	Exon (C825 T)	AF	Candidate gene	AF	97
$I_{to,fast}$	KCND3	rs2798334	Intron	PR	Genome-wide	General population	98
I_{Ks}	KCNQ1	rs12296050	Intron	QTc	Genome-wide	General population	95
		rs12576239	Intron	QTc	Genome-wide	General population	99
		rs2074238	Intron	QTc	Genome-wide	General population	99
		rs757092	Intron	QTc	Candidate genes	General population	100
		rs2074238	Intron	QTc	Candidate genes	LQTS	93
		rs2283222	Intron	SCD	Candidate genes	General population	101
		rs2519184	3'UTR	QTc/symptoms	Candidate genes	LQTS type 1	94
		rs8234	3'UTR	QTc/symptoms	Candidate genes	LQTS type 1	94
		rs10798	3'UTR	QTc/symptoms	Candidate genes	LQTS type 1	94
	KCNE1	rs1805128	Exon (D85 N)	QTc	Genome-wide	General population	99
				QTc	Candidate genes	General population	102
				QTc	Candidate genes	LQTS	91
				QTc	Whole exome	Drug-induced LQTS	103
		rs74315445	Exon (D76 N)	QTc	Whole exome	Drug-induced LQTS	103
		rs727957	Intergenic	QTc	Candidate genes	General population	100
		rs1805127	Exon (S38 G)	AF	Candidate genes	AF	104
	AKAP9	rs2961024	Intron	QTc	Candidate genes	LQTS type 1	105
		rs11772585	Intron	Symptoms	Candidate genes	LQTS type 1	105
		rs7808587	Intron	Symptoms	Candidate genes	LQTS type 1	105
I_{kr}	KCNH2	rs2968863	Intergenic	QTc	Genome-wide	General population	95
		rs4725982	Intergenic	QTc	Genome-wide	General population	99
		rs1805123	Exon (K897 T)	QTc	Candidate genes	General population	100,102,106
				TPE	Candidate genes	General population	107
				AF	Candidate genes	AF	108
				QTc	Candidate genes	LQTS type 2	92
				QTc	Candidate genes	General population	100,102,106
		rs3807375	Intron	QTc	Candidate genes	General population	102,106
		rs3815459	Intron	QTc	Candidate genes	General population	100
I_{kCa}	KCNN3	rs13376333	Intron	AF	Genome-wide	AF	34
		rs6666258	Intron	AF	Genome-wide	AF	35

Abbreviations: PR, PR interval; SCD, sudden cardiac death; TPE, T-peak to T-end interval.
Data from Refs.[34,35,92,94–108]

KCNE1, encoding a β-subunit of the I_{Ks} channel (higher risk for AF)[104]; (3) K897 T, the coding variant in *KCNH,2* which is also recognized as a phenotypic modifier in LQT2 (higher risk for AF)[108]; and (4) and 2 intronic variants in *KCNN3*, encoding the α-subunit of the Ca^{2+}-activated $K_{Ca}2.3$ channel (higher AF risk).[34,35] The precise role of these variants in the complex pathogenesis of AF remains to be elucidated.

Cardiac K⁺ Channel Genes as Modifiers of Phenotype in the General Population

Both candidate gene studies and GWAS have discovered significant associations between common variants in K⁺ channel genes and the risk of sudden cardiac death or ECG indices of conduction (PR) and repolarization (QTc) in the general population (see **Table 4**). These studies have

Table 5
MicroRNAs regulating the expression of cardiac K⁺ channels

Current	Gene	Subunit	MicroRNA	Effect	Reference
I_{K1}	KCNJ2	Kir2.1	miR-1	Reduced miR-1 levels in AF is associated with increased I_{K1} (humans).	111
			miR-1	Overexpression of miR-1 leads to decreased Kir2.1 and I_{K1} levels (rat model).	114
			miR-26	Reduced miR-26 levels in AF is associated with increased Kir2.1 and I_{K1} (humans).	112
			miR-26	Overexpression of miR-26 leads to decreased Kir2.1 and I_{K1} levels (rat model).	112
			mi-212	Overexpression of miR-212 leads to decreased Kir2.1 and I_{K1} levels (in vitro).	115
		Cav3	miR-22	Increased miR-22 levels leads to decreased Cav3 levels (mouse model).	116
I_{KATP}	ABCC9	SUR2	miR-9a-3p	Increased miR-9a-3p levels leads to decreased SUR2B levels (in vitro).	117
$I_{to,fast}$	KCND2	$K_v4.2$	miR-1	Deletion of miR-1 leads to decreased expression of *KCND2*, effect mediated via transcription factor Irx5, which represses *KCND2* (mouse model).	118
			miR-301a	Increased miR-301a levels is associated with decreased $K_v4.2$ levels (mouse model).	119
			miR-301a	Overexpression of miR-301a leads to decreased $K_v4.2$ levels (in vitro).	119
	KCNIP2	KChIP2	miR-133	Overexpression of miR-133 leads to decreased $I_{to,fast}$ probably by decreasing the expression of *KCNIP2* through an indirect mechanism (mouse model).	120
I_{Ks}	KCNQ1	$K_v7.1$	miR-1 and miR-133	Increased miR-1 and miR-133 levels leads to decreased $K_v7.1$, minK and I_{Ks} levels (in vitro).	121
	KCNE1	minK	miR-1	Increased miR-1 levels leads to decreased minK levels and increased I_{Ks} levels (rabbit model).	122
I_{Kr}	KCNH2	$K_v11.1$	miR-133	Overexpression of miR-133 leads to decreased $K_v11.1$ and I_{Kr} levels (guinea pig model).	123
I_{KCa3}	KCNN3	$K_{Ca}2.3$	miR-499	Increased miR-499 levels in AF is associated with decreased $K_{Ca}2.3$ (humans).	113
				Overexpression of miR-499 leads to decreased $K_{Ca}2.3$ levels (in vitro).	113
I_{TASK-1}	KCNK3	$K_{2p}3.1$	miR-34a and miR-124a	Overexpression of miR-34a or miR-124a levels leads to decreased $K_{2p}3.1$ levels (in vitro).	124

Data from Refs.[111,112,114–124]

also found an association between D85 N and K897 T (variants that are recognized as modifiers of phenotype in LQTS) and QTc in the general population.[99,100,102,106] This finding emphasizes the importance of these variants in modulating human repolarization. In addition, GWAS have uncovered novel associations between QTc in the general population and common variants in genomic loci harboring other important cardiac genes, such as *SCN5A* and *NOS1AP*.[95,99] The modifying impact of *NOS1AP*, encoding the nitric oxide synthase 1 adaptor protein, on QTc duration has recently been confirmed in LQTS cohorts.[109,110] In this way, GWAS provide a valuable source of common variants that can serve as novel genetic modifiers of phenotype in heritable arrhythmia syndromes.

CARDIAC K⁺ CHANNEL GENES AND MICRORNAS

Recently, the discovery of microRNAs (miRNAs) has inspired researchers to pay more attention to genetic variations outside the open reading frame of a gene, especially the 3′UTR. The 3′UTR starts immediately after the stop codon of the coding region and contains binding sites for miRNAs, which are small noncoding RNAs. MiRNAs bind to the 3′UTR of their target mRNAs, leading to degradation or repression of the translation of the mRNAs. As a result of these repressive effects of miRNAs, the 3′UTR determines in a *cis*-regulatory manner whether and to what extent mRNA is translated to protein. Several miRNAs have been proposed as regulating the translation of different cardiac K⁺ channels (**Table 5**). Because miRNAs can bind to multiple mRNA, some miRNAs (eg, miR-1 and miR-133) are linked to the regulation of different K⁺ channels. Changes in expression levels of some miRNA during disease (eg, AF, ischemia, and heart failure) have been reported, and these changes are expected to influence the translation of the cardiac K⁺ channels that are regulated by these miRNAs.[111–113] In this way, miRNAs may play an important role in the occurrence of arrhythmias during disease conditions. Next to changes in miRNA levels, genetic variations within miRNA binding sites in the 3′UTR also may influence the magnitude of the repressive effects of miRNAs on translation.[94] The authors have associated SNPs in miRNA binding sites in *KCNQ1*'s 3′UTR with QTc duration and cardiac symptoms in LQT1 patients in an allele-specific manner. Patients with the minor SNP alleles on their mutated *KCNQ1* gene had shorter QTc and fewer symptoms, whereas patients with the minor SNP alleles on their healthy *KCNQ1* gene had significantly longer QTc and more symptoms. The authors' in vitro studies suggested that the minor SNP alleles reduce the expression levels of K$_v$7.1, the α-subunit of the I$_{Ks}$ channel. Thus, the authors' data suggested that suppressive 3′UTR SNPs in *cis* (on the same allele) to the mutation attenuate disease severity by lowering the abundance of mutated K$_v$7.1 proteins, whereas suppressive 3′UTR SNPs in *trans* (on the opposite allele) to the mutation worsen the clinical outcome by reducing the expression of the normal *KCNQ1* allele. The role of variations in the 3′UTR as allele-specific modifiers of phenotype, however, awaits replication in other independent cohorts.

SUMMARY

Approximately 80 genes in the human genome are known to code for pore-forming α-subunits of K⁺ channels, which, in the heart, play a crucial role in cardiac excitability and repolarization. A rapidly growing number of variants in these genes have been implicated in the etiology (rare variants) or clinical manifestation (common variants) of heritable arrhythmia syndromes (eg, LQTS, SQTS, BrS, and AF). The increasing availability and analysis of the continuously expanding data on human genome, however, have led to the notion that many of the rare variants previously linked to heritable arrhythmia syndromes, in particular BrS, ERS, and AF, may not be pathogenic and that at least some heritable arrhythmia syndromes may not be monogenic heritable diseases but oligogenic or polygenic diseases. Thus, the overwhelming number of publications on genetic variants and their possible functional role in health and disease and increasing knowledge of the human genome make the already complex genetic cardiac diseases even more complex and complicate the understanding of their underlying pathophysiologic mechanisms. It is, therefore, of utmost importance to systematically collect and analyze all available data to build a large and up-to-date genetic database that may help, in the future, draw more definite conclusions regarding the causative link between any genetic variant and a certain phenotype. For now, extreme caution is required when a genetic variant is designated as a pathogenic mutation, because this may have major impacts on risk stratification and therapy in mutation carriers and their family members.

REFERENCES

1. Papazian DM, Schwarz TL, Tempel BL, et al. Cloning of genomic and complementary DNA from

Shaker, a putative potassium channel gene from Drosophila. Science 1987;237:749–53.

2. Coetzee W, Amarillo Y, Chiu J, et al. Molecular diversity of K⁺ channels. Ann N Y Acad Sci 1999; 868:233–85.

3. Curran ME, Splawski I, Timothy KW, et al. A molecular basis for cardiac arrhythmia: HERG mutations cause long QT syndrome. Cell 1995;80: 795–803.

4. Wang Q, Curran ME, Splawski I, et al. Positional cloning of a novel potassium channel gene: KVLQT1 mutations cause cardiac arrhythmias. Nat Genet 1996;12:17–23.

5. Schmitt N, Grunnet M, Olesen SP. Cardiac potassium channel subtypes: new roles in repolarization and arrhythmia. Physiol Rev 2014;94:609–53.

6. Kolder IC, Tanck MW, Bezzina CR. Common genetic variation modulating cardiac ECG parameters and susceptibility to sudden cardiac death. J Mol Cell Cardiol 2012;52:620–9.

7. Alexander SPH, Benson HE, Faccenda E, et al, CGTP Collaborators. The Concise Guide to PHARMACOLOGY 2013/14: ion channels. Br J Pharmacol 2013;170:1607–51.

8. Hibino H, Inanobe A, Furutani K, et al. Inwardly rectifying potassium channels: their structure, function, and physiological roles. Physiol Rev 2010;90: 291–366.

9. Raab-Graham KF, Radeke CM, Vandenberg CA. Molecular cloning and expression of a human heart inward rectifier potassium channel. Neuroreport 1994;5:2501–5.

10. Stoffel M, Espinosa R III, Powell KL, et al. Human G-protein-coupled inwardly rectifying potassium channel (GIRK1) gene (KCNJ3): localization to chromosome 2 and identification of a simple tandem repeat polymorphism. Genomics 1994;21: 254–6.

11. Spauschus A, Lentes KU, Wischmeyer E, et al. A G-protein-activated inwardly rectifying K⁺ channel (GIRK4) from human hippocampus associates with other GIRK channels. J Neurosci 1996;6: 930–8.

12. Krapivinsky G, Krapivinsky L, Wickman K, et al. Gβγ binds directly to the G protein-gated K⁺ channel, I_{KACh}. J Biol Chem 1995;270:29059–62.

13. Inagaki N, Inazawa J, Seino S. cDNA sequence, gene structure, and chromosomal localization of the human ATP-sensitive potassium channel, uK_{ATP}-1, gene (KCNJ8). Genomics 1995;30:102–4.

14. Inagaki N, Gonoi T, Clement JPIV, et al. Reconstitution of I_{KATP}: an inward rectifier subunit plus the sulfonylurea receptor. Science 1995;270:1166–70.

15. Inagaki N, Gonoi T, Clement JP, et al. A family of sulfonylurea receptors determines the pharmacological properties of ATP-sensitive K⁺ channels. Neuron 1996;16:1011–7.

16. Flagg TP, Enkvetchakul D, Koster JC, et al. Muscle K_{ATP} channels: recent insights to energy sensing and myoprotection. Physiol Rev 2010;90:799–829.

17. Zhang XD, Lieu DK, Chiamvimonvat N. Small-conductance Ca^{2+}-activated K⁺ channels and cardiac arrhythmias. Heart Rhythm 2015;12:1845–51.

18. Gessler M, Grupe A, Grzechik KH, et al. The potassium channel gene HK1 maps to human chromosome 11p14.1, close to the FSHB gene. Hum Genet 1992;90:319–21.

19. Xiao L, Koopmann TT, Ördög B, et al. Unique cardiac Purkinje fiber transient outward current β-subunit composition: a potential molecular link to idiopathic ventricular fibrillation. Circ Res 2013; 112:1310–22.

20. Isbrandt D, Leicher T, Waldschütz R, et al. Gene structures and expression profiles of three human KCND (Kv4) potassium channels mediating A-type currents I_{TO} and I_{SA}. Genomics 2000;64: 144–54.

21. Gaborit N, Le Bouter S, Szuts V, et al. Regional and tissue specific transcript signatures of ion channel genes in the non-diseases human heart. J Physiol 2007;582(pt 2):675–93.

22. Kim LA, Furst J, Butler MH, et al. I_{to} channels are octameric complexes with four subunits of each Kv4.2 and K+ channel-interacting protein 2. J Biol Chem 2004;279:5549–54.

23. Rosati B, Pan Z, Lypen S, et al. Regulation of KChIP2 potassium channel β subunit gene expression underlies the gradient of transient outward current in canine and human ventricle. J Physiol 2001; 533:119–25.

24. Landes GM, Curran ME, Keating MT. Molecular characterization and refined genomic localization of three human potassium ion channel genes. Cytogenet Cell Genet 1995;70:280–4.

25. Abbott GW, Sesti F, Splawski I, et al. MiRP1 forms I_{Kr} potassium channels with HERG and is associated with cardiac arrhythmia. Cell 1999; 97:175–87.

26. Pourrier M, Zicha S, Ehrlich J, et al. Canine ventricular KCNE2 expression resides predominantly in Purkinje fibers. Circ Res 2003;93:189–91.

27. Jonsson MKB, Van der Heyden MAG, Van Veen TAB. Deciphering hERG channels: molecular basis of the rapid component of the delayed recitifer current. J Mol Cell Cardiol 2012;53:369–74.

28. Korostowski L, Raval A, Breuer G, et al. Enhancer-driven chromatin interactions during development promote escape from silencing by a long noncoding RNA. Epigenetics Chromatin 2011;4:21–32.

29. Litt M, LaMorticella D, Bond CT, et al. Gene structure and chromosome mapping of the human small-conductance calcium-activated potassium channel SK1 gene (KCNN1). Cytogenet Cell Genet 1999;86(1):70–3.

30. Xu Y, Tuteja D, Zhang Z, et al. Molecular identification and functional roles of a Ca^{2+}-activated K^+ channel in human and mouse hearts. J Biol Chem 2003;278:49085–94.

31. Sun G, Tomita H, Shakottai VG, et al. Genomic organization and promoter analysis of human *KCNN3* gene. J Hum Genet 2001;46:463–70.

32. Feliciangeli S, Chatelain FC, Bichet D, et al. The family of K_{2P} channels: salient structural and functional properties. J Physiol 2015;593:2587–603.

33. Friedrich C, Rinné S, Zumhagen S, et al. Gain-of-function mutation in TASK-4 channels and severe cardiac conduction disorder. EMBO Mol Med 2014;6:937–51.

34. Ellinor PT, Lunetta KL, Glazer N, et al. Common variants in *KCNN3* are associated with lone atrial fibrillation. Nat Genet 2010;42:240–4.

35. Ellinor PT, Lunetta KL, Albert CM, et al. Meta-analysis identifies six new susceptibility loci for atrial fibrillation. Nat Genet 2012;44:670–5.

36. Abriel H, Rougier JS, Jalife J. Ion channel macromolecular complexes in cardiomyocytes: roles in sudden cardiac death. Circ Res 2015;116:1971–88.

37. Risgaard B, Jabbari R, Refsgaard L, et al. High prevalence of genetic variants previously associated with Brugada syndrome in new exome data. Clin Genet 2013;84:489–95.

38. Le Scouarnec S, Karakachoff M, Gourraud JB, et al. Testing the burden of rare variation in arrhythmia-susceptibility genes provides new insights into molecular diagnosis for Brugada syndrome. Hum Mol Genet 2015;24:2757–63.

39. Kapplinger JD, Giudicessi JR, Ye D, et al. Enhanced classification of Brugada syndrome-associated and long-QT syndrome-associated genetic variants in the *SCN5A*-encoded $Na_v1.5$ cardiac sodium channel. Circ Cardiovasc Genet 2015;8:582–95.

40. Amin AS, Pinto YM, Wilde AA. Long QT syndrome: beyond the causal mutation. J Physiol 2013;591:4125–39.

41. Plaster NM, Tawil R, Tristani-Firouzi M, et al. Mutations in Kir2.1 cause the developmental and episodic electrical phenotypes of Andersen's syndrome. Cell 2001;105:511–9.

42. Priori SG, Pandit SV, Rivolta I, et al. A novel form of short QT syndrome (SQT3) is caused by a mutation in the *KCNJ2* gene. Circ Res 2005;96:800–7.

43. Xia M, Jin Q, Bendahhou S, et al. Kir 2.1 gain-of-function mutation underlies familial atrial fibrillation. Biochem Biophys Res Commun 2005;332:1012–9.

44. Yang Y, Yang Y, Liang B, et al. Identification of a Kir3.4 mutation in congenital long QT syndrome. Am J Hum Genet 2010;86:872–80.

45. Calloe K, Ravn LS, Schmitt N, et al. Characterizations of a loss-of-function mutation in the Kir3.4

channel subunit. Biochem Biophys Res Commun 2007;364:889–95.

46. Barajas-Martínez H, Hu D, Ferrer T, et al. Molecular genetic and functional association of Brugada and early repolarization syndromes with S422L missense mutation in *KCNJ8*. Heart Rhythm 2012;9:548–55.

47. Haïssaguerre M, Chatel S, Sacher F, et al. Ventricular fibrillation with prominent early repolarization associated with a rare variant of $KCNJ8/K_{ATP}$ channel. J Cardiovasc Electrophysiol 2009;20:93–8.

48. Hu D, Barajas-Martinez H, Terzic A, et al. *ABCC9* is a novel Brugada and early repolarization syndrome susceptibility gene. Int J Cardiol 2014;171:431–42.

49. Olson TM, Alekseev AE, Moreau C, et al. K_{ATP} channel mutation confers risk for vein of Marshall adrenergic atrial fibrillation. Nat Clin Pract Cardiovasc Med 2007;4:110–6.

50. Perrin MJ, Adler A, Green S, et al. Evaluation of genes encoding for the transient outward current (Ito) identifies the *KCND2* gene as a cause of J-wave syndrome associated with sudden cardiac death. Circ Cardiovasc Genet 2014;7:782–9.

51. Giudicessi JR, Ye D, Tester DJ, et al. Transient outward current (I_{to}) gain-of-function mutations in the *KCND3*-encoded Kv4.3 potassium channel and Brugada syndrome. Heart Rhythm 2011;8:1024–32.

52. Olesen MS, Refsgaard L, Holst AG, et al. A novel *KCND3* gain of-function mutation associated with early-onset of persistent lone atrial fibrillation. Cardiovasc Res 2013;98:488–95.

53. Delpón E, Cordeiro JM, Núñez L, et al. Functional effects of KCNE3 mutation and its role in the development of Brugada syndrome. Circ Arrhythm Electrophysiol 2008;1:209–18.

54. Lundby A, Ravn LS, Svendsen JH, et al. KCNE3 mutation V17M identified in a patient with lone atrial fibrillation. Cell Physiol Biochem 2008;21:47–54.

55. Ohno S, Zankov DP, Ding WG, et al. KCNE5 (*KCNE1L*) variants are novel modulators of Brugada syndrome and idiopathic ventricular fibrillation. Circ Arrhythm Electrophysiol 2011;4:352–61.

56. Olson TM, Alekseev AE, Liu XK, et al. Kv1.5 channelopathy due to *KCNA5* loss-of-function mutation causes human atrial fibrillation. Hum Mol Genet 2006;15:2185–91.

57. Neyroud N, Tesson F, Denjoy I, et al. A novel mutation in the potassium channel gene *KVLQT1* causes the Jervell and Lange-Nielsen cardioauditory syndrome. Nat Genet 1997;15:186–9.

58. Bellocq C, van Ginneken ACG, Bezzina CR, et al. Mutation in the *KCNQ1* gene leading to the short QT-interval syndrome. Circulation 2004;109:2394–7.

59. Chen YH, Xu SJ, Bendahhou S, et al. *KCNQ1* gain-of-function mutation in familial atrial fibrillation. Science 2003;299:251–4.

60. Splawski I, Tristani-Firouzi M, Lehmann MH, et al. Mutations in the hminK gene cause long QT syndrome and suppress I_{Ks} function. Nat Genet 1997;17:338–40.

61. Schulze-Bahr E, Wang Q, Wedekind H, et al. *KCNE1* mutations cause jervell and Lange-Nielsen syndrome. Nat Genet 1997;17:267–8.

62. Olesen MS, Bentzen BH, Nielsen JB, et al. Mutations in the potassium channel subunit KCNE1 are associated with early-onset familial atrial fibrillation. BMC Med Genet 2012;13:24.

63. Yang Y, Xia M, Jin Q, et al. Identification of a KCNE2 gain-of-function mutation in patients with familial atrial fibrillation. Am J Hum Genet 2004; 75:899–905.

64. Ohno S, Toyoda F, Zankov DP, et al. Novel *KCNE3* mutation reduces repolarizing potassium current and associated with long QT syndrome. Hum Mutat 2009;30:557–63.

65. Ravn LS, Aizawa Y, Pollevick GD, et al. Gain of function in I_{Ks} secondary to a mutation in *KCNE5* associated with atrial fibrillation. Heart Rhythm 2008;5:427–35.

66. Chen L, Marquardt ML, Tester DJ, et al. Mutation of an A-kinase-anchoring protein causes long-QT syndrome. Proc Natl Acad Sci U S A 2007;104: 20990–5.

67. Brugada R, Hong K, Dumaine R, et al. Sudden death associated with short-QT syndrome linked to mutations in HERG. Circulation 2004;109:30–5.

68. Wang Q, Ohno S, Ding WG, et al. Gain-of-function *KCNH2* mutations in patients with Brugada syndrome. J Cardiovasc Electrophysiol 2014;25: 522–30.

69. Liang B, Soka M, Christensen AH, et al. Genetic variation in the two-pore domain potassium channel, TASK-1, may contribute to an atrial substrate for arrhythmogenesis. J Mol Cell Cardiol 2014;67: 69–76.

70. Tester DJ, Ackerman MJ. Genetic testing for potentially lethal, highly treatable inherited cardiomyopathies/channelopathies in clinical practice. Circulation 2011;123:1021–37.

71. Shimizu W, Horie M. Phenotypic manifestations of mutations in genes encoding subunits of cardiac potassium channels. Circ Res 2011;109:97–109.

72. Moss AJ, Shimizu W, Wilde AA, et al. Clinical aspects of type-1 long-QT syndrome by location, coding type, and biophysical function of mutations involving the KCNQ1 gene. Circulation 2007;115: 2481–9.

73. Shimizu W, Moss AJ, Wilde AA, et al. Genotype-phenotype aspects of type 2 long QT syndrome. J Am Coll Cardiol 2009;54:2052–62.

74. Kapplinger JD, Tester DJ, Salisbury BA, et al. Spectrum and prevalence of mutations from the first 2,500 consecutive unrelated patients referred for the FAMILION long QT syndrome genetic test. Heart Rhythm 2009;6:1297–303.

75. Barc J, Briec F, Schmitt S, et al. Screening for copy number variation in genes associated with the long QT syndrome. J Am Coll Cardiol 2011;57:40–7.

76. Kapa S, Tester DJ, Salisbury BA, et al. Genetic testing for long-QT syndrome: distinguishing pathogenic mutations from benign variants. Circulation 2009;120:1752–60.

77. Schwartz PJ, Spazzolini C, Crotti L, et al. The Jervell and Lange-Nielsen syndrome: natural history, molecular basis, and clinical outcome. Circulation 2006;113:783–90.

78. Anderson CL, Delisle BP, Anson BD, et al. Most LQT2 mutations reduce Kv11.1 (hERG) current by a class 2 (trafficking-deficient) mechanism. Circulation 2006;113:365–73.

79. Gong Q, Zhang L, Vincent GM, et al. Nonsense mutations in hERG cause a decrease in mutant mRNA transcripts by nonsense-mediated mRNA decay in human long-QT syndrome. Circulation 2007;116:17–24.

80. Tristani-Firouzi M, Jensen JL, Donaldson MR, et al. Functional and clinical characterization of *KCNJ2* mutations associated with LQT7 (Andersen syndrome). J Clin Invest 2002;110:381–8.

81. Patel C, Yan GX, Antzelevitch C. Short QT syndrome: from bench to bedside. Circ Arrhythm Electrophysiol 2010;3:401–8.

82. Gussak I, Brugada P, Brugada J, et al. Idiopathic short QT interval: a new clinical syndrome? Cardiology 2000;94:99–102.

83. Gaita F, Giustetto C, Bianchi F, et al. Short QT syndrome: a familial cause of sudden death. Circulation 2003;108:965–70.

84. Junttila MJ, Sager SJ, Tikkanen JT, et al. Clinical significance of variants of J-points and J-waves: early repolarization patterns and risk. Eur Heart J 2012;33:2639–43.

85. Antzelevitch C, Yan GX. J wave syndromes. Heart Rhythm 2010;7:549–58.

86. Veeramah KR, Karafet TM, Wolf D, et al. The KCNJ8-S422L variant previously associated with J-wave syndromes is found at an increased frequency in Ashkenazi Jews. Eur J Hum Genet 2014;22:94–8.

87. Andrade J, Khairy P, Dobrev D, et al. The clinical profile and pathophysiology of atrial fibrillation: relationships among clinical features, epidemiology, and mechanisms. Circ Res 2014;114:1453–68.

88. Vincent GM, Timothy KW, Leppert M, et al. The spectrum of symptoms and QT intervals in carriers of the gene for the long-QT syndrome. N Engl J Med 1992;327:846–52.

89. Priori SG, Napolitano C, Schwartz PJ. Low penetrance in the long-QT syndrome: clinical impact. Circulation 1999;99:529–33.

90. Westenskow P, Splawski I, Timothy KW, et al. Compound mutations: a common cause of severe long-QT syndrome. Circulation 2004;109:1834–41.

91. Nishio Y, Makiyama T, Itoh H, et al. D85N, a KCNE1 polymorphism, is a disease-causing gene variant in long QT syndrome. J Am Coll Cardiol 2009;54:812–9.

92. Crotti L, Lundquist AL, Insolia R, et al. KCNH2-K897T is a genetic modifier of latent congenital long-QT syndrome. Circulation 2005;112:1251–8.

93. Duchatelet S, Crotti L, Peat RA, et al. Identification of a KCNQ1 polymorphism acting as a protective modifier against arrhythmic risk in long-QT syndrome. Circ Cardiovasc Genet 2013;6:354–61.

94. Amin AS, Giudicessi JR, Tijsen AJ, et al. Variants in the 3' untranslated region of the KCNQ1-encoded $K_V7.1$ potassium channel modify disease severity in patients with type 1 long QT syndrome in an allele-specific manner. Eur Heart J 2010;33:714–23.

95. Pfeufer A, Sanna S, Arking DE, et al. Common variants at ten loci modulate the QT interval duration in the QTSCD Study. Nat Genet 2009;41:407–14.

96. Marjamaa A, Oikarinen L, Porthan K, et al. A common variant near the KCNJ2 gene is associated with T-peak to T-end interval. Heart Rhythm 2012;9:1099–103.

97. Schreieck J, Dostal S, von Beckerath N, et al. C825T polymorphism of the G-protein β3 subunit gene and atrial fibrillation: association of the TT genotype with a reduced risk for atrial fibrillation. Am Heart J 2004;148:545–50.

98. Verweij N, Mateo Leach I, van den Boogaard M, et al. Genetic determinants of P wave duration and PR segment. Circ Cardiovasc Genet 2014;7:475–81.

99. Newton-Cheh C, Eijgelsheim M, Rice KM, et al. Common variants at ten loci influence QT interval duration in the QTGEN Study. Nat Genet 2009;41:399–406.

100. Pfeufer A, Jalilzadeh S, Perz S, et al. Common variants in myocardial ion channel genes modify the QT interval in the general population: results from the KORA study. Circ Res 2005;96:693–701.

101. Albert CM, MacRae CA, Chasman DI, et al. Common variants in cardiac ion channel genes are associated with sudden cardiac death. Circ Arrhythm Electrophysiol 2010;3:222–9.

102. Marjamaa A, Newton-Cheh C, Porthan K, et al. Common candidate gene variants are associated with QT interval duration in the general population. J Intern Med 2009;265:448–58.

103. Weeke P, Mosley JD, Hanna D, et al. Exome sequencing implicates an increased burden of rare potassium channel variants in the risk of drug-induced long QT interval syndrome. J Am Coll Cardiol 2014;63:1430–7.

104. Fatini C, Sticchi E, Genuardi M, et al. Analysis of minK and eNOS genes as candidate loci for predisposition to non-valvular atrial fibrillation. Eur Heart J 2006;27:1712–8.

105. de Villiers CP, van der Merwe L, Crotti L, et al. AKAP9 is a genetic modifier of congenital long-QT syndrome type 1. Circ Cardiovasc Genet 2014;7:599–606.

106. Newton-Cheh C, Guo CY, Larson MG, et al. Common genetic variation in KCNH2 is associated with QT interval duration: the Framingham Heart Study. Circulation 2007;116:1128–36.

107. Porthan K, Marjamaa A, Viitasalo M, et al. Relationship of common candidate gene variants to electrocardiographic T-wave peak to T-wave end interval and T-wave morphology parameters. Heart Rhythm 2010;7:898–903.

108. Sinner MF, Pfeufer A, Akyol M, et al. The non-synonymous coding I_{Kr}-channel variant KCNH2-K897T is associated with atrial fibrillation: results from a systematic candidate gene-based analysis of KCNH2 (HERG). Eur Heart J 2008;29:907–14.

109. Tomàs M, Napolitano C, De Giuli L, et al. Polymorphisms in the NOS1AP gene modulate QT interval duration and risk of arrhythmias in the long QT syndrome. J Am Coll Cardiol 2010;55:2745–52.

110. Crotti L, Monti MC, Insolia R, et al. NOS1AP is a genetic modifier of the long-QT syndrome. Circulation 2009;120:1657–63.

111. Girmatsion Z, Biliczki P, Bonauer A, et al. Changes in microRNA-1 expression and I_{K1} up-regulation in human atrial fibrillation. Heart Rhythm 2009;6:1802–9.

112. Luo X, Dong D, Zhang Y, et al. MicroRNA-26 governs profibrillatory inward-rectifier potassium current changes in atrial fibrillation. J Clin Invest 2013;123:1939–51.

113. Ling TY, Wang XL, Chai Q, et al. Regulation of the SK3 channel by microRNA-449-Potential role in atrial fibrillation. Heart Rhythm 2013;10:1001–9.

114. Yang B, Lin H, Xiao J, et al. The muscle-specific microRNA miR-1 causes cardiac arrhythmias by targeting GJA1 and KCNJ2 genes. Nat Med 2007;13:486–91.

115. Goldoni D, Yarham JM, McGahon MK, et al. A novel dual-fluorescence strategy for functionally validating microRNA targets in 3' untranslated regions: regulation of the inward rectifier potassium channel $K_{ir}2.1$ by miR-212. Biochem J 2012;448:103–13.

116. Chen Z, Qi Y, Gao C. Cardiac myocyte-protective effect of microRNA-22 during ischemia and reperfusion through disrupting the caveolin-3/eNOS signaling. Int J Clin Exp Pathol 2015;8:4614–26.

117. Li SS, Wu Y, Jin X, et al. The SUR2B subunit of rat vascular K_{ATP} channel is targeted by miR-9a-3p induced by prolonged exposure to methylglyoxal. Am J Physiol Cell Physiol 2015;308: C139–45.

118. Zhao Y, Ransom JF, Li A, et al. Dysregulation of cardiogenesis, cardiac conduction, and cell cycle in mice lacking miRNA-1-2. Cell 2007;129:303–17.

119. Panguluri SK, Tur J, Chapalamadugu KC, et al. MicroRNA-301a mediated regulation of Kv4.2 in diabetes: identification of key modulators. PLoS One 2013;8:e60545.

120. Matkovich SJ, Wang W, Tu Y, et al. MicroRNA-133a protects against myocardial fibrosis and modulates electrical repolarization without affecting hypertrophy in pressure-overloaded adult hearts. Circ Res 2010;106:166–75.

121. Li Y, Yang CM, Xi Y, et al. MicroRNA-1/133 targeted dysfunction of potassium channels KCNE1 and KCNQ1 in human cardiac progenitor cells with simulated hyperglycemia. Int J Cardiol 2013;167:1076–8.

122. Jia X, Zheng S, Xie X, et al. MicroRNA-1 accelerates the shortening of atrial effective refractory period by regulating KCNE1 and KCNB2 expression: an atrial tachypacing rabbit model. PLoS One 2013;8:e85639.

123. Shan H, Zhang Y, Cai B, et al. Upregulation of microRNA-1 and microRNA-133 contributes to arsenic-induced cardiac electrical remodeling. Int J Cardiol 2013;167:2798–805.

124. Farberov L, Herzig E, Modai S, et al. Micro-RNA-mediated regulation of p21 and TASK1 cellular restriction factor enhances HIV-1 infection. J Cell Sci 2015;128:1607–16.

Cardiac Delayed Rectifier Potassium Channels in Health and Disease

Lei Chen, PhD, Kevin J. Sampson, PhD, Robert S. Kass, PhD*

KEYWORDS

- Delayed rectifiers • I_{Ks} • I_{Kr} • I_{Kur} • Long QT Syndrome • Short QT Syndrome • Atrial fibrillation

KEY POINTS

- Cardiac delayed rectifier potassium channels conduct outward potassium currents during the plateau phase of action potentials and play pivotal roles in cardiac repolarization.
- The rapid progress in molecular biology and genetics in the 1990s resulted in the discoveries of the molecular identities and architecture of I_{Kr} and I_{Ks} channel complexes.
- Inherited mutations or drug block of the delayed rectifier channels cause cardiac arrhythmias.
- Delayed rectifier potassium channels may be used as therapeutic targets.

DELAYED RECTIFIERS IN THE HEART: I_{KS}, I_{KR}, AND I_{KUR}

Cardiac action potentials are characterized by an initial depolarization followed by a prolonged depolarization, or plateau phase, before a return to the resting potential. In these cells, sodium channels provide large inward currents that drive rapid depolarization (phase 0) followed by subsequent minor repolarization (phase 1) resulting from transition of sodium channels into a nonconducting inactivated state, as well as activation of transient outward potassium currents (I_{to}). The plateau phase of the action potential, a period in which membrane potentials become relatively stable for up to several hundred milliseconds, follows. During the plateau phase (phase 2), calcium entry via L-type calcium channels triggers contraction. Counterbalancing the calcium influx, potassium ions pass through the membrane in the outward direction: the plateau phase is thus a balance of inward and outward currents. Unlike the I_{to} currents that terminate quickly, the slower potassium channel currents persist during the plateau phase,

contribute to the repolarization of the cell, and eventually terminate the action potential (phase 3) as the balance of currents tips in the outward direction[1] (**Fig. 1**). Early electrophysiologists noticed such outward potassium conductance that lasts throughout the plateau phase, and referred to these currents as "delayed rectifier" currents. The delayed rectifiers, in concert with other ion channels, essentially determine the waveform as well as action potential duration (APD), and thus play critical roles in cardiac physiology and pathophysiology. Disruption of the normal functions of delayed rectifier channels renders the heart susceptible to abnormal electrical activity, and ultimately predisposes the heart to arrhythmia.

The identities of the delayed rectifiers, however, remained elusive because of a lack of proper pharmacologic tools and knowledge of ion channels as functional proteins in cell membrane. It was not until 1969 that Noble and Tsien[2,3] using an elegant quantitative approach, demonstrated the existence of 2 distinct components (which they called I_{x1} and I_{x2}) of the outward currents in the plateau potentials in cardiac Purkenje fibers. The 2

Department of Pharmacology, College of Physicians & Surgeons of Columbia University, 630 West 168th Street, New York, NY 10032, USA
* Corresponding author.
E-mail address: rsk20@columbia.edu

Card Electrophysiol Clin 8 (2016) 307–322
http://dx.doi.org/10.1016/j.ccep.2016.01.004

cardiacEP.theclinics.com

Atrium   Ventricle

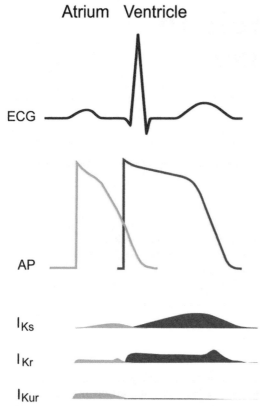

Fig. 1. Schematics of waveforms of ECG, cardiac action potentials and delayed rectifier potassium currents. *Top panel*: ECG waveforms showing P wave (atrial depolarization), QRS complex (ventricle depolarization), and T wave (ventricle repolarization). *Middle panel*: Cardiac action potential from atrium (*green*) and ventricle (*red*). *Lower panels*: Delayed rectifier currents from I_{Ks}, I_{Kr}, and I_{Kur} during cardiac repolarization and their tissue (atrial in *green* and ventricle in *red*) distributions.

components differ mainly in activation kinetics, one rapid and one slow. Noble and Tsien's[2,3] formalism was disputed by some investigators based on technical issues with the preparations used and the basis of delayed rectification remained controversial. Twenty years later, Sanguinetti and Jurkiewicz[4] confirmed Noble and Tsien's[2,3] seminal findings by pharmacologically separating the 2 components with the use of E4031, a benzene sulfonamide antiarrhythmic agent that selectively blocked the rapid component, which they named I_{Kr} accordingly. The remaining slow component was given the name I_{Ks}. The terms I_{Ks} and I_{Kr} have since been widely used to describe the delayed rectifier currents in cardiac myocytes of various species.[4–10] In the atria, an additional ultrarapid component, I_{Kur}, is prominent during the plateau phase.[11–15]

The rapid progress in molecular biology and genetics in the 1990s resulted in the discoveries of the molecular identities and architecture of I_{Kr} and I_{Ks} channel complexes, defined previously only through pharmacology. Remarkably, these discoveries were all associated with studies of the congenital Long QT Syndromes (LQTS), cardiac rhythm disorders caused by mutations in genes coding for ion channels or channel-associated proteins with a common functional phenotype: prolongation of cellular APD and QT interval of the electrocardiogram. Loss-of-function mutations of the 2 prominent delayed rectifiers I_{Ks} and I_{Kr} with dysfunctional trafficking or channel-gating properties have been shown to cause congenital LQTS, underscoring the critical importance of the delayed rectifiers in cardiac physiology.

I_{Ks}, I_{Kr}, and I_{Kur} channels all fall into the superfamily of voltage-gated potassium channels. These channels are formed from tetramers of membrane-spanning proteins that possess a voltage-sensing domain (VSD) as well as a pore domain. I_{Ks} channels are activated slowly by depolarizing voltages during the plateau phase. The pore-forming subunit is KCNQ1 (also known as KvLQT1 or Kv7.1), first identified by positional cloning and its linkage to LQTS variant 1 (LQT1).[16] Like other voltage-gated potassium channels, it has 6 transmembrane domains and is composed of a voltage-sensing domain (S1–4) and a pore domain (S5 and S6), as well as the intracellular N- and C-termini. Four such subunits form a functional channel. However, it is KCNE1 (also known as minK), a single transmembrane protein,[17] that co-assembles with KCNQ1 and imparts to the KCNQ1 channel its unique slow kinetics similar to that of the native I_{Ks} recorded in cardiac myocytes.[18,19] Thus, the physiologically relevant activity of the I_{Ks} channel requires co-assembly of both KCNQ1 and KCNE1. Like KCNQ1, mutations in KCNE1 are also associated with LQTS variant 5 (LQT5).[20,21] I_{Kr} currents are conducted by hERG channels (also known as Kv11.1 or KCNH2),[22] which was first cloned in the brain as a homolog of the *Drosophila* "ether-a-go-go" (EAG) potassium channel,[23] and was later shown to link to LQTS variant 2 (LQT2).[24] Similar to I_{Ks} channels, the hERG channel is a tetramer of 4 identical subunits, each with 6 transmembrane domains that form the VSD and the pore. MiRP1 (or KCNE2), a single transmembrane protein homologous to KCNE1, was shown to associate with hERG channels and alter its biophysical properties, and was linked to LQTS variant 6 (LQT6).[25] However, the exact role of MiRP1 in the molecular composition of I_{Kr} channels is disputed.[26] I_{Kur} channels have more recently been identified to be composed of Kv1.5 alpha subunits[27,28] encoded by KCNA5 and are a major contributor to atrial repolarization (**Fig. 2**).

Although both are activated by depolarizing voltages during the plateau phase of cardiac action potentials, I_{Ks} and I_{Kr} channels differ biophysically in many respects.[4] Their different functions can be studied using selective blockers for these currents, E4031 for I_{Kr}[4] and Chromanol 293B for I_{Ks}.[29] I_{Kr} plays the largest role in repolarization in normal conditions and is characterized by prominent inward rectification caused by voltage-dependent inactivation. That is, at more positive potentials during the plateau phase, the channels are inactivated and conduct smaller outward current. As repolarization progresses, I_{Kr} channels recover from inactivation and produce a large resurgent outward current that repolarizes the membrane potential. I_{Ks} channels, however, have little inactivation and activate slowly and gradually impact cellular repolarization (see **Fig. 2**). The role of I_{Ks} is heightened under certain stressors, including adrenergic stimulation wherein I_{Ks} currents are larger, more rapidly activate, and slowly deactivate to allow for shortened action potentials that can maintain adequate diastolic filling times even in the face of accelerated heart rate. Under conditions of I_{Kr} blockade, the role of I_{Ks} also increases and can become the largest contributor to cellular repolarization. Together, these channels are critical determinants of the duration and morphology of cardiac action potentials, and consequently impact the QT interval measured in the electrocardiogram (ECG). Inhibition of these channels resulting from either inherited mutations or drug block can lead to LQTS associated with increased risk of life-threatening arrhythmias.

Following the groundbreaking discoveries of the roles of I_{Kr} and I_{Ks} in LQTS, it has now become clear that these channels also underlie other cardiac rhythm disorders, such as Short QT Syndrome (SQTS) and familial atrial fibrillation (AF).[30–33] In recent years, genome-wide association studies have revealed that KCNQ1, KCNE1, and hERG were among the common variant loci associated with QT-interval variations,[34,35] thus highlighting again the significance of delayed rectifier channels in cardiac function. The search for precise pharmacologic regulation of these channels has now expanded in seeking therapeutic approaches to manage a wide range of clinical disorders.

DELAYED RECTIFIERS AND CARDIAC RHYTHM DISORDERS
Congenital and Acquired Long QT Syndromes

Congenital LQTSs are genetic cardiac rhythm disorders of a common clinical phenotype: delayed repolarization that manifests on body surface ECG as prolonged QT intervals. As a result, abnormal electrical activity, such as early afterdepolarizations (EAD) can trigger severe ventricular tachycardia (very often in the form of Torsade de Pointes, or TdP), leading to syncope or sudden death. Clinically, congenital LQTS includes the autosomal recessive Romano Ward Syndrome, which affects approximately 1 in 7000 people, and the very rare Jervell and Lange-Nielsen syndrome, which is accompanied by hearing loss and is autosomal dominant. Most cases of

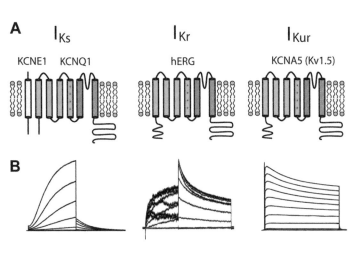

A I_{Ks} I_{Kr} I_{Kur}

KCNE1 KCNQ1   hERG   KCNA5 (Kv1.5)

B

Fig. 2. Cardiac delayed rectifier channels include I_{Ks}, I_{Kr}, and the atrial-specific I_{Kur} channels and are all voltage-gated potassium channels. (*A*) Molecular composition and architecture of cardiac delayed rectifier channels. I_{Ks} channels are composed of pore-forming KCNQ1 and auxiliary KCNE1 subunits. I_{Kr} channels are composed of hERG subunits. I_{Kur} channels are composed of KCNA5 (Kv1.5) subunits. Each α-subunit has 6 transmembrane helices (S1-6). S1-4 is the voltage sensing domain with positively charged residues on S4 as the voltage sensor. S5-6 is the pore domain that conducts ionic currents. (*B*) Recordings of current voltage relationships of I_{Ks}, I_{Kr}, and I_{Kur} channels. I_{Kur} current traces. (*Adapted from* Decher N, Pirard B, Bundis F, et al. Molecular basis for Kv1.5 channel block: conservation of drug binding sites among voltage-gated K+ channels. J Biol Chem 2004;279(1):395.)

congenital LQTS are caused by loss-of-function mutations in either KCNQ1 or hERG channels (LQT1 and LQT2, respectively). Less frequent but with marked severity is LQT3, which is due to gain-of-function (because of impaired inactivation) mutations in SCN5A, the gene coding for the Nav1.5 cardiac sodium channel alpha subunit. Rare genotypes include mutations in KCNE1, inward rectifiers, calcium channels, adaptor protein AKAP9, and so forth.[36–44] LQTS may also be induced by drugs. In this case, it is the hERG channels that are most often blocked. In the following sections, we discuss the different types of congenital LQTS caused by dysfunctional delayed rectifier channels and their associating binding partners, including KCNE1 and AKAP9, as well drug-induced LQTS caused by hERG block.

KCNQ1 and long QT1
Loss-of-function KCNQ1 mutations contribute to 42% to 49% of all long QT genotypes.[45,46] At the cellular level, mutations exert negative impact on I_{Ks} channel function through various mechanisms.[47,48] Some mutations may cause reduction in current densities at physiologically relevant voltages through biophysical effects on the gating of I_{Ks}.[49] Deficiency in membrane trafficking of mutant channel subunits is a common mechanism and may lead to fewer functional channels on the cell surface and in turn a reduction of repolarization reserve.[50–54] Mutations may also affect I_{Ks} channel tetramerization and assembly.[55] Some mutations occur at sites critical for interaction with key molecules involved in functional modulation. For example, clusters of basic residues (R190, R195, R243, H258, R259, K352, R360 and K362) located in the intracellular linker or proximal C-terminus are critical for PIP2 regulation. Mutations of most of them are associated with LQT1.[48,56–58] A leucine zipper motif located in the KCNQ1 C-terminus is responsible for coassembly with the adaptor molecule Yotiao (also known as AKAP9) that recruits PKA and protein phosphatase 1 (PP1) to the I_{Ks} macromolecular complex. Thus, this macromolecular complex allows for precise and rapid adrenergic modulation of the channel. Mutation within the leucine zipper at residue G589 was shown to minimize PKA-dependent phosphorylation of the I_{Ks} channel and is linked to LQT1.[59] Unraveling this pathway provided mechanistic insight into the known risk of cardiac events of LQT1 patients during exercise, when sympathetic nerve activity is elevated. When coexpressed with wild-type KCNQ1 to mimic the heterogeneity of LQT1, some mutants show a propensity for a dominant negative effect, whereas others do not affect the function of wild-type

channels.[51,60] Not surprisingly, patients who carry dominant negative mutations (functional expression reduced >50%) show longer QTc and significantly higher risk for cardiac events, compared with those who carry mutations with haploinsufficiency phenotypes (functional expression reduced <50%).[61]

The locations of mutations on KCNQ1 correlate with clinical phenotypes and therapeutic responses. To date, more than 200 genetic variations have been identified in KCNQ1 to cause LQT1. LQT1 mutations have been found in the KCNQ1 C-terminus (32%), pore (29%, S5-6), intracellular linkers (20%), voltage-sensing domain (11%), extracellular link (6%), and N-terminus (2%) (**Fig. 3**A).[62] In 2 separate studies, Shimizu and colleagues[63] and Moss and colleagues[61] found that cumulative probability of cardiac events was significantly higher in patients who carry mutations in the KCNQ1 transmembrane domains than those who carry mutations in the C-terminus (**Fig. 3**B). Patients with missense mutation in the cytoplasmic loops of KCNQ1 exhibit the highest risks for cardiac events and the best response to β-blockers.[64]

KCNE1 and long QT syndrome variant 5
KCNE1 coassembles with KCNQ1 and alters the biophysical properties of the channel profoundly. It slows both activation and deactivation kinetic, shifts activation voltage dependence in the positive direction, and significantly increases current amplitude.[18,19] Coexpression of KCNQ1 and KCNE1 results in functional channels with biophysical properties similar to the native I_{Ks} channels.[18,19] Loss-of-function mutations of KCNE1 lead to congenital LQTS variant 5 (LQT5) in the forms of both Romano-Ward and Jervell and Lange-Nielsen syndromes,[21] albeit at much lower prevalence (1.7%–3.0% of all LQTS)[45,46] compared with LQT1, LQT2, and LQT3. Approximately 20 KCNE1 mutations have been identified to cause LQT5. Most of them are located in either the transmembrane domain or the cytoplasmic C-terminus.[65] At the cellular level, LQT5 disease pathogenesis involves various mechanisms. For example, KCNE1 L51H, a JLN mutation, does not express on the cell membrane, and does not functionally interact with KCNQ1. Other KCNE1 mutations, such as V47F, D76N, and W87R, undergo normal trafficking to the cell membrane, but exert distinct impacts on coexpressed KCNQ1: both V47F and W87R functionally interact with KCNQ1 and alter I_{Ks} gating, whereas D76N is a dominant negative mutation that severely suppresses current amplitude.[66,67] Seebohm and colleagues[68] found that serum- and

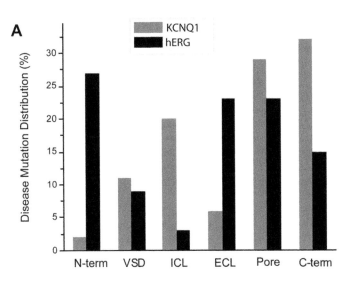

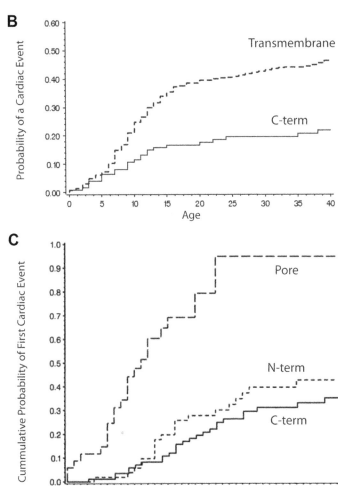

Fig. 3. (*A*) Locations of LQTS mutations in KCNQ1 (*gray bars*) and hERG (*black bars*). C-term, C-terminus; ECL, extracellular loops; ICL, intracellular loops; N-term, N-terminus; Pore, channel pore (S5-6); VSD, voltage-sensing domain (S1-4). (*B*) Comparison of probability of a cardiac event in patients with LQT1 with mutations in KCNQ1 transmembrane domain and C-terminus. (*C*) Comparison of cumulative probability of first cardiac event in patients with LQT2 with mutations in hERG pore domain, N- and C-terminus. (*Data from* Refs.[61,62,108])

glucocorticoid-inducible kinase 1 (SGK1) upregulate I_{Ks} currents by facilitating exocytosis of KCNQ1 channel in a RAB-11–dependent manner. KCNE1 D76N disrupts this mechanism and results in lower functional expression of I_{Ks} current.[68]

Much progress has been made in determining the mechanisms underlying KCNE1 effects on the biophysical properties of KCNQ1. KCNE1 makes extensive contact with different parts of the KCNQ1 channel, including the pore domain,[69–72] extracellular domain,[73–75] and the voltage-sensing domain.[76] The physiologically critical stoichiometry of KCNQ1 and KCNE1 remains to be confirmed. KCNQ1/KCNE1 ratios of 4:2 and 4:4[77–80] have been reported. KCNE1 has been shown to alter the movement of the KCNQ1 voltage sensor using various methods, such as substituted cysteine accessibility methods[73] and voltage clamp fluorometry.[81–83]

AKAP9 and long QT syndrome variant 11

Patients with LQT1 are more likely to experience cardiac events (68% of all events) during exercise or periods of elevated sympathetic nervous system activity.[84] The autonomic modulation of delayed rectifier potassium channel and its potential roles in the etiology of LQTs have long been recognized. Walsh and Kass[85] first reported that the I_{Ks} channel is regulated by PKA at physiological temperatures.[85] Marx and colleagues[59] later demonstrated that such regulation requires Yotiao (or AKAP9), an A-kinase anchoring protein, which functions as an adaptor that presents PKA and PP1 to the I_{Ks} channel so that the channel phosphorylation state can be finely controlled by adrenergic pathways. Subsequent studies have revealed that AKAP9 plays a central role in regulating the cAMP/PKA levels in the compartmentalized microenvironment surrounding the I_{Ks} channels.[86,87] AKAP9 coordinates the actions of 2 pairs of enzymes: PKA and protein phosphatase 1 (PP1) that phosphorylate or dephosphorylate the channel, respectively, and adenylyl cyclase and phosphodiesterase that synthesize or hydrolyze cAMP, respectively, which in turn stimulate PKA.[88] As a result, the phosphorylation level of I_{Ks} channels is tightly regulated by the macromolecular signaling complex anchored by AKAP9. During sympathetic activation, which increases heart rate subsequent to physical or emotional stressors, I_{Ks} channel activity is enhanced by PKA to shorten QTc accordingly and to allow for sufficient diastolic filling time as heart rate increases. LQT11 is an LQTS variant associated with mutations in AKAP9. A role of AKAP9 in LQTS was discovered in a study of a patient with suspected LQTS who was found to carry a mutation (S1570L) located in a region on AKAP9 critical for interaction with I_{Ks} channels. The proband's family members were also found to carry the same mutation and had a history of LQTS. In vitro analysis showed that this AKAP9 mutation reduced the response of I_{Ks} channels to cAMP and associated with LQT,[89] and thus, like LQT1 and LQT5, arrhythmia risk is increased during exercise. A recent study suggested that AKAP9 is a genetic modifier of QT intervals in people who carry the LQT1 mutation, confirming the role of AKAP9 in cardiac electrophysiology.[90]

hERG and long QT syndrome variant 2

Of all LQTSs, 39% to 45% have been attributed to loss-of-function mutations in hERG.[45,46] To date, nearly 500 hERG variations have been found to associate with LQT2.[91] Both haploinsufficiency and dominant negative phenotypes have been found in hERG mutants. Deletion mutants such as ΔI500-F508, or frameshift mutants such as Δbp1261, do not form functional channels by themselves and do not coassemble with wild-type subunits. As a result, hERG channel expression is reduced drastically (haploinsufficiency) as only tetramers of the remaining wild-type channels can pass current. On the other hand, some missense mutations, such as N470D, A561V, and G628S, suppress the function of wild-type channel, causing dominant negative effects.[92] At the molecular and cellular levels, many LQT2 mutations in hERG lead to reduction in membrane trafficking associated with protein misfolding, endoplasmic reticulum (ER) retention, and subsequent protein degradation.[93–95] A recent comprehensive analysis confirmed that trafficking deficiency contributes to loss-of-function phenotypes for most LQT2 mutations in hERG.[91] Therefore, pharmacologic agents such as thapsigargin[96] and fexofenadine,[97] which restore normal trafficking, offer a potential therapy for LQT2.[98–101] Although trafficking defects are common, LQT2 mutations may also reduce total I_{Kr} by affecting channel gating. For example, G584S was shown to enhance inactivation,[102] whereas a series of mutations (F29L, N33T, G53R, R56Q, C66G, H70R, A78P, L86R)[103] in the hERG N-terminal PAS domain,[104] a hotspot for channel regulation and LQT2 mutations, was shown to accelerate deactivation. Mutations that affect both gating and trafficking have also been reported.[105] Loss-of-function can also occur as a consequence of altered gene transcription.[106,107] Whatever the underlying mechanism, loss of I_{Kr} contributes to a reduction in net outward current during the repolarization phase of cardiac action potentials, and hence QT prolongation in the ECG.

Compared with LQT1 mutations that are largely clustered in the KCNQ1 pore, intracellular linker and C-terminus, LQT2 mutations are more widely distributed throughout the protein with a significant presence in the extracellular linker and the N-terminus. Twenty-one percent of all LQT2 mutations were found in the N-terminal PAS domain, 23% in the pore region, 23% in the extracellular linkers, and 15% in the C-terminus (see **Fig. 3**A).[62] Locations of the mutations not only correlate with cellular phenotypes, but also clinical risks. Most pore mutations exert dominant negative effects on wild-type channels.[91] As such, patients with missense mutations in the channel pore region (S5-pore-S6) carry the highest risk of arrhythmia (**Fig. 3**C).[108,109]

hERG and drug-induced long QT

A significant number of patients (estimates range from 2%–8.8%) who receive antiarrhythmic agents develop drug-induced arrhythmia.[110] This problem is most pronounced with the use of Class III antiarrhythmic drugs such as dofetilide, E-4031, and MK-499.[111–113] These drugs are known to block hERG channels with a high affinity, thus causing drug-induced loss of hERG channel function. The QT interval prolongation that results[114,115] predisposes patients to ventricular arrhythmia, including TdP, in a manner that parallels clinical manifestation of congenital LQTS. It is now abundantly clear that drug-induced arrhythmia is not limited to antiarrhythmic agents.[110] As examples, drugs including antibiotics (such as clarithromycin, erythromycin), antipsychotics (such as chlorpromazine, haloperidol, pimozide, thioridazine), antihistamines (such as astemizole, terfenadine), and gastric prokinetics (such as cisapride) have all been linked to hERG block and TdP.[116] Because of the widespread off-target inhibition of hERG channels, virtually all drug development programs must include testing for hERG channel inhibition over drug concentrations that are proposed for clinical regimens.

Reminiscent of delayed rectifier blockade by quaternary ammonium described by Armstrong,[117] most of the hERG blockers require an open channel to gain access to the channel pore.[111,114,118,119] The binding of the blockers to their receptor sites inside the channel pore is state dependent: blockers bind to the open channels and dissociate from the closed channel. However, the closing of the channel gates may trap the dissociated blockers inside the closed channels, if the size of the blocker is small enough to fit the limited space of the inner cavities of the channel. Such "drug trapping" causes extremely slow recovery from channel block.[114,118] Mitcheson and

colleagues[120] observed that MK499, a *methanesulphonanilide* derivative with size too large to fit the cavity of Shaker and KcsA channels, was trapped inside closed hERG, suggesting that the inner cavity of hERG is probably larger than that of Shaker or KcsA. The larger cavity is one potential reason for the unique susceptibility of hERG to blockade by small molecules. Multiple receptor sites for hERG blockers have been determined and are all located on the S6: a pair of polar residues (Thr 623 and Ser 624) sit just below the selectivity filter and a pair of aromatic residues (Tyr 652 and Phe 656) in the lower part of the S6 helix.[121–123] Apart from direct channel block, some drugs also may cause inhibition of membrane trafficking of hERG subunits.[124,125] Arsenic trioxide,[126] geldanamycin,[127] pentamidine,[128,129] and probucol[130,131] have been shown to inhibit trafficking without causing channel block. Other reports also have suggested that some previously described hERG blockers may cause additional inhibition of trafficking and are thus termed dual inhibitors.[124]

Short QT Syndrome

Algra and colleagues[132] first noticed that patients with shortened QT interval (<400 ms) had risks of sudden deaths as high as those with prolonged QT. Since then, cases of sporadic and familial SQTS have been reported.[133–135] Current diagnostic criteria for short QT is 330 to 370 ms (QTc).[136,137] Patients with SQTS may develop AF, syncope, polymorphic ventricular tachycardia, ventricular fibrillation, and sudden death. To date, 4 gain-of-function mutations of hERG have been reported to cause SQTS variant 1 (SQT1). Both N558K[138,139] and T618I[140] cause reduction in hERG inactivation, abolish rectification, and subsequently produce greater current during the plateau phase of cardiac action potentials. R1135H causes slower deactivation, which in turn may cause greater "resurgent" current during phase 3 of action potential and results in shortened repolarization. An ECG of a patient with R1135H showed not only shortened QT, but also a Brugada pattern.[141,142] I560T significantly increased peak current density and shifted inactivation curve to a more positive voltage range.[143] Mutations in KCNQ1 are associated with SQTS variant 2 (SQT2) and lead to gain of function of I_{Ks} by multiple mechanisms. For example, V307L accelerated activation kinetics and left-shifted voltage-dependent activation, thus resulting in gain of function.[144] The F279I mutation was shown to decrease the association with KCNE1, and thus accelerate activation and left shift voltage-dependent activation.[145] Also, R259H increased current density and caused slower deactivation and faster activation.[146] Drugs that reduce outward potassium currents, such as hydroquinidine,[147,148] dysopyramide,[149,150] and propafenone[151] have been shown effective for SQT1.

Familial Atrial Fibrillation

Familial aggregation is common among patients with idiopathic AF (or lone AF) without underlying cardiovascular diseases. Up to 30% of these patients have a positive family history.[30,152–155] The relative risk of AF is significantly higher in individuals with a positive family history.[156] These findings suggest a strong genetic predisposition for familial AF. Mutations in all 3 delayed rectifier channels (I_{Ks}, I_{Kr}, and I_{Kur}) have been associated with familial AF in single-gene Mendelian fashion[155,157–172] (see **Table 1** for a list of AF mutations identified in KCNQ1, hERG, and Kv1.5). Followed by the first report of S140G mutation in KCNQ1[159] in 2003, multiple mutations of KCNQ1 have been identified to associate with AF. Most of them are gain-of-function mutations that are located in the voltage-sensing domain and patients have both familial AF and SQTS. The biophysical properties of KCNQ1 S140G and V141M have been studied extensively. The 2 affected residues are located in the S1 domain. Both mutations cause extremely slow deactivation and negative shift of voltage-dependent activation.[160] The mutant channels slow deactivation such that insufficient time passes during diastolic intervals for channels to fully deactivate. Over a series of beats, this results in a high percentage of channels accumulating in the open state, leading to a large, seemingly time-independent outward current. Most of the identified gain-of-function KCNQ1 mutations associated with AF show similar slowed deactivation kinetics to various degrees.[163–165,167,168] Intriguingly, although most AF mutations identified in KCNQ1 demonstrate gain of function, a few loss-of-function mutations have also been found. For example, A302V is retained in the ER, conducts very small current,[158] and was previously shown as an LQT mutation.[173] Two hERG mutations, N588K[138,174] and K897T,[169] have also been shown to associate with AF.

Table 1
List of AF mutations identified in KCNQ1, hERG, and Kv1.5 channels

Channel	Mutation	Location	Function	Clinical Phenotype	Reference
KCNQ1	A46T	N	Gain	Normal or long QT, AF	158
	S140G	S1	Gain	Normal or long QT, AF	159,160
	V141M	S1	Gain	Short QT, AF	160,161
	Q147R	S1	Loss	Long QT, AF	162
	R195W	Intracellular	Gain	Normal or long QT, AF	158
	S209P	S3	Gain	Normal QT, AF	163
	G229D	S4	Gain	Normal QT, AF	164
	R231C	S4	Gain	Normal or long QT, AF	165,166
	R231H	S4	Gain	Normal or long QT, AF	167
	V241F	S4	Gain	Normal QT, AF	168
	A302V	pore	Loss	long QT, AF	158
	R670K	C	Gain	Normal QT, AF	158
hERG	N588K	pore	Gain	Short QT, AF	138,174
	K897T	C	Loss/Gain	Long or short QT, AF	169
Kv1.5	71–81del	N	Loss	AF	155
	E48G	N	Gain	AF	170
	Y155C	N	Loss	AF	170
	A305T	S1-2	Gain	AF	170
	D322H	S1-2	Gain	AF	170
	E375X	S4	Loss	AF	171
	D469E	Pore	Loss	AF	170
	P488S	Pore	Loss	AF	170
	T527M	Pore	Loss	AF	172
	A576V	C	Loss	AF	172
	E610K	C	Loss	AF	172

Abbreviation: AF, atrial fibrillation.
Data from Refs.[138,158–172]

More recently, more than 10 mutations in Kv1.5 (KCNA5), the alpha subunit of the atrial-specific I_{Kur} channel, have been identified in patients with familial and idiopathic AF.[155,170–172] Olson and colleagues[171] first reported in 2006 that a mutation (E375X) in the S4 domain led to truncation and loss of function of Kv1.5 and was associated with idiopathic AF. Yang and colleagues[155] identified an 11–amino acid residue deletion in Kv1.5 in 2 probands with strong family history of AF. The mutant channel conducted smaller currents. However, the deletion occurred in a functional motif for tyrosine kinase signaling and rendered the channel insensitive to Src tyrosine kinase regulation, important for stretch response. This may disrupt the physiological response to stretch and result in shortening of APD.[155] In a recent study, a series of nonsynonymous mutations (E48G, Y155C, A305T, D322H, D469E, and P488S) were identified in patients with lone AF. These include both gain-of-function (E48G, A305T, and D322H) and loss-of-function (Y155C, D469E and P488S) mutations that are distributed on all major functional domains of Kv1.5.[170] Conceptually, increased function of potassium channels may lead to shortening of the effective refractory period (ERP) and increased propensity for reentrant arrhythmia such as AF.[175] This supports the findings that most of the mutations found in patients with AF showed gain-of-function phenotype. On the other hand, recent studies have revealed that multiple loss-of-function mutations in both I_{Ks} and I_{Kur} channels are linked to AF. The exact mechanism is still unclear. It was shown that Kv1.5 dysfunction in human atrial myocyte caused prolonged APD associated with a propensity of early after depolarizations and rendered the atria prone to arrhythmogenesis.[171]

DELAYED RECTIFIER CHANNELS AS THERAPEUTIC TARGETS FOR CARDIAC ARRHYTHMIA

Given their pivotal roles in cardiac repolarization as well as various rhythm disorders, delayed rectifier channels have long been considered promising therapeutic targets for cardiac arrhythmia. Class III antiarrhythmic agents, such as amiodarone, sotalol, and dronedarone, primarily block these channels and prolong APD. These drugs are used for both ventricular and atrial arrhythmias. Activators of both hERG and KCNQ1 channels have been sought after as potential therapies to correct LQT. Several molecules have been identified to upregulate hERG or KCNQ1 function,[176] but their clinical efficacies have yet to be confirmed.

More recently, pharmaceutical companies have attempted to develop atrial-specific therapy for AF using Kv1.5 as target. The primary pharmacologic approach to treat reentrant arrhythmia such as AF is to stop the reentry circuit by lengthening the ERP, which is essentially determined by APD.[175] Blockers of delayed rectifiers prolong APD and are thus common therapy for AF. Clinically, sotalol (I_{Kr} blocker) and amiodarone (multichannel blocker) are effective agents that are able to convert AF to and maintain sinus rhythm.[177,178] However, blocking delayed rectifier channels such as I_{Kr} that are expressed in the ventricles may cause drug-induced LQTS, TdP, and mortality.[179] As a result, development of atrial-specific therapy for AF has received much attention in recent years. Because of its unique atrial-specific expression, Kv1.5 is an ideal pharmacologic target for AF treatment that may avoid the undesired proarrhythmic activities.[180] Numerous Kv1.5 blockers have been in development, but to date, most of them have failed to reach clinical trials for various reasons.[181] Vernakalant developed by Cardiome (Vancouver, Canada) has been shown effective to convert acute-onset AF to sinus rhythm and was approved in Europe. Vernakalant inhibits 2 atrial-specific potassium channels, I_{Kur} (Kv1.5) and I_{KAch} (Kir3.1/3.4), at low concentration, but is able to block I_{to} and I_{Na} at higher concentration.[182] Recent study suggests its efficacy is likely due to its rapid unbinding sodium channel blockade.[183] XEN-D0101 developed by Xention (Cambridge, UK) is another selective Kv1.5 inhibitor[184] and was show effective for AF in animal models.[176]

SUMMARY AND FUTURE DIRECTIONS

Delayed rectifier channels conduct outward currents during the plateau phase of cardiac action potentials and play critical roles in the timing of cardiac repolarization. Extensive studies on the biophysical properties of these channels closely combined with molecular genetics and clinical medicine have established a clear "central dogma" that causally connects dysfunctional ion channels, abnormal repolarization, and arrhythmia. This is especially true in the field of congenital LQTS, in which there is a large body of literature describing hundreds of mutations in the I_{Ks} and I_{Kr} channels as well as their cellular and clinical phenotypes. In recent years, new evidence has emerged to associate mutations in these channels with other inherited cardiac rhythm disorders, such as familial fibrillation and SQTSs. In these disorders, many questions remain unanswered. For example, although most KCNQ1 mutations associated with AF cause gain of function, a few loss-of-function mutations have been identified in patients with familial AF. It is curious that both gain- and loss-of-function mutations in the same channel may result in the same type of arrhythmia. Overlap in clinical phenotypes is another intriguing phenomenon. For example, hERG R1135H was first identified in a patient with SQTS, whose ECG also showed a Brugada pattern.[141,142,185] To understand these questions, it is imperative to understand the functional consequences of gene mutations in multiple systems that include, but are not limited to, heterologous expression systems, animal models, and the use of patient-specific–induced pluripotent stem cells. Great challenges also remain in the search for safe therapy of cardiac arrhythmia using delayed rectifiers as targets. Despite the effort to develop channel-specific or region-specific therapies, proarrhythmic activity still poses major hurdles and causes major safety concerns. With growing knowledge of potassium channel structure-function relationships, the application of high-throughput screening using automated patch clamp system, and expanded roles of human-induced pluripotent stem cell–derived myocytes as pharmacologic profiling platforms, we expect more molecules may emerge to modulate channel function with better specificity and safety profiles.

REFERENCES

1. Nerbonne JM, Kass RS. Molecular physiology of cardiac repolarization. Physiol Rev 2005;85(4): 1205–53.
2. Noble D, Tsien RW. Reconstruction of the repolarization process in cardiac Purkinje fibres based on voltage clamp measurements of membrane current. J Physiol 1969;200(1):233–54.
3. Noble D, Tsien RW. Outward membrane currents activated in the plateau range of potentials in cardiac Purkinje fibres. J Physiol 1969;200(1): 205–31.
4. Sanguinetti MC, Jurkiewicz NK. Two components of cardiac delayed rectifier K+ current. Differential sensitivity to block by class III antiarrhythmic agents. J Gen Physiol 1990;96(1):195–215.
5. Wang Z, Fermini B, Nattel S. Rapid and slow components of delayed rectifier current in human atrial myocytes. Cardiovasc Res 1994;28(10):1540–6.
6. Liu DW, Antzelevitch C. Characteristics of the delayed rectifier current (IKr and IKs) in canine ventricular epicardial, midmyocardial, and endocardial myocytes. A weaker IKs contributes to the longer action potential of the M cell. Circ Res 1995;76(3): 351–65.
7. Balser JR, Bennett PB, Roden DM. Time-dependent outward current in guinea pig ventricular myocytes. Gating kinetics of the delayed rectifier. J Gen Physiol 1990;96(4):835–63.
8. Walsh KB, Arena JP, Kwok WM, et al. Delayed-rectifier potassium channel activity in isolated membrane patches of guinea pig ventricular myocytes. Am J Physiol 1991;260(4 Pt 2):H1390–3.
9. Li GR, Feng J, Yue L, et al. Evidence for two components of delayed rectifier K+ current in human ventricular myocytes. Circ Res 1996;78(4): 689–96.
10. Apkon M, Nerbonne JM. Characterization of two distinct depolarization-activated K+ currents in isolated adult rat ventricular myocytes. J Gen Physiol 1991;97(5):973–1011.
11. Bou-Abboud E, Nerbonne JM. Molecular correlates of the calcium-independent, depolarization-activated K+ currents in rat atrial myocytes. J Physiol 1999;517(Pt 2):407–20.
12. Boyle WA, Nerbonne JM. A novel type of depolarization-activated K+ current in isolated adult rat atrial myocytes. Am J Physiol 1991;260(4 Pt 2):H1236–47.
13. Boyle WA, Nerbonne JM. Two functionally distinct 4-aminopyridine-sensitive outward K+ currents in rat atrial myocytes. J Gen Physiol 1992;100(6): 1041–67.
14. Wang Z, Fermini B, Nattel S. Sustained depolarization-induced outward current in human atrial myocytes. Evidence for a novel delayed rectifier K+ current similar to Kv1.5 cloned channel currents. Circ Res 1993;73(6):1061–76.
15. Wang Z, Fermini B, Nattel S. Delayed rectifier outward current and repolarization in human atrial myocytes. Circ Res 1993;73(2):276–85.
16. Wang Q, Curran ME, Splawski I, et al. Positional cloning of a novel potassium channel gene: KVLQT1 mutations cause cardiac arrhythmias. Nat Genet 1996;12(1):17–23.
17. Takumi T, Ohkubo H, Nakanishi S. Cloning of a membrane protein that induces a slow voltage-gated potassium current. Science 1988; 242(4881):1042–5.
18. Barhanin J, Lesage F, Guillemare E, et al. K(V)LQT1 and IsK (minK) proteins associate to form the I(Ks) cardiac potassium current. Nature 1996;384(6604): 78–80.
19. Sanguinetti MC, Curran ME, Zou A, et al. Coassembly of K(V)LQT1 and minK (IsK) proteins to form cardiac I(Ks) potassium channel. Nature 1996; 384(6604):80–3.
20. Schulze-Bahr E, Wang Q, Wedekind H, et al. KCNE1 mutations cause Jervell and Lange-Nielsen syndrome. Nat Genet 1997;17(3):267–8.
21. Splawski I, Tristani-Firouzi M, Lehmann MH, et al. Mutations in the hminK gene cause long QT syndrome and suppress IKs function. Nat Genet 1997;17(3):338–40.

22. Sanguinetti MC, Jiang C, Curran ME, et al. A mechanistic link between an inherited and an acquired cardiac arrhythmia: HERG encodes the IKr potassium channel. Cell 1995;81(2):299–307.

23. Warmke JW, Ganetzky B. A family of potassium channel genes related to eag in *Drosophila* and mammals. Proc Natl Acad Sci U S A 1994;91(8): 3438–42.

24. Curran ME, Splawski I, Timothy KW, et al. A molecular basis for cardiac arrhythmia: HERG mutations cause long QT syndrome. Cell 1995; 80(5):795–803.

25. Abbott GW, Sesti F, Splawski I, et al. MiRP1 forms IKr potassium channels with HERG and is associated with cardiac arrhythmia. Cell 1999;97(2): 175–87.

26. Weerapura M, Nattel S, Chartier D, et al. A comparison of currents carried by HERG, with and without coexpression of MiRP1, and the native rapid delayed rectifier current. Is MiRP1 the missing link? J Physiol 2002;540(Pt 1):15–27.

27. Feng J, Wible B, Li GR, et al. Antisense oligodeoxynucleotides directed against Kv1.5 mRNA specifically inhibit ultrarapid delayed rectifier K+ current in cultured adult human atrial myocytes. Circ Res 1997;80(4):572–9.

28. Rampe D, Wang Z, Fermini B, et al. Voltage- and time-dependent block by perhexiline of K+ currents in human atrium and in cells expressing a Kv1.5-type cloned channel. J Pharmacol Exp Ther 1995;274(1):444–9.

29. Busch AE, Suessbrich H, Waldegger S, et al. Inhibition of IKs in guinea pig cardiac myocytes and guinea pig IsK channels by the chromanol 293B. Pflugers Arch 1996;432(6):1094–6.

30. Andalib A, Brugada R, Nattel S. Atrial fibrillation: evidence for genetically determined disease. Curr Opin Cardiol 2008;23(3):176–83.

31. Tucker NR, Ellinor PT. Emerging directions in the genetics of atrial fibrillation. Circ Res 2014;114(9): 1469–82.

32. Giudicessi JR, Ackerman MJ. Potassium-channel mutations and cardiac arrhythmias–diagnosis and therapy. Nat Rev Cardiol 2012;9(6):319–32.

33. Abriel H, Zaklyazminskaya EV. Cardiac channelopathies: genetic and molecular mechanisms. Gene 2013;517(1):1–11.

34. Pfeufer A, Sanna S, Arking DE, et al. Common variants at ten loci modulate the QT interval duration in the QTSCD Study. Nat Genet 2009;41(4):407–14.

35. Arking DE, Pulit SL, Crotti L, et al. Genetic association study of QT interval highlights role for calcium signaling pathways in myocardial repolarization. Nat Genet 2014;46(8):826–36.

36. Bezzina CR, Lahrouchi N, Priori SG. Genetics of sudden cardiac death. Circ Res 2015;116(12): 1919–36.

37. Mizusawa Y, Horie M, Wilde AA. Genetic and clinical advances in congenital long QT syndrome. Circ J 2014;78(12):2827–33.

38. Tester DJ, Ackerman MJ. Genetics of long QT syndrome. Methodist Debakey Cardiovasc J 2014; 10(1):29–33.

39. Schwartz PJ, Ackerman MJ. The long QT syndrome: a transatlantic clinical approach to diagnosis and therapy. Eur Heart J 2013;34(40): 3109–16.

40. Crotti L, Celano G, Dagradi F, et al. Congenital long QT syndrome. Orphanet J Rare Dis 2008;3:18.

41. Cummings S, Priori S. Genetics of cardiac arrhythmias. Minerva Med 2011;102(3):209–22.

42. Keating MT, Sanguinetti MC. Molecular and cellular mechanisms of cardiac arrhythmias. Cell 2001; 104(4):569–80.

43. Goldenberg I, Moss AJ. Long QT syndrome. J Am Coll Cardiol 2008;51(24):2291–300.

44. Towbin JA, Vatta M. Molecular biology and the prolonged QT syndromes. Am J Med 2001;110(5): 385–98.

45. Splawski I, Shen J, Timothy KW, et al. Spectrum of mutations in long-QT syndrome genes. KVLQT1, HERG, SCN5A, KCNE1, and KCNE2. Circulation 2000;102(10):1178–85.

46. Napolitano C, Priori SG, Schwartz PJ, et al. Genetic testing in the long QT syndrome: development and validation of an efficient approach to genotyping in clinical practice. JAMA 2005;294(23):2975–80.

47. Peroz D, Rodriguez N, Choveau F, et al. Kv7.1 (KCNQ1) properties and channelopathies. J Physiol 2008;586(7):1785–9.

48. Dvir M, Peretz A, Haitin Y, et al. Recent molecular insights from mutated IKS channels in cardiac arrhythmia. Curr Opin Pharmacol 2014;15:74–82.

49. Eldstrom J, Xu H, Werry D, et al. Mechanistic basis for LQT1 caused by S3 mutations in the KCNQ1 subunit of IKs. J Gen Physiol 2010; 135(5):433–48.

50. Dahimene S, Alcoléa S, Naud P, et al. The N-terminal juxtamembranous domain of KCNQ1 is critical for channel surface expression: implications in the Romano-Ward LQT1 syndrome. Circ Res 2006;99(10):1076–83.

51. Sato A, Arimura T, Makita N, et al. Novel mechanisms of trafficking defect caused by KCNQ1 mutations found in long QT syndrome. J Biol Chem 2009;284(50):35122–33.

52. Schmitt N, Calloe K, Nielsen NH, et al. The novel C-terminal KCNQ1 mutation M520R alters protein trafficking. Biochem Biophys Res Commun 2007; 358(1):304–10.

53. Gouas L, Bellocq C, Berthet M, et al. New KCNQ1 mutations leading to haploinsufficiency in a general population; defective trafficking of a KvLQT1 mutant. Cardiovasc Res 2004;63(1):60–8.

54. Wilson AJ, Quinn KV, Graves FM, et al. Abnormal KCNQ1 trafficking influences disease pathogenesis in hereditary long QT syndromes (LQT1). Cardiovasc Res 2005;67(3):476–86.

55. Schmitt N, Schwarz M, Peretz A, et al. A recessive C-terminal Jervell and Lange-Nielsen mutation of the KCNQ1 channel impairs subunit assembly. EMBO J 2000;19(3):332–40.

56. Matavel A, Medei E, Lopes CM. PKA and PKC partially rescue long QT type 1 phenotype by restoring channel-PIP2 interactions. Channels (Austin) 2010;4(1):3–11.

57. Thomas AM, Harmer SC, Khambra T, et al. Characterization of a binding site for anionic phospholipids on KCNQ1. J Biol Chem 2011; 286(3):2088–100.

58. Zaydman MA, Silva JR, Delaloye K, et al. Kv7.1 ion channels require a lipid to couple voltage sensing to pore opening. Proc Natl Acad Sci U S A 2013; 110(32):13180–5.

59. Marx SO, Kurokawa J, Reiken S, et al. Requirement of a macromolecular signaling complex for beta adrenergic receptor modulation of the KCNQ1-KCNE1 potassium channel. Science 2002; 295(5554):496–9.

60. Bianchi L, Priori SG, Napolitano C, et al. Mechanisms of I(Ks) suppression in LQT1 mutants. Am J Physiol Heart Circ Physiol 2000;279(6): H3003–11.

61. Moss AJ, Shimizu W, Wilde AA, et al. Clinical aspects of type-1 long-QT syndrome by location, coding type, and biophysical function of mutations involving the KCNQ1 gene. Circulation 2007; 115(19):2481–9.

62. Jackson HA, Accili EA. Evolutionary analyses of KCNQ1 and HERG voltage-gated potassium channel sequences reveal location-specific susceptibility and augmented chemical severities of arrhythmogenic mutations. BMC Evol Biol 2008;8:188.

63. Shimizu W, Horie M, Ohno S, et al. Mutation site-specific differences in arrhythmic risk and sensitivity to sympathetic stimulation in the LQT1 form of congenital long QT syndrome: multicenter study in Japan. J Am Coll Cardiol 2004;44(1):117–25.

64. Barsheshet A, Goldenberg I, O-Uchi J, et al. Mutations in cytoplasmic loops of the KCNQ1 channel and the risk of life-threatening events: implications for mutation-specific response to beta-blocker therapy in type 1 long-QT syndrome. Circulation 2012;125(16):1988–96.

65. Hedley PL, Jørgensen P, Schlamowitz S, et al. The genetic basis of long QT and short QT syndromes: a mutation update. Hum Mutat 2009; 30(11):1486–511.

66. Bianchi L, Shen Z, Dennis AT, et al. Cellular dysfunction of LQT5-minK mutants: abnormalities of IKs, IKr and trafficking in long QT syndrome. Hum Mol Genet 1999;8(8):1499–507.

67. Harmer SC, Tinker A. The role of abnormal trafficking of KCNE1 in long QT syndrome 5. Biochem Soc Trans 2007;35(Pt 5):1074–6.

68. Seebohm G, Strutz-Seebohm N, Ureche ON, et al. Long QT syndrome-associated mutations in KCNQ1 and KCNE1 subunits disrupt normal endosomal recycling of IKs channels. Circ Res 2008; 103(12):1451–7.

69. Melman YF, Um SY, Krumerman A, et al. KCNE1 binds to the KCNQ1 pore to regulate potassium channel activity. Neuron 2004;42(6):927–37.

70. Melman YF, Domènech A, de la Luna S, et al. Structural determinants of KvLQT1 control by the KCNE family of proteins. J Biol Chem 2001; 276(9):6439–44.

71. Melman YF, Krumerman A, McDonald TV. A single transmembrane site in the KCNE-encoded proteins controls the specificity of KvLQT1 channel gating. J Biol Chem 2002;277(28):25187–94.

72. Nakajo K, Nishino A, Okamura Y, et al. KCNQ1 subdomains involved in KCNE modulation revealed by an invertebrate KCNQ1 orthologue. J Gen Physiol 2011;138(5):521–35.

73. Nakajo K, Kubo Y. KCNE1 and KCNE3 stabilize and/ or slow voltage sensing S4 segment of KCNQ1 channel. J Gen Physiol 2007;130(3):269–81.

74. Xu X, Jiang M, Hsu KL, et al. KCNQ1 and KCNE1 in the IKs channel complex make state-dependent contacts in their extracellular domains. J Gen Physiol 2008;131(6):589–603.

75. Chung DY, Chan PJ, Bankston JR, et al. Location of KCNE1 relative to KCNQ1 in the I(KS) potassium channel by disulfide cross-linking of substituted cysteines. Proc Natl Acad Sci U S A 2009;106(3): 743–8.

76. Nakajo K, Kubo Y. Nano-environmental changes by KCNE proteins modify KCNQ channel function. Channels (Austin) 2011;5(5):397–401.

77. Chen H, Kim LA, Rajan S, et al. Charybdotoxin binding in the I(Ks) pore demonstrates two MinK subunits in each channel complex. Neuron 2003; 40(1):15–23.

78. Morin TJ, Kobertz WR. Counting membrane-embedded KCNE beta-subunits in functioning K+ channel complexes. Proc Natl Acad Sci U S A 2008;105(5):1478–82.

79. Plant LD, Xiong D, Dai H, et al. Individual IKs channels at the surface of mammalian cells contain two KCNE1 accessory subunits. Proc Natl Acad Sci U S A 2014;111(14):E1438–46.

80. Nakajo K, Ulbrich MH, Kubo Y, et al. Stoichiometry of the KCNQ1-KCNE1 ion channel complex. Proc Natl Acad Sci U S A 2010;107(44):18862–7.

81. Osteen JD, Gonzalez C, Sampson KJ, et al. KCNE1 alters the voltage sensor movements necessary to

open the KCNQ1 channel gate. Proc Natl Acad Sci U S A 2010;107(52):22710–5.

82. Ruscic KJ, Miceli F, Villalba-Galea CA, et al. IKs channels open slowly because KCNE1 accessory subunits slow the movement of S4 voltage sensors in KCNQ1 pore-forming subunits. Proc Natl Acad Sci U S A 2013;110(7): E559–66.

83. Barro-Soria R, Rebolledo S, Liin SI, et al. KCNE1 divides the voltage sensor movement in KCNQ1/KCNE1 channels into two steps. Nat Commun 2014;5:3750.

84. Schwartz PJ, Priori SG, Spazzolini C, et al. Genotype-phenotype correlation in the long-QT syndrome: gene-specific triggers for life-threatening arrhythmias. Circulation 2001;103(1):89–95.

85. Walsh KB, Kass RS. Regulation of a heart potassium channel by protein kinase A and C. Science 1988;242(4875):67–9.

86. Terrenoire C, Houslay MD, Baillie GS, et al. The cardiac IKs potassium channel macromolecular complex includes the phosphodiesterase PDE4D3. J Biol Chem 2009;284(14):9140–6.

87. Li Y, Chen L, Kass RS, et al. The A-kinase anchoring protein Yotiao facilitates complex formation between adenylyl cyclase type 9 and the IKs potassium channel in heart. J Biol Chem 2012; 287(35):29815–24.

88. Chen L, Kass RS. A-kinase anchoring protein 9 and IKs channel regulation. J Cardiovasc Pharmacol 2011;58(5):459–513.

89. Chen L, Marquardt ML, Tester DJ, et al. Mutation of an A-kinase-anchoring protein causes long-QT syndrome. Proc Natl Acad Sci U S A 2007; 104(52):20990–5.

90. de Villiers CP, van der Merwe L, Crotti L, et al. AKAP9 is a genetic modifier of congenital long-QT syndrome type 1. Circ Cardiovasc Genet 2014;7(5):599–606.

91. Anderson CL, Kuzmicki CE, Childs RR, et al. Large-scale mutational analysis of Kv11.1 reveals molecular insights into type 2 long QT syndrome. Nat Commun 2014;5:5535.

92. Sanguinetti MC, Curran ME, Spector PS, et al. Spectrum of HERG K+-channel dysfunction in an inherited cardiac arrhythmia. Proc Natl Acad Sci U S A 1996;93(5):2208–12.

93. Zhou Z, Gong Q, Epstein ML, et al. HERG channel dysfunction in human long QT syndrome. Intracellular transport and functional defects. J Biol Chem 1998;273(33):21061–6.

94. Anderson CL, Delisle BP, Anson BD, et al. Most LQT2 mutations reduce Kv11.1 (hERG) current by a class 2 (trafficking-deficient) mechanism. Circulation 2006;113(3):365–73.

95. Gong Q, Jones MA, Zhou Z. Mechanisms of pharmacological rescue of trafficking-defective hERG

mutant channels in human long QT syndrome. J Biol Chem 2006;281(7):4069–74.

96. Delisle BP, Anderson CL, Balijepalli RC, et al. Thapsigargin selectively rescues the trafficking defective LQT2 channels G601S and F805C. J Biol Chem 2003;278(37):35749–54.

97. Rajamani S, Anderson CL, Anson BD, et al. Pharmacological rescue of human K(+) channel long-QT2 mutations: human ether-a-go-go-related gene rescue without block. Circulation 2002; 105(24):2830–5.

98. Mehta A, Sequiera GL, Ramachandra CJ, et al. Re-trafficking of hERG reverses long QT syndrome 2 phenotype in human iPS-derived cardiomyocytes. Cardiovasc Res 2014;102(3):497–506.

99. Smith JL, Reloj AR, Nataraj PS, et al. Pharmacological correction of long QT-linked mutations in KCNH2 (hERG) increases the trafficking of Kv11.1 channels stored in the transitional endoplasmic reticulum. Am J Physiol Cell Physiol 2013;305(9):C919–30.

100. Ayon RJ, Fernandez RA, Yuan JX. Mutant hERG channel traffic jam. Focus on "Pharmacological correction of long QT-linked mutations in KCNH2 (hERG) increases the trafficking of Kv11.1 channels stored in the transitional endoplasmic reticulum". Am J Physiol Cell Physiol 2013;305(9): C916–8.

101. Robertson GA, January CT. HERG trafficking and pharmacological rescue of LQTS-2 mutant channels. Handb Exp Pharmacol 2006;(171):349–55.

102. Zhao JT, Hill AP, Varghese A, et al. Not all hERG pore domain mutations have a severe phenotype: G584S has an inactivation gating defect with mild phenotype compared to G572S, which has a dominant negative trafficking defect and a severe phenotype. J Cardiovasc Electrophysiol 2009; 20(8):923–30.

103. Chen J, Zou A, Splawski I, et al. Long QT syndrome-associated mutations in the Per-Arnt-Sim (PAS) domain of HERG potassium channels accelerate channel deactivation. J Biol Chem 1999;274(15):10113–8.

104. Morais Cabral JH, Lee A, Cohen SL, et al. Crystal structure and functional analysis of the HERG potassium channel N terminus: a eukaryotic PAS domain. Cell 1998;95(5):649–55.

105. Balijepalli SY, Lim E, Concannon SP, et al. Mechanism of loss of Kv11.1 K+ current in mutant T421M-Kv11.1-expressing rat ventricular myocytes: interaction of trafficking and gating. Circulation 2012;126(24):2809–18.

106. Gong Q, Zhang L, Vincent GM, et al. Nonsense mutations in hERG cause a decrease in mutant mRNA transcripts by nonsense-mediated mRNA decay in human long-QT syndrome. Circulation 2007;116(1):17–24.

107. Gong Q, Zhang L, Moss AJ, et al. A splice site mutation in hERG leads to cryptic splicing in human long QT syndrome. J Mol Cell Cardiol 2008;44(3):502–9.

108. Moss AJ, Zareba W, Kaufman ES, et al. Increased risk of arrhythmic events in long-QT syndrome with mutations in the pore region of the human ether-a-go-go-related gene potassium channel. Circulation 2002;105(7):794–9.

109. Shimizu W, Moss AJ, Wilde AA, et al. Genotype-phenotype aspects of type 2 long QT syndrome. J Am Coll Cardiol 2009;54(22):2052–62.

110. Haverkamp W, Breithardt G, Camm AJ, et al. The potential for QT prolongation and pro-arrhythmia by non-anti-arrhythmic drugs: clinical and regulatory implications. Report on a Policy Conference of the European Society of Cardiology. Cardiovasc Res 2000;47(2):219–33.

111. Spector PS, Curran ME, Keating MT, et al. Class III antiarrhythmic drugs block HERG, a human cardiac delayed rectifier K+ channel. Open-channel block by methanesulfonanilides. Circ Res 1996;78(3):499–503.

112. Tseng GN. I(Kr): the hERG channel. J Mol Cell Cardiol 2001;33(5):835–49.

113. Baskin EP, Lynch JJ Jr. Comparative effects of increased extracellular potassium and pacing frequency on the class III activities of methanesulfonanilide IKr blockers dofetilide, D-sotalol, E-4031, and MK-499. J Cardiovasc Pharmacol 1994;24(2):199–208.

114. Carmeliet E. Voltage- and time-dependent block of the delayed K+ current in cardiac myocytes by dofetilide. J Pharmacol Exp Ther 1992;262(2):809–17.

115. Kiehn J, Lacerda AE, Wible B, et al. Molecular physiology and pharmacology of HERG. Single-channel currents and block by dofetilide. Circulation 1996;94(10):2572–9.

116. Hancox JC, McPate MJ, El Harchi A, et al. The hERG potassium channel and hERG screening for drug-induced torsades de pointes. Pharmacol Ther 2008;119(2):118–32.

117. Armstrong CM. Interaction of tetraethylammonium ion derivatives with the potassium channels of giant axons. J Gen Physiol 1971;58(4):413–37.

118. Yang T, Snyders DJ, Roden DM. Ibutilide, a methanesulfonanilide antiarrhythmic, is a potent blocker of the rapidly activating delayed rectifier K+ current (IKr) in AT-1 cells. Concentration-, time-, voltage-, and use-dependent effects. Circulation 1995;91(6):1799–806.

119. Kiehn J, Wible B, Lacerda AE, et al. Mapping the block of a cloned human inward rectifier potassium channel by dofetilide. Mol Pharmacol 1996;50(2):380–7.

120. Mitcheson JS, Chen J, Sanguinetti MC. Trapping of a methanesulfonanilide by closure of the HERG potassium channel activation gate. J Gen Physiol 2000;115(3):229–40.

121. Lees-Miller JP, Duan Y, Teng GQ, et al. Molecular determinant of high-affinity dofetilide binding to HERG1 expressed in Xenopus oocytes: involvement of S6 sites. Mol Pharmacol 2000;57(2):367–74.

122. Mitcheson JS, Chen J, Lin M, et al. A structural basis for drug-induced long QT syndrome. Proc Natl Acad Sci U S A 2000;97(22):12329–33.

123. Vandenberg JI, Perry MD, Perrin MJ, et al. hERG K(+) channels: structure, function, and clinical significance. Physiol Rev 2012;92(3):1393–478.

124. Nogawa H, Kawai T. hERG trafficking inhibition in drug-induced lethal cardiac arrhythmia. Eur J Pharmacol 2014;741:336–9.

125. Dennis A, Wang L, Wan X, et al. hERG channel trafficking: novel targets in drug-induced long QT syndrome. Biochem Soc Trans 2007;35(Pt 5):1060–3.

126. Ficker E, Kuryshev YA, Dennis AT, et al. Mechanisms of arsenic-induced prolongation of cardiac repolarization. Mol Pharmacol 2004;66(1):33–44.

127. Ficker E, Dennis AT, Wang L, et al. Role of the cytosolic chaperones Hsp70 and Hsp90 in maturation of the cardiac potassium channel HERG. Circ Res 2003;92(12):e87–100.

128. Cordes JS, Sun Z, Lloyd DB, et al. Pentamidine reduces hERG expression to prolong the QT interval. Br J Pharmacol 2005;145(1):15–23.

129. Kuryshev YA, Ficker E, Wang L, et al. Pentamidine-induced long QT syndrome and block of hERG trafficking. J Pharmacol Exp Ther 2005;312(1):316–23.

130. Guo J, Li X, Shallow H, et al. Involvement of caveolin in probucol-induced reduction in hERG plasma-membrane expression. Mol Pharmacol 2011;79(5):806–13.

131. Guo J, Massaeli H, Li W, et al. Identification of IKr and its trafficking disruption induced by probucol in cultured neonatal rat cardiomyocytes. J Pharmacol Exp Ther 2007;321(3):911–20.

132. Algra A, Tijssen JG, Roelandt JR, et al. QT interval variables from 24 hour electrocardiography and the two year risk of sudden death. Br Heart J 1993;70(1):43–8.

133. Gussak I, Brugada P, Brugada J, et al. Idiopathic short QT interval: a new clinical syndrome? Cardiology 2000;94(2):99–102.

134. Gussak I, Bjerregaard P. Short QT syndrome–5 years of progress. J Electrocardiol 2005;38(4):375–7.

135. Gaita F, Giustetto C, Bianchi F, et al. Short QT Syndrome: a familial cause of sudden death. Circulation 2003;108(8):965–70.

136. Priori SG, Wilde AA, Horie M, et al. HRS/EHRA/APHRS expert consensus statement on the diagnosis and management of patients with inherited primary arrhythmia syndromes: document endorsed

by HRS, EHRA, and APHRS in May 2013 and by ACCF, AHA, PACES, and AEPC in June 2013. Heart Rhythm 2013;10(12):1932–63.

137. Gollob MH, Redpath CJ, Roberts JD. The short QT syndrome: proposed diagnostic criteria. J Am Coll Cardiol 2011;57(7):802–12.

138. Brugada R, Hong K, Dumaine R, et al. Sudden death associated with short-QT syndrome linked to mutations in HERG. Circulation 2004;109(1):30–5.

139. Cordeiro JM, Brugada R, Wu YS, et al. Modulation of I(Kr) inactivation by mutation N588K in KCNH2: a link to arrhythmogenesis in short QT syndrome. Cardiovasc Res 2005;67(3):498–509.

140. Sun Y, Quan XQ, Fromme S, et al. A novel mutation in the KCNH2 gene associated with short QT syndrome. J Mol Cell Cardiol 2011;50(3):433–41.

141. Itoh H, Sakaguchi T, Ashihara T, et al. A novel KCNH2 mutation as a modifier for short QT interval. Int J Cardiol 2009;137(1):83–5.

142. Wilders R, Verkerk AO. Role of the R1135H KCNH2 mutation in Brugada syndrome. Int J Cardiol 2010;144(1):149–51.

143. Harrell DT, Ashihara T, Ishikawa T, et al. Genotype-dependent differences in age of manifestation and arrhythmia complications in short QT syndrome. Int J Cardiol 2015;190:393–402.

144. Bellocq C, van Ginneken AC, Bezzina CR, et al. Mutation in the KCNQ1 gene leading to the short QT-interval syndrome. Circulation 2004;109(20):2394–7.

145. Moreno C, Oliveras A, de la Cruz A, et al. A new KCNQ1 mutation at the S5 segment that impairs its association with KCNE1 is responsible for short QT syndrome. Cardiovasc Res 2015;107(4):613–23.

146. Wu ZJ, Huang Y, Fu YC, et al. Characterization of a Chinese KCNQ1 mutation (R259H) that shortens repolarization and causes short QT syndrome 2. J Geriatr Cardiol 2015;12(4):394–401.

147. Gaita F, Giustetto C, Bianchi F, et al. Short QT syndrome: pharmacological treatment. J Am Coll Cardiol 2004;43(8):1494–9.

148. Giustetto C, Schimpf R, Mazzanti A, et al. Long-term follow-up of patients with short QT syndrome. J Am Coll Cardiol 2011;58(6):587–95.

149. Dumaine R, Antzelevitch C. Disopyramide: although potentially life-threatening in the setting of long QT, could it be life-saving in short QT syndrome? J Mol Cell Cardiol 2006;41(3):421–3.

150. McPate MJ, Duncan RS, Witchel HJ, et al. Disopyramide is an effective inhibitor of mutant HERG K+ channels involved in variant 1 short QT syndrome. J Mol Cell Cardiol 2006;41(3):563–6.

151. Bjerregaard P, Gussak I. Short QT syndrome: mechanisms, diagnosis and treatment. Nat Clin Pract Cardiovasc Med 2005;2(2):84–7.

152. Darbar D, Herron KJ, Ballew JD, et al. Familial atrial fibrillation is a genetically heterogeneous disorder. J Am Coll Cardiol 2003;41(12):2185–92.

153. Ellinor PT, Yoerger DM, Ruskin JN, et al. Familial aggregation in lone atrial fibrillation. Hum Genet 2005;118(2):179–84.

154. Patton KK, Zacks ES, Chang JY, et al. Clinical subtypes of lone atrial fibrillation. Pacing Clin Electrophysiol 2005;28(7):630–8.

155. Yang T, Yang P, Roden DM, et al. Novel KCNA5 mutation implicates tyrosine kinase signaling in human atrial fibrillation. Heart Rhythm 2010;7(9):1246–52.

156. Fox CS, Parise H, D'Agostino RB Sr, et al. Parental atrial fibrillation as a risk factor for atrial fibrillation in offspring. JAMA 2004;291(23):2851–5.

157. Mahida S, Lubitz SA, Rienstra M, et al. Monogenic atrial fibrillation as pathophysiological paradigms. Cardiovasc Res 2011;89(4):692–700.

158. Steffensen AB, Refsgaard L, Andersen MN, et al. IKs gain- and loss-of-function in early-onset lone atrial fibrillation. J Cardiovasc Electrophysiol 2015;26(7):715–23.

159. Chen YH, Xu SJ, Bendahhou S, et al. KCNQ1 gain-of-function mutation in familial atrial fibrillation. Science 2003;299(5604):251–4.

160. Restier L, Cheng L, Sanguinetti MC. Mechanisms by which atrial fibrillation-associated mutations in the S1 domain of KCNQ1 slow deactivation of IKs channels. J Physiol 2008;586(Pt 17):4179–91.

161. Hong K, Piper DR, Diaz-Valdecantos A, et al. De novo KCNQ1 mutation responsible for atrial fibrillation and short QT syndrome in utero. Cardiovasc Res 2005;68(3):433–40.

162. Lundby A, Ravn LS, Svendsen JH, et al. KCNQ1 mutation Q147R is associated with atrial fibrillation and prolonged QT interval. Heart Rhythm 2007;4(12):1532–41.

163. Das S, Makino S, Melman YF, et al. Mutation in the S3 segment of KCNQ1 results in familial lone atrial fibrillation. Heart Rhythm 2009;6(8):1146–53.

164. Hasegawa K, Ohno S, Ashihara T, et al. A novel KCNQ1 missense mutation identified in a patient with juvenile-onset atrial fibrillation causes constitutively open IKs channels. Heart Rhythm 2014;11(1):67–75.

165. Bartos DC, Duchatelet S, Burgess DE, et al. R231C mutation in KCNQ1 causes long QT syndrome type 1 and familial atrial fibrillation. Heart Rhythm 2011;8(1):48–55.

166. Henrion U, Zumhagen S, Steinke K, et al. Overlapping cardiac phenotype associated with a familial mutation in the voltage sensor of the KCNQ1 channel. Cell Physiol Biochem 2012;29(5–6):809–18.

167. Bartos DC, Anderson JB, Bastiaenen R, et al. A KCNQ1 mutation causes a high penetrance for familial atrial fibrillation. J Cardiovasc Electrophysiol 2013;24(5):562–9.

168. Ki CS, Jung CL, Kim HJ, et al. A KCNQ1 mutation causes age-dependant bradycardia and persistent atrial fibrillation. Pflugers Arch 2014;466(3):529–40.

169. Sinner MF, Pfeufer A, Akyol M, et al. The non-synonymous coding IKr-channel variant KCNH2-K897T is associated with atrial fibrillation: results from a systematic candidate gene-based analysis of KCNH2 (HERG). Eur Heart J 2008;29(7):907–14.

170. Christophersen IE, Olesen MS, Liang B, et al. Genetic variation in KCNA5: impact on the atrial-specific potassium current IKur in patients with lone atrial fibrillation. Eur Heart J 2013;34(20): 1517–25.

171. Olson TM, Alekseev AE, Liu XK, et al. Kv1.5 channelopathy due to KCNA5 loss-of-function mutation causes human atrial fibrillation. Hum Mol Genet 2006;15(14):2185–91.

172. Yang Y, Li J, Lin X, et al. Novel KCNA5 loss-of-function mutations responsible for atrial fibrillation. J Hum Genet 2009;54(5):277–83.

173. Yang T, Chung SK, Zhang W, et al. Biophysical properties of 9 KCNQ1 mutations associated with long-QT syndrome. Circ Arrhythm Electrophysiol 2009;2(4):417–26.

174. Hong K, Bjerregaard P, Gussak I, et al. Short QT syndrome and atrial fibrillation caused by mutation in KCNH2. J Cardiovasc Electrophysiol 2005;16(4): 394–6.

175. Nattel S. New ideas about atrial fibrillation 50 years on. Nature 2002;415(6868):219–26.

176. Wulff H, Castle NA, Pardo LA. Voltage-gated potassium channels as therapeutic targets. Nat Rev Drug Discov 2009;8(12):982–1001.

177. Roy D, Talajic M, Dorian P, et al. Amiodarone to prevent recurrence of atrial fibrillation. Canadian trial of atrial fibrillation investigators. N Engl J Med 2000;342(13):913–20.

178. Qin D, Leef G, Alam MB, et al. Comparative effectiveness of antiarrhythmic drugs for rhythm control of atrial fibrillation. J Cardiol 2015. [Epub ahead of print].

179. Waldo AL, Camm AJ, deRuyter H, et al. Effect of d-sotalol on mortality in patients with left ventricular dysfunction after recent and remote myocardial infarction. The SWORD Investigators. Survival with oral d-sotalol. Lancet 1996;348(9019):7–12.

180. Ravens U, Poulet C, Wettwer E, et al. Atrial selectivity of antiarrhythmic drugs. J Physiol 2013; 591(Pt 17):4087–97.

181. Ford JW, Milnes JT. New drugs targeting the cardiac ultra-rapid delayed-rectifier current (I Kur): rationale, pharmacology and evidence for potential therapeutic value. J Cardiovasc Pharmacol 2008; 52(2):105–20.

182. Vizzardi E, Salghetti F, Bonadei I, et al. A new anti-arrhythmic drug in the treatment of recent-onset atrial fibrillation: vernakalant. Cardiovasc Ther 2013;31(5):e55–62.

183. Comtois P, Sakabe M, Vigmond EJ, et al. Mechanisms of atrial fibrillation termination by rapidly unbinding Na+ channel blockers: insights from mathematical models and experimental correlates. Am J Physiol Heart Circ Physiol 2008;295(4): H1489–504.

184. Ford J, Milnes J, Wettwer E, et al. Human electrophysiological and pharmacological properties of XEN-D0101: a novel atrial-selective Kv1.5/IKur inhibitor. J Cardiovasc Pharmacol 2013; 61(5):408–15.

185. Wang Q, Ohno S, Ding WG, et al. Gain-of-function KCNH2 mutations in patients with Brugada syndrome. J Cardiovasc Electrophysiol 2014;25(5): 522–30.

Adenosine Triphosphate-Sensitive Potassium Currents in Heart Disease and Cardioprotection

Colin G. Nichols, PhD

KEYWORDS

• SUR2 • Kir6.1 • Kir6.2 • Cantu • Vasodilation • Edema • Arrhythmia

KEY POINTS

- Cardiac KATP is not a single channel, but a family of channels made up of variable complexes of Kir6.1, Kir6.2, SUR1 and SUR2 subunits.
- Although the potential cardiac KATP conductance is large, animal studies reveal tolerance for both loss and gain of function.
- Such studies reveal complex compensation including alterations of Ca^{2+} currents.
- KATP channel mutations have been associated with multiple cardiac pathologies, but causal linkage is generally still not clear. However, the association of gain-of-function mutations in Kir6.1 and SUR2 with Cantu Syndrome is now very strong.
- Cardiovascular complications resulting from altered KATP activity are manifold and still poorly understood, but in future will inform the role of cardiac KATP and potential for therapeutic manipulation.

ADENOSINE TRIPHOSPHATE-SENSITIVE POTASSIUM CHANNEL AND CARDIOVASCULAR DISEASE: THE THEORETIC CASE

Cardiovascular Adenosine Triphosphate-Sensitive Potassium Channel and Cardioprotection

Since their discovery in cardiac myocytes more than 30 years ago, it has been recognized that adenosine triphosphate-sensitive potassium (K_{ATP}) channels provide a very large potential ionic conductance in the surface membranes of all muscle cells. Under normal metabolic conditions, cardiac K_{ATP} channels are predominantly closed, and they do not significantly contribute to cell excitability. However, these channels can open when exposed to a severe metabolic stress such as anoxia, metabolic inhibition, or ischemia. By shortening the action potential, K_{ATP} activation will reduce Ca^{2+} entry and inhibit contractility,[1] thereby reducing energy consumption, potentially protecting the cell. Such a preservation 'strategy' is naturally self-limiting; if too many myocytes stop contracting, the heart will stop pumping and the animal will die, but it has always been a reasonable notion that temporary protection of a small number of cells, or region of the heart,

Citation of Financial Support for the Author: Our own experimental work has been supported by NIH grants HL45742 and HL95010, and a grant from the Children's Discovery Institute at Washington University (to C.G. Nichols [CH-MI-II-2015-488]).
Disclosures: None.
Department of Cell Biology and Physiology, Center for the Investigation of Membrane Excitability Diseases, Washington University School of Medicine, 660 South Euclid Avenue, St Louis, MO 63110, USA
E-mail address: cnichols@wustl.edu

Card Electrophysiol Clin 8 (2016) 323–335
http://dx.doi.org/10.1016/j.ccep.2016.01.005
1877-9182/16/$ – see front matter

against the damage of Ca^{2+} overload during ischemia, is a likely beneficial consequence of K_{ATP} channel activation.

In the vasculature, activation of K_{ATP} channels will hyperpolarize the membrane potential, leading to inhibition of voltage-sensitive Ca^{2+} channels and lowering of intracellular Ca^{2+}, resulting in vasodilation.[2]

Cardiac Adenosine Triphosphate-Sensitive Potassium Channels and Arrhythmia

The opening of cardiac K_{ATP} channels both shortens the action potential and reduces the refractory period, such that channel activation could establish an arrhythmogenic substrate supporting reentry. Hence, inhibition of K_{ATP} could be a way to stop or even prevent arrhythmias. Because K_{ATP} channels tend to open only when cell metabolism is inhibited, any agents that inhibit K_{ATP} activity should specifically target channels only during ischemia, leaving nonischemic myocardium unaffected. In contrast, activation of cardiac K_{ATP} channels has consistently been shown to protect the heart from damage during ischemia, by limiting Ca^{2+} entry.

THE MOLECULAR BASIS OF ADENOSINE TRIPHOSPHATE-SENSITIVE POTASSIUM CHANNELS

K_{ATP} channels are heterooctameric complexes of 4 pore-forming Kir6 channel-forming subunits, each associated with one regulatory SUR subunit. Two Kir6 genes, *KCNJ8* (Kir6.1) and *KCNJ11* (Kir6.2),[3,4] and 2 SUR genes, ABCC8 (SUR1) and ABCC9 (SUR2)[4–6] encode mammalian K_{ATP} subunits, but alternative RNA splicing can give rise to multiple SUR protein variants (eg, SUR2A and SUR2B) that confer distinct physiologic and pharmacologic properties on the channel complex.[7,8] Interestingly, the genes for Kir6.2 and SUR1 are located next to each other on human chromosome 11p15.1,[4] suggesting an as yet unrecognized coregulation at the gene level. In addition, the genes for Kir6.1 and SUR2 are also adjacent to one another on chromosome 12p12.1,[4,6] implicating an evolutionary duplication. In heterologous expression, both Kir6.2 and SUR1 subunits coassemble in a 4:4 stoichiometry[4] to generate the functional K_{ATP} channel.[9–11] Similarly, biochemical studies confirm that the SUR2 protein variants, SUR2A and SUR2B, also coassemble with Kir6 subunits,[3,12–14] presumably in a similar octameric arrangement.

Crystallographic studies of bacterial and eukaryotic Kir channels[15,16] demonstrate a conserved architecture of Kir channels with 2 transmembrane helices (M1, M2) bridged by an extracellular loop that generates the narrow portion of the pore and controls ion selectivity. As with other ABCC proteins, SURs contain two 6-helix transmembrane domains, TMD1 and TMD2 and 2 cytoplasmic nucleotide binding folds, but also contain an additional *N*-terminal TMD0 domain that is critical for trafficking and gating of the channel complex.[17] The details of the physical connection between Kir6 and SUR subunits remains unclear, but electron micrography and intersubunit FRET studies of complete K_{ATP} complexes suggest an intimate packing of 4 SUR and 4 Kir6.x subunits.[18,19]

The key regulatory features of K_{ATP} channels are rapid and reversible closure by cytoplasmic ATP, and activation by nucleotide triphosphates and diphosphates.[20] In the absence of other nucleotides, the free [ATP] that causes half-maximal channel inhibition is in the micromolar range. Because intracellular ATP concentrations are in the low millimolar range and change little under physiologic conditions, [ATP] is probably always sufficient to almost fully inhibit channel activity. The channel activation then arises from the activating effects of Mg-nucleotides, particularly MgADP, on the SUR subunit.[21] Nucleotide regulation is probably the key molecular regulator of K_{ATP} channel activities, although other second messenger systems and regulators[22] may be involved in control of channel activity and channel-dependent pathologies.

CARDIOVASCULAR TISSUE DISTRIBUTION OF ADENOSINE TRIPHOSPHATE-SENSITIVE POTASSIUM CHANNEL SUBUNITS

From studies in heterologous expression systems where SUR and Kir6 subunit expression can be controlled, it is apparent that all possible subunit combinations can and do occur. Posttranslational quality control mechanisms have been described that ensure the appropriate octameric composition of the channel,[23,24] yet there is no evidence that these mechanisms discriminate between subunits. There have been relatively few studies to examine the transcriptional regulation of K_{ATP} subunits and still little is known about what specific factors might control K_{ATP} structure, although members of the forkhead transcription factor family and heat inducible factor-1α have been shown to regulate the expression of some subunits (as well as metabolic enzymes).[25,26]

Kir6.1 and Kir6.2, as well as SUR2 and SUR1, are all expressed in the heart.[3,27–29] There is now good evidence that, in mouse hearts, SUR1 and Kir6.2 are major constituents of the atrial myocyte sarcolemmal K$_{ATP}$, whereas SUR2A and Kir6.2 generate ventricular K$_{ATP}$.[30,31] However, in hearts of larger animals, including humans, both SUR1 and SUR2A subunits probably contribute to sarcolemmal channels in both atrial and ventricular myocytes[32] (**Fig. 1**). The situation may be more complex in critical subregions of the heart, including nodal and conduction cells. K$_{ATP}$ channel currents have been detected throughout the pacemaking and conduction systems.[33–35] Low K$_{ATP}$ single channel conductances in rabbit sinoatrial node cells and mouse conduction cells[33] suggests a role for Kir6.1 in generating the channel pore in these tissues, yet sarcolemmal K$_{ATP}$ is abolished in Kir6.2$^{-/-}$ sinoatrial node cells,[36] indicating a necessary requirement for Kir6.2. The identity of the SUR component of K$_{ATP}$ in conducting and pacemaker tissues is unknown, although K$_{ATP}$ channels in nodal cells do respond to the relatively SUR2-specific openers cromakalim and pinacidil, suggesting a major role for SUR2.[33–35]

K$_{ATP}$ channel density is relatively low in vascular smooth muscle (VSM) compared with cardiac myocytes[37,38] and the biophysical and pharmacologic properties are quite variable, reflecting variable expression of K$_{ATP}$ subtypes between vascular beds.[39–46] There is considerable variation in reported single channel conductances,[42,43,47–51] although low-conductance channels (unitary conductances from 20 to 50 pS) may represent the predominant K$_{ATP}$ channel subtype, with a more limited distribution of medium- and high conductance K$_{ATP}$ channels (50–70 pS and >200 pS, respectively).[52] Importantly, and unlike classic K$_{ATP}$ channels of the heart[3,53] or pancreas,[4,54] the predominant VSM K$_{ATP}$ conductances are inactive in isolated membrane patches, and require nucleotide diphosphates (adenosine

diphosphate, uridine 5'-diphosphate, guanosine 5'-diphosphate) in the presence of Mg^{2+} to open, leading to their functional designation as 'nucleotide-dependent' K$^+$ channels, or K$_{NDP}$ channels.[44,45,50] Heterologously expressed Kir6.1/SUR2B channels recapitulate many of these biophysical properties of native VSM K$_{ATP}$/K$_{NDP}$.[4,12,55–58] Thus, the Kir6.1/SUR2B channel may represent the predominant VSM K$_{ATP}$, but other subtypes are also likely to be expressed in specific vascular beds, separately or in combination with Kir6.1/SUR2B subunits[50] (see **Fig. 1**).

Finally, K$_{ATP}$ channels are also prominent in lymphatic muscle. Although the classical understanding was that fluid flow in the lymphatic system was passive, it is now clear that lymphatic vessels are lined by smooth muscle. Contractility of these vessels is clearly sensitive to K$_{ATP}$ activation,[59] with a pharmacologic profile that is consistent with the major subunits expressed in lymphatic muscle being Kir6.1 and SUR2.[60]

CARDIOVASCULAR DISEASE AND ADENOSINE TRIPHOSPHATE-SENSITIVE POTASSIUM CHANNEL MUTATIONS
Predictions from Genetically Modified Animals

Murine knockout models of each of the 4 K$_{ATP}$ channel genes have been generated and analyzed extensively. Knockout of Kir6.2 or SUR1 results in a loss of glucose-dependent insulin secretion, modeling features of hyperinsulinism in humans.[61,62] Conversely, knockout of Kir6.1 or SUR2 leads to a vascular hypercontractility phenotype.[29,63] The key features are baseline hypertension, coronary artery vasospasm and sudden cardiac death. SUR2$^{-/-}$ mice treated with

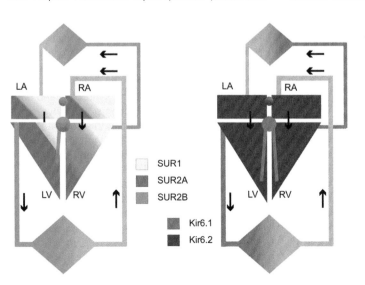

Fig. 1. Cardiovascular adenosine triphosphate-sensitive potassium (K$_{ATP}$) channel distribution. Schematic representation of K$_{ATP}$ channel subunit distribution in the cardiovascular system. SUR2A and to a lesser extent SUR1 are prominent in ventricular chambers (left ventricle [LV], right ventricle [RV]), whereas SUR1 is more prominent in atrial chambers (left atrium [LA], right atrium [RA]), and SUR2B is prominent throughout the vasculature. Arrows indicate flow direction in systemic and pulmonary circulation. Kir6.2 is found throughout the myocardium, with Kir6.1 more prominent in conducting tissue and in the vasculature.

the Ca^{2+} channel blocker nifedipine exhibit a reduction in coronary artery vasospasm, implicating abnormally elevated $[Ca^{2+}]_i$ owing to loss of hyperpolarizing K_{ATP} current as causal in the hypercontractility.[63] Collectively, these K_{ATP}-null mice recapitulate clinical features of the human disorder of Prinzmetal (or variant) angina, but several studies have failed to demonstrate any association of human coronary vasospasm or hypertension with loss-of-function (LOF) mutations in Kir6.1 or SUR2,[64,65] even though linkage analysis indicates that there are associated genes within the same locus as Kir6.1 and SUR2.[66]

We have explored extensively the potential for K_{ATP} gain-of-function (GOF) action in the heart and vasculature by transgenic introduction of mutant Kir6.1 and Kir6.2 channels that are insensitive to closure by ATP.[67–69] Under alpha myosin heavy chain control, GOF subunits expressed in the heart generate channels that still remain closed under all but extreme circumstances, and cause little overt malfunction, with no decrease in cardiac action potential duration or decrease in contractility.[67,69] Curiously, we find that in ventricular myocytes from these animals there is actually dramatically enhanced Ca^{2+} current,[70] which may be a compensatory response to an initial or local action potential shortening. These studies also reveal that overexpressing the SUR1 isoform in the myocardium has an effect to prolong the PR interval,[71] and that when Kir6.2 GOF is expressed together with SUR1, second- and third-degree atrioventricular block results, progressing to ventricular and supraventricular arrhythmias and death.[71,72]

Although the phenotype of animals expressing K_{ATP} GOF in the heart is complex, expression of Kir6.1 GOF mutants in smooth muscle (under smooth muscle heavy chain promoter control) leads to enhanced K_{ATP} activity in VSM, and a clear reduction of systolic and diastolic blood pressures,[68] paralleling the effects of potassium channel openers in human hypertensive patients.

Adenosine Triphosphate-Sensitive Potassium Channel–Associated Human Disease

Thus, animal studies have provided a clear prediction of hypertensive or hypotensive consequences for K_{ATP} LOF or GOF, respectively, in smooth muscle, but rather complex and contradictory predictions regarding K_{ATP} mutations in the heart. This may help to explain why, until recently, there has been little evidence for human cardiovascular disease resulting from K_{ATP} gene mutations (**Table 1**). GOF and loss-of function mutations in *KCNJ11* (Kir6.2) and *ABCC8* (SUR1), which encode the predominant K_{ATP} channel subunits in pancreatic β-cells and in neurons,[73] are now well-understood to underlie neonatal diabetes and congenital hyperinsulinism, respectively.[74] However, and despite evidence for expression of these subunits in cardiac myocytes, there is no published evidence for any cardiovascular problems in these patients.

Sequence analysis of DNA from necropsy tissue on sudden infant death syndrome cases identified coding mutations in *KCNJ8* (Kir6.1), an in-frame deletion (E332del), and a missense mutation (V346I), both in the distal C-terminus of Kir6.1. Reduced channel activity was reported from expressed mutant channels, leading the authors to conclude that LOF mutations in Kir6.1 may be one cause of sudden infant death syndrome,[75] through as yet unexplained mechanisms. There have also been 2 reports of SUR2 LOF mutations leading to cardiac disease.[76,77] In each case, the mutations were identified in the C-terminal exons and would therefore lead to a disruption of the second nucleotide binding fold of SUR2A, and hence reduction of nucleotide stimulation of channel activity, without affecting SUR2B. In the first report, the single patient with the mutation presented with long-standing atrial fibrillation originating in the vein of Marshall, with normal cardiac morphology and contractile features.[77] In the second report, 2 individuals with 2 distinct mutations presented with heart failure owing to idiopathic dilated cardiomyopathy.[76] There have been no subsequent reports of similar genetic defects, and further evidence for causal association of Kir6.1 or SUR2 LOF mutations with disease is lacking.

Several studies reported a single *KCNJ8* mutation (encoding S422L in Kir6.1) protein to be associated with the 'J-wave' phenomenon, characterized by abnormalities in the J-point of the electrocardiograph and early repolarization syndrome. First reported by Haissaguerre and colleagues,[78] subsequent studies have reported association of this variant with atrial fibrillation,[79] as well as additional Brugada syndrome and early repolarization syndrome patients.[80,81] However, a recent study has reported that this variant is relatively common in individuals of Ashkenazi Jewish origin and it remains unclear whether the reported associations are causal.[82]

More recently, it has become clear that mutations in both *ABCC9* (encoding SUR1) and *KCNJ8* (Kir6.1) are associated with Cantu syndrome[83] (MIM 239850), or hypertrichosis–osteochondrodysplasia–cardiomegaly syndrome, a distinctive multiorgan disease.[84–87] In many cases, the mutations are de novo, but autosomal-

Table 1
Reported association of disease with adenosine triphosphate-sensitive potassium channel mutations

Gene	Clinical Condition	Features	No. of Reported Affected Individuals	Refs
KCNJ8 (Kir6.1)	J-wave syndrome	S422L mutation. Reportedly GOF. Abnormalities in the J-point of the electrocardiogram, and including Brugada syndrome and early repolarization syndrome, including VF and AF.	9	[78–80]
	SIDS	In-frame deletion (E332del) and LOF mutation (V346I), through as yet unexplained mechanisms.	2	[75]
	Cantu syndrome	GOF mutations associated with complex multiorgan disease (see **Box 1**).	2	[86,87]
KCNJ11 (Kir6.2)	Neonatal diabetes	Multiple GOF mutations cause inhibition of insulin secretion. No cardiovascular phenotype.	>100	[124]
	Congenital hyperinsulinism	LOF mutations cause hypersecretion of insulin. No cardiovascular phenotype.	>10	[74,124]
ABCC8 (SUR1)	Neonatal diabetes	Multiple GOF mutations cause inhibition of insulin secretion. No cardiovascular phenotype	>100	[124]
	Congenital hyperinsulinism	Multiple LOF mutations cause hypersecretion of insulin. No cardiovascular phenotype.	>100	[74,124]
ABCC9 (SUR2)	AF	Isolated case of LOF mutation associated with AF originating in the vein of Marshal.	1	[77]
	Idiopathic dilated cardiomyopathy	Two cases with distinct LOF mutations associated with heart failure owing to idiopathic dilated cardiomyopathy.	2	[76]
	Cantu syndrome	GOF mutations associated with complex multiorgan disease (see **Box 1**).	>25	[84,85]

Abbreviations: AF, atrial fibrillation; GOF, gain-of-function; LOF, loss-of-function; SIDS, sudden infant death syndrome; VF, ventricular fibrillation.
   Data from Refs.[74–80,84–87,124]

dominant inheritance also occurs.[88] The conclusion that these mutations all lead to GOF K$_{ATP}$ channel function has been confirmed in several studies,[84,86,89] which demonstrate decreased sensitivity to ATP inhibition or enhanced activation by MgADP in each case.

Cantu Syndrome: Multiple Tissue Symptoms

Perhaps most striking about this recent discovery is that so many of the features of Cantu syndrome are not trivially predictable, and in the heart, the resultant phenotypes are even counter to any naïve predictions. Since first being recognized as a unique syndrome in 1982,[83] a constellation of features has been described in Cantu syndrome patients[88,90–97] (**Box 1**). Multiple cardiovascular complications include cardiac enlargement, concentric hypertrophy of the ventricles, and pericardial effusion. Some patients have required

pericardiocentesis and even pericardial stripping to prevent reaccumulation of the pericardial effusion. Multiple vascular consequences include pulmonary hypertension secondary to partial pulmonary venous obstruction has been reported, associated with severe mitral valve regurgitation that spontaneously resolved.[92] A significant number of patients have had patent ductus arteriosus requiring surgical closure, as well as bicuspid aortic valves with and without stenosis. Lymphedema involving the lower extremities may develop over time, and in 1 patient, lymphangiogram demonstrated dilated lymphatic vessels in the legs with delayed lymphatic drainage.[91] Interestingly, diazoxide, Minoxidil, and other related K$_{ATP}$ channel openers that are used to treat severe refractory hypertension can also result in similar features as unexplained side effects, including hypertrichosis, pericardial effusion, edema, and even coarsening of the facial features.[98,99]

Box 1
Major clinical features of Cantu syndrome

Neonatal features
Neonatal macrosomia
Maternal polyhydramnios
Macrocephaly

Craniofacial dysmorphology
Coarse facial appearance (can be confused with a storage disorder)
Epicanthal folds
Broad nasal bridge
Anteverted nostrils
Long philtrum
Wide mouth with full lips
Macroglossia
High or narrow palate
Gingival hyperplasia

Hair
Congenital generalized hirsutism
Thick scalp hair
Thick and/or curly eyelashes
Excessive hair growth on forehead, face, back and limbs

Cardiovascular
Cardiomegaly
Concentric hypertrophy of the ventricles
Normal ventricular contractility
Pericardial effusion
Pulmonary hypertension
Partial pulmonary venous obstruction
Mitral valve regurgitation
Congenital anomalies
    Patent ductus arteriosus
    Bicuspid and/or stenotic aortic valve

Skeletal abnormalities
Thickened calvarium
Narrow shoulders and thorax
Pectus carinatum
Broad ribs
Platyspondyly and ovoid vertebral bodies
Hypoplastic ischium and pubic bones
Erlenmeyer-flask-like long bones with metaphyseal flaring
Delayed bone age

Skin and joints
Loose and/or wrinkled skin, especially in neonates

Deep palmar and plantar creases

Persistent fingertip pads

Hyperextensibility of joints

Lymphatic system

Lymphedema, onset usually in adolescence or adulthood

Gastrointestinal

Pyloric stenosis

Increased risk for upper gastrointestinal bleeding

Teratogenic effects of minoxidil, including marked hypertrichosis, dysmorphic facial features, low blood pressure, and transposition of the great vessels and pulmonary bicuspid valvular stenosis, have been reported in the offspring of minoxidil-treated mothers.[100,101] These observations first led to the suggestion that Cantu syndrome might result from GOF mutations in K^+ channel activity.[88]

Normally, an abrupt increase in oxygen tension and falling prostaglandin E2 and prostacyclin levels lead to inhibition of voltage-gated K channels and contraction of smooth muscle fibers in the ductus arteriosus, resulting in wall thickening and lumen obliteration after birth. Persistence of the patent ductus arteriosus in Cantu syndrome patients may thus be explained readily as a consequence of maintained vessel dilation owing to K_{ATP} overactivity. More generally, mechanisms of persistent patent ductus arteriosus are not clear,[102] but the enhancement of a K current in smooth muscle presents an obvious potential explanation in patients with Cantu syndrome. Altered vascular tone may also underlie pericardial effusion, but the reason for cardiomegaly is not obvious. Cardiomegaly reported in most cases of Cantu syndrome is owing to increased myocardial mass (hypertrophy) with larger cardiac chambers but with normal systolic function; this does not fit the diagnostic criteria of dilated or hypertrophic cardiomyopathy,[103] and may be a secondary response to reduced vascular tone.[104] Similarly, the reason for osteochondrodysplasia and facial dysmorphology is not obvious, and the mechanism by which minoxidil causes hair growth has remained controversial.[105] Although Cantu syndrome patients show no evidence of problems with orthostatic blood pressure, systematic analysis of patient blood pressures does show that these are physiologically below the norm for age (G.K. Singh, M.D. Levin, D.K. Grange, C.G. Nichols, unpublished data, 2014). Through opening vascular K channels and dilation of blood vessels, the supply of oxygen, blood and nutrients to the hair follicle may be increased, causing follicles in the telogen phase to shed and be replaced by new thicker hairs in a new anagen phase. However, there is also evidence that SUR2 isoforms are present in follicular dermal papillae[106] and, although the new realization definitively ties the hair growth to an action on K_{ATP} channels, it does not immediately prove where the action is.

ADENOSINE TRIPHOSPHATE-SENSITIVE POTASSIUM CHANNEL MANIPULATION IN HEART DISEASE

Perhaps no other channel in the heart carries more potential and promise than do K_{ATP} channels for breaking the link between myocardial ischemia and cardiac arrhythmia. Since the first report detailing the presence of K_{ATP} in cardiac myocytes was published,[107] the possibility that this channel (1) determines the electrical behavior of the heart during ischemia and (2) might protect the heart has been well recognized. Nevertheless, efforts to exploit cardiac K_{ATP} channels to ameliorate arrhythmia and moderate damage of the myocardium during ischemia have yet to mature.

As genetic variation in humans, and manipulation in animals, has made clear, cardiac sarcolemmal K_{ATP} channels are normally predominantly closed in physiologic conditions, and application of channel-blocking sulfonylureas generally has little or no effect on the ventricular action potential.[108] Because K_{ATP} channels in different regions of the heart have different composition, it is likely that they will be operative under different conditions in vivo. For example, shortening of the Purkinje action potential may be greater than that of the ventricular action potential at the same ATP/adenosine diphosphate ratio, given that SUR2B and Kir6.1 may be prominent in these cells.[109] K_{ATP} channels composed of SUR1 and Kir6.2, as in the mouse atrium,[31] will have still different activating conditions.

When metabolism is inhibited, the action potential can shorten markedly and contraction can be inhibited as a result of K_{ATP} activation.[1,110,111] K_{ATP} activation during ischemia is likely to be cardioprotective, because reduction of action potential duration and contraction may preserve ATP stores that would otherwise be consumed during the contractile cycle. In support of this idea, treatment with the K_{ATP} opener pinacidil during ischemia increases cellular ATP and energy stored as creatine phosphate.[112] Conversely, AP shortening is absent in Kir6.2$^{-/-}$ hearts, and the time to contractile failure is prolonged but the time to onset of rigor contracture is decreased.[113] Diastolic Ca^{2+} overload, myocardial damage, and increased mortality are also observed in isoproterenol-challenged Kir6.2$^{-/-}$ myocytes.[114] In addition to highlighting the acute protective effect of K_{ATP} activation, Kir6.2$^{-/-}$ animals show increased mortality and exaggerated hypertrophy in response to pressure overload,[115,116] and to mineralocorticoid/salt challenge.[117] Together, these studies suggest that decreased K_{ATP}, by stopping the protective 'unloading' that K_{ATP} activation leads to, should tend to cause Ca overload and perhaps hasten the transition to heart failure under stressed conditions. However, other studies seem to contradict a cardioprotective role. Both SUR2- (SUR2$^{-/-}$) and SUR1-knockout (SUR1$^{-/-}$) mice were found to be more tolerant of global ischemia–reperfusion than control mice, with reduced infarct sizes.[118,119] Because the SUR2$^{-/-}$ mice have a marked reduction of ventricular sarcolemmal K_{ATP} channels, the enhanced cardioprotection is opposite the expected phenotype (ie, impaired protection). Cardioprotection in SUR2$^{-/-}$ mice might conceivably be owing to concomitant loss of the SUR2B component of vascular K_{ATP} channels, but similar cardioprotection in SUR1$^{-/-}$ mice[119] could not be explained by such a mechanism.

Potential for Therapeutic Modulation of Cardiovascular Adenosine Triphosphate-Sensitive Potassium Channel Activity

There is tremendous potential for modulation of K_{ATP} channel activity in general and more important, perhaps, in a tissue-specific manner, because there is already a rich pharmacology, not only of channel inhibitors but also potassium channel openers. Potassium channel openers have been used in 2 major clinical settings: (1) to block insulin secretion in conditions of hyperinsulinema and (2) as antihypertensives.

Sulfonylureas have seen widespread use as glucose-lowering agents in type 2 diabetes. K_{ATP} channel inhibitory drugs have not reached clinical acceptance in the cardiovascular arena, the

expectation being that blockade of cardiac K_{ATP} channels may be detrimental in conditions of myocardial ischemia, during which these channels can open and are presumed to be protective, as discussed. This debate is still not resolved.[120,121] The association of Cantu syndrome with K_{ATP} GOF holds the promise that sulfonylureas or other blockers should be an effective therapy for this disease. It is generally accepted that most sulfonylureas are physiologically more potent inhibitors of SUR1-dependent K_{ATP} than SUR2A-dependent channels, although there has also been little careful comparison of effect on SUR1- versus SUR2B-dependent channels. There has been a long-standing dogma that the drug HMR1098 is a cardiac specific K_{ATP} blocker, although direct head-to-head comparison confirms that it is also a more effective blocker of SUR1-dependent than SUR2A-dependent K_{ATP} channels.[30,31,122] Relative efficacies of HMR1098 versus other sulfonylureas under specific physiologic conditions may be important to understand, because it is conceivable that specific K_{ATP} inhibitors could successfully counteract the symptoms of Cantu syndrome, without significantly affecting blood glucose control, a key issue if K_{ATP} channel inhibition is to be a viable treatment for the disease.

Further Implications and Future Prospects

It is now recognized that the subunit makeup of the family of K_{ATP} channels is more complex and labile than originally thought.[14,123] The growing association of Kir6.1 and SUR2 variants with specific cardiovascular electrical and contractile derangements and the clear association with Cantu syndrome firmly establish the importance of appropriate activity in normal function of the heart and vasculature. Further studies of such patients will reveal new mutations in K_{ATP} subunits and perhaps in proteins that regulate K_{ATP} synthesis, trafficking, or location, all of which may ultimately benefit therapeutically from the unique pharmacology of K_{ATP} channels.

REFERENCES

1. Lederer WJ, Nichols CG, Smith GL. The mechanism of early contractile failure of isolated rat ventricular myocytes subjected to complete metabolic inhibition. J Physiol 1989;413:329–49.
2. Nelson MT, Quayle JM. Physiological roles and properties of potassium channels in arterial smooth muscle. Am J Physiol 1995;268:C799–822.
3. Inagaki N, Gonoi T, Clement JP, et al. A family of sulfonylurea receptors determines the pharmacological properties of ATP-sensitive K+ channels. Neuron 1996;16:1011–7.

4. Inagaki N, Gonoi T, Clement JP, et al. Reconstitution of IK$_{ATP}$: an inward rectifier subunit plus the sulfonylurea receptor. Science 1995;270:1166–70 [see comments].

5. Aguilar-Bryan L, Nichols CG, Wechsler SW, et al. Cloning of the beta cell high-affinity sulfonylurea receptor: a regulator of insulin secretion. Science 1995;268:423–6.

6. Chutkow WA, Simon MC, Le Beau MM, et al. Cloning, tissue expression, and chromosomal localization of SUR2, the putative drug-binding subunit of cardiac, skeletal muscle, and vascular KATP channels. Diabetes 1996;45:1439–45.

7. Shi NQ, Ye B, Makielski JC. Function and distribution of the SUR isoforms and splice variants. J Mol Cell Cardiol 2005;39:51–60.

8. Chutkow WA, Makielski JC, Nelson DJ, et al. Alternative splicing of sur2 Exon 17 regulates nucleotide sensitivity of the ATP-sensitive potassium channel. J Biol Chem 1999;274:13656–65.

9. Shyng S, Nichols CG. Octameric stoichiometry of the K$_{ATP}$ channel complex. J Gen Physiol 1997; 110:655–64.

10. Clement JP, Kunjilwar K, Gonzalez G, et al. Association and stoichiometry of K(ATP) channel subunits. Neuron 1997;18:827–38.

11. Inagaki N, Gonoi T, Seino S. Subunit stoichiometry of the pancreatic beta-cell ATP-sensitive K+ channel. FEBS Lett 1997;409:232–6.

12. Yamada M, Isomoto S, Matsumoto S, et al. Sulphonylurea receptor 2B and Kir6.1 form a sulphonylurea-sensitive but ATP-insensitive K+ channel. J Physiol 1997;499:715–20.

13. Okuyama Y, Yamada M, Kondo C, et al. The effects of nucleotides and potassium channel openers on the SUR2A/Kir6.2 complex K+ channel expressed in a mammalian cell line, HEK293T cells. Pflugers Arch 1998;435:595–603.

14. Babenko AP, Gonzalez G, Aguilar-Bryan L, et al. Reconstituted human cardiac K$_{ATP}$ channels: functional identity with the native channels from the sarcolemma of human ventricular cells. Circ Res 1998;83:1132–43.

15. Kuo A, Gulbis JM, Antcliff JF, et al. Crystal structure of the potassium channel KirBac1.1 in the closed state. Science 2003;300:1922–6.

16. Tao X, Avalos JL, Chen J, et al. Crystal structure of the eukaryotic strong inward-rectifier K+ channel Kir2.2 at 3.1 A resolution. Science 2009;326: 1668–74.

17. Bryan J, Vila-Carriles WH, Zhao G, et al. Toward linking structure with function in ATP-sensitive K+ channels. Diabetes 2004;53(Suppl 3):S104–12.

18. Mikhailov MV, Campbell JD, de Wet H, et al. 3-D structural and functional characterization of the purified K$_{ATP}$ channel complex Kir6.2-SUR1. EMBO J 2005;24:4166–75.

19. Wang S, Makhina EN, Masia R, et al. Domain organization of the ATP-sensitive potassium channel complex examined by FRET. J Biol Chem 2013; 288(6):4378–88.

20. Nichols CG. K$_{ATP}$ channels as molecular sensors of cellular metabolism. Nature 2006;440:470–6.

21. Nichols CG, Shyng SL, Nestorowicz A, et al. Adenosine diphosphate as an intracellular regulator of insulin secretion. Science 1996;272:1785–7.

22. Beguin P, Nagashima K, Nishimura M, et al. PKA-mediated phosphorylation of the human K(ATP) channel: separate roles of Kir6.2 and SUR1 subunit phosphorylation. EMBO J 1999; 18:4722–32.

23. Zerangue N, Schwappach B, Jan YN, et al. A new ER trafficking signal regulates the subunit stoichiometry of plasma membrane K(ATP) channels. Neuron 1999;22:537–48.

24. Heusser K, Yuan H, Neagoe I, et al. Scavenging of 14-3-3 proteins reveals their involvement in the cell-surface transport of ATP-sensitive K+ channels. J Cell Sci 2006;119:4353–63.

25. Isidoro Tavares N, Philip-Couderc P, Papageorgiou I, et al. Expression and function of ATP-dependent potassium channels in late post-infarction remodeling. J Mol Cell Cardiol 2007;42:1016–25.

26. Raeis-Dauve V, Philip-Couderc P, Faggian G, et al. Increased expression of adenosine triphosphate-sensitive K+ channels in mitral dysfunction: mechanically stimulated transcription and hypoxia-induced protein stability? J Am Coll Cardiol 2011;59:390–6.

27. Morrissey A, Parachuru L, Leung M, et al. Expression of ATP-sensitive K+ channel subunits during perinatal maturation in the mouse heart. Pediatr Res 2005;58:185–92.

28. Morrissey A, Rosner E, Lanning J, et al. Immunolocalization of K$_{ATP}$ channel subunits in mouse and rat cardiac myocytes and the coronary vasculature. BMC Physiol 2005;5:1.

29. Miki T, Suzuki M, Shibasaki T, et al. Mouse model of Prinzmetal angina by disruption of the inward rectifier Kir6.1. Nat Med 2002;8:466–72.

30. Glukhov AV, Flagg TP, Fedorov VV, et al. Differential K(ATP) channel pharmacology in intact mouse heart. J Mol Cell Cardiol 2009;48:152–60.

31. Flagg TP, Kurata HT, Masia R, et al. Differential structure of atrial and ventricular K$_{ATP}$: atrial KATP channels require SUR1. Circ Res 2008; 103:1458–65.

32. Fedorov VV, Glukhov AV, Ambrosi CM, et al. Effects of K$_{ATP}$ channel openers diazoxide and pinacidil in coronary-perfused atria and ventricles from failing and non-failing human hearts. J Mol Cell Cardiol 2011;51:215–25.

33. Han X, Light PE, Giles WR, et al. Identification and properties of an ATP-sensitive K+ current in rabbit

sino-atrial node pacemaker cells. J Physiol 1996; 490:337–50.

34. Kakei M, Noma A. Adenosine-5'-triphosphate-sensitive single potassium channel in the atrioventricular node cell of the rabbit heart. J Physiol 1984; 352:265–84.

35. Light PE, Cordeiro JM, French RJ. Identification and properties of ATP-sensitive potassium channels in myocytes from rabbit Purkinje fibres. Cardiovasc Res 1999;44:356–69.

36. Fukuzaki K, Sato T, Miki T, et al. Role of sarcolemmal ATP-sensitive K+ channels in the regulation of sinoatrial node automaticity: an evaluation using Kir6.2-deficient mice. J Physiol 2008;586: 2767–78.

37. Dart C, Standen NB. Adenosine-activated potassium current in smooth muscle cells isolated from the pig coronary artery. J Physiol 1993; 471:767–86.

38. Nichols CG, Lederer WJ. The regulation of ATP-sensitive K+ channel activity in intact and permeabilized rat ventricular myocytes. J Physiol 1990; 423:91–110.

39. Blanco-Rivero J, Gamallo C, Aras-Lopez R, et al. Decreased expression of aortic KIR6.1 and SUR2B in hypertension does not correlate with changes in the functional role of K(ATP) channels. Eur J Pharmacol 2008;587:204–8.

40. Cui Y, Tran S, Tinker A, et al. The molecular composition of K(ATP) channels in human pulmonary artery smooth muscle cells and their modulation by growth. Am J Respir Cell Mol Biol 2002; 26:135–43.

41. Standen NB, Quayle JM, Davies NW, et al. Hyperpolarizing vasodilators activate ATP-sensitive K+ channels in arterial smooth muscle. Science 1989;245:177–80.

42. Miyoshi Y, Nakaya Y, Wakatsuki T, et al. Endothelin blocks ATP-sensitive K+ channels and depolarizes smooth muscle cells of porcine coronary artery. Circ Res 1992;70:612–6.

43. Ottolia M, Toro L. Reconstitution in lipid bilayers of an ATP-sensitive K+ channel from pig coronary smooth muscle. J Membr Biol 1996;153: 203–9.

44. Beech DJ, Zhang H, Nakao K, et al. K channel activation by nucleotide diphosphates and its inhibition by glibenclamide in vascular smooth muscle cells. Br J Pharmacol 1993;110:573–82.

45. Kajioka S, Kitamura K, Kuriyama H. Guanosine diphosphate activates an adenosine 5'-triphosphate-sensitive K+ channel in the rabbit portal vein. J Physiol 1991;444:397–418.

46. Kamouchi M, Kitamura K. Regulation of ATP-sensitive K+ channels by ATP and nucleotide diphosphate in rabbit portal vein. Am J Physiol 1994;266:H1687–98.

47. Miyoshi Y, Nakaya Y. Angiotensin II blocks ATP-sensitive K+ channels in porcine coronary artery smooth muscle cells. Biochem Biophys Res Commun 1991;181:700–6.

48. Wakatsuki T, Nakaya Y, Inoue I. Vasopressin modulates K(+)-channel activities of cultured smooth muscle cells from porcine coronary artery. Am J Physiol 1992;263:H491–6.

49. Furspan PB, Webb RC. Decreased ATP sensitivity of a K+ channel and enhanced vascular smooth muscle relaxation in genetically hypertensive rats. J Hypertens 1993;11:1067–72.

50. Zhang HL, Bolton TB. Two types of ATP-sensitive potassium channels in rat portal vein smooth muscle cells. Br J Pharmacol 1996;118:105–14.

51. Cole WC, Malcolm T, Walsh MP, et al. Inhibition by protein kinase C of the K(NDP) subtype of vascular smooth muscle ATP-sensitive potassium channel. Circ Res 2000;87:112–7.

52. Cole WC, Clement-Chomienne O. ATP-sensitive K+ channels of vascular smooth muscle cells. J Cardiovasc Electrophysiol 2003;14:94–103.

53. Aguilar-Bryan L, Nichols CG, Rajan AS, et al. Co-expression of sulfonylurea receptors and K_{ATP} channels in hamster insulinoma tumor (HIT) cells. Evidence for direct association of the receptor with the channel. J Biol Chem 1992;267:14934–40.

54. Ashcroft FM, Harrison DE, Ashcroft SJ. Glucose induces closure of single potassium channels in isolated rat pancreatic beta-cells. Nature 1984;312: 446–8.

55. Farzaneh T, Tinker A. Differences in the mechanism of metabolic regulation of ATP-sensitive K+ channels containing Kir6.1 and Kir6.2 subunits. Cardiovasc Res 2008;79:621–31.

56. Isomoto S, Kondo C, Yamada M, et al. A novel sulfonylurea receptor forms with BIR (Kir6.2) a smooth muscle type ATP-sensitive K+ channel. J Biol Chem 1996;271:24321–4.

57. Satoh E, Yamada M, Kondo C, et al. Intracellular nucleotide-mediated gating of SUR/Kir6.0 complex potassium channels expressed in a mammalian cell line and its modification by pinacidil. J Physiol 1998;511:663–74.

58. Babenko AP, Bryan J. A conserved inhibitory and differential stimulatory action of nucleotides on K(IR)6.0/SUR complexes is essential for excitation-metabolism coupling by K(ATP) channels. J Biol Chem 2001;276:49083–92.

59. von der Weid PY, Lee S, Imtiaz MS, et al. Electrophysiological properties of rat mesenteric lymphatic vessels and their regulation by stretch. Lymphat Res Biol 2014;12:66–75.

60. Telinius N, Kim S, Pilegaard H, et al. The contribution of K(+) channels to human thoracic duct contractility. Am J Physiol Heart Circ Physiol 2014;307:H33–43.

61. Seino S, Iwanaga T, Nagashima K, et al. Diverse roles of K(ATP) channels learned from Kir6.2 genetically engineered mice. Diabetes 2000;49:311–8.

62. Remedi MS, Nichols CG. Hyperinsulinism and diabetes: genetic dissection of beta cell metabolism-excitation coupling in mice. Cell Metab 2009;10: 442–53.

63. Chutkow WA, Pu J, Wheeler MT, et al. Episodic coronary artery vasospasm and hypertension develop in the absence of Sur2 K(ATP) channels. J Clin Invest 2002;110:203–8 [see comment].

64. Ellis JA, Lamantia A, Chavez R, et al. Genes controlling postural changes in blood pressure: comprehensive association analysis of ATP-sensitive potassium channel genes KCNJ8 and ABCC9. Physiol Genomics 2009;40:184–8.

65. Duan R, Cui W, Wang H. Mutational analysis of the Kir6.1 gene in Chinese hypertensive patients treated with the novel ATP-sensitive potassium channel opener iptakalim. Exp Ther Med 2011;2: 757–60.

66. Harrap SB, Cui JS, Wong ZY, et al. Familial and genomic analyses of postural changes in systolic and diastolic blood pressure. Hypertension 2004; 43:586–91.

67. Koster JC, Knopp A, Flagg TP, et al. Tolerance for ATP-insensitive K(ATP) channels in transgenic mice. Circ Res 2001;89:1022–9.

68. Li A, Knutsen RH, Zhang H, et al. Hypotension due to Kir6.1 gain-of-function in vascular smooth muscle. J Am Heart Assoc 2013;2:e000365.

69. Levin MD, Zhang H, Uchida K, et al. Electrophysiologic consequences of K$_{ATP}$ gain of function in the heart: conduction abnormalities in Cantu syndrome. Heart Rhythm 2015;12:2316–24.

70. Flagg TP, Charpentier F, Manning-Fox J, et al. Remodeling of excitation-contraction coupling in transgenic mice expressing ATP-insensitive sarcolemmal K$_{ATP}$ channels. Am J Physiol Heart Circ Physiol 2004;286:H1361–9.

71. Flagg TP, Patton B, Masia R, et al. Arrhythmia susceptibility and premature death in transgenic mice overexpressing both SUR1 and Kir6.2[DeltaN30,K185Q] in the heart. Am J Physiol Heart Circ Physiol 2007;293:H836–45.

72. Toib A, Zhang HX, Broekelmann TJ, et al. Cardiac specific ATP-sensitive K(+) channel (K(ATP)) overexpression results in embryonic lethality. J Mol Cell Cardiol 2012;53:437–45.

73. Miki T, Seino S. Roles of K$_{ATP}$ channels as metabolic sensors in acute metabolic changes. J Mol Cell Cardiol 2005;38:917–25.

74. Nichols CG, Koster JC, Remedi MS. beta-cell hyperexcitability: from hyperinsulinism to diabetes. Diabetes Obes Metab 2007;9(Suppl 2):81–8.

75. Tester DJ, Tan BH, Medeiros-Domingo A, et al. Loss-of-function mutations in the KCNJ8-encoded Kir6.1 K(ATP) channel and sudden infant death syndrome. Circ Cardiovasc Genet 2011;4:510–5.

76. Bienengraeber M, Olson TM, Selivanov VA, et al. ABCC9 mutations identified in human dilated cardiomyopathy disrupt catalytic K$_{ATP}$ channel gating. Nat Genet 2004;36:382–7.

77. Olson TM, Alekseev AE, Moreau C, et al. K$_{ATP}$ channel mutation confers risk for vein of Marshall adrenergic atrial fibrillation. Nat Clin Pract Cardiovasc Med 2007;4:110–6.

78. Haissaguerre M, Chatel S, Sacher F, et al. Ventricular fibrillation with prominent early repolarization associated with a rare variant of KCNJ8/ K$_{ATP}$ channel. J Cardiovasc Electrophysiol 2009;20:93–8.

79. Delaney JT, Muhammad R, Blair MA, et al. A KCNJ8 mutation associated with early repolarization and atrial fibrillation. Europace 2012;14:1428–32.

80. Medeiros-Domingo A, Tan BH, Crotti L, et al. Gain-of-function mutation S422L in the KCNJ8-encoded cardiac K(ATP) channel Kir6.1 as a pathogenic substrate for J-wave syndromes. Heart Rhythm 2010;7:1466–71.

81. Barajas-Martinez H, Hu D, Ferrer T, et al. Molecular genetic and functional association of Brugada and early repolarization syndromes with S422L missense mutation in KCNJ8. Heart Rhythm 2011;9:548–55.

82. Veeramah KR, Karafet TM, Wolf D, et al. The KCNJ8-S422L variant previously associated with J-wave syndromes is found at an increased frequency in Ashkenazi Jews. Eur J Hum Genet 2014;22(1):94–8.

83. Cantu JM, Garcia-Cruz D, Sanchez-Corona J, et al. A distinct osteochondrodysplasia with hypertrichosis- Individualization of a probable autosomal recessive entity. Hum Genet 1982;60:36–41.

84. Harakalova M, van Harssel JJ, Terhal PA, et al. Dominant missense mutations in ABCC9 cause Cantu syndrome. Nat Genet 2012;44:793–6.

85. van Bon BW, Gilissen C, Grange DK, et al. Cantu syndrome is caused by mutations in ABCC9. Am J Hum Genet 2012;90:1094–101.

86. Cooper PE, Reutter H, Woelfle J, et al. Cantu syndrome resulting from activating mutation in the KCNJ8 gene. Hum Mutat 2014;35:809–13.

87. Brownstein CA, Towne MC, Luquette LJ, et al. Mutation of KCNJ8 in a patient with Cantu syndrome with unique vascular abnormalities - support for the role of K(ATP) channels in this condition. Eur J Med Genet 2013;56:678–82.

88. Grange DK, Lorch SM, Cole PL, et al. Cantu syndrome in a woman and her two daughters: further confirmation of autosomal dominant inheritance and review of the cardiac manifestations. Am J Med Genet A 2006;140:1673–80.

89. Cooper PE, Sala-Rabanal M, Lee SJ, et al. Differential mechanisms of Cantu syndrome-associated

gain of function mutations in the ABCC9 (SUR2) subunit of the K$_{ATP}$ channel. J Gen Physiol 2015; 146:527–40.

90. Scurr I, Wilson L, Lees M, et al. Cantu syndrome: report of nine new cases and expansion of the clinical phenotype. Am J Med Genet A 2011;155A: 508–18.

91. Garcia-Cruz D, Mampel A, Echeverria MI, et al. Cantu syndrome and lymphoedema. Clin Dysmorphol 2011;20:32–7.

92. Kobayashi D, Cook AL, Williams DA. Pulmonary hypertension secondary to partial pulmonary venous obstruction in a child with Cantu syndrome. Pediatr Pulmonol 2010;45:727–9.

93. Engels H, Bosse K, Ehrbrecht A, et al. Further case of Cantu syndrome: exclusion of cryptic subtelomeric chromosome aberrations. Am J Med Genet 2002;111:205–9.

94. Lazalde B, Sanchez-Urbina R, Nuno-Arana I, et al. Autosomal dominant inheritance in Cantu syndrome (congenital hypertrichosis, osteochondrodysplasia, and cardiomegaly). Am J Med Genet 2000;94:421–7.

95. Concolino D, Formicola S, Camera G, et al. Congenital hypertrichosis, cardiomegaly, and osteochondrodysplasia (Cantu syndrome): a new case with unusual radiological findings. Am J Med Genet 2000;92:191–4.

96. Robertson SP, Kirk E, Bernier F, et al. Congenital hypertrichosis, osteochondrodysplasia, and cardiomegaly: Cantu syndrome. Am J Med Genet 1999;85:395–402.

97. Rosser EM, Kaariainen H, Hurst JA, et al. Three patients with the osteochondrodysplasia and hypertrichosis syndrome–Cantu syndrome. Clin Dysmorphol 1998;7:79–85.

98. Pennisi AJ, Takahashi M, Bernstein BH, et al. Minoxidil therapy in children with severe hypertension. J Pediatr 1977;90:813–9.

99. Mehta PK, Mamdani B, Shansky RM, et al. Severe hypertension. Treatment with minoxidil. JAMA 1975;233:249–52.

100. Kaler SG, Patrinos ME, Lambert GH, et al. Hypertrichosis and congenital anomalies associated with maternal use of minoxidil. Pediatrics 1987;79: 434–6.

101. Rosa FW, Idanpaan-Heikkila J, Asanti R. Fetal minoxidil exposure. Pediatrics 1987;80:120.

102. Schneider DJ, Moore JW. Patent ductus arteriosus. Circulation 2006;114:1873–82.

103. Richardson P, McKenna W, Bristow M, et al. Report of the 1995 World Health Organization/International Society and Federation of Cardiology Task Force on the Definition and Classification of cardiomyopathies. Circulation 1996;93:841–2.

104. Mehta PA, Dubrey SW. High output heart failure. QJM 2009;102:235–41.

105. Rossi A, Cantisani C, Melis L, et al. Minoxidil use in dermatology, side effects and recent patents. Recent Pat Inflamm Allergy Drug Discov 2012;6:130–6.

106. Shorter K, Farjo NP, Picksley SM, et al. Human hair follicles contain two forms of ATP-sensitive potassium channels, only one of which is sensitive to minoxidil. FASEB J 2008;22:1725–36.

107. Noma A. ATP-regulated K+ channels in cardiac muscle. Nature 1983;305:147–8.

108. Faivre JF, Findlay I. Effects of tolbutamide, glibenclamide and diazoxide upon action potentials recorded from rat ventricular muscle. Biochim Biophys Acta 1989;984:1–5.

109. Bao L, Kefaloyianni E, Lader J, et al. Unique properties of the ATP-sensitive K channel in the mouse ventricular cardiac conduction system. Circ Arrhythm Electrophysiol 2011;4:926–35.

110. Cole WC, McPherson CD, Sontag D. ATP-regulated K+ channels protect the myocardium against ischemia/reperfusion damage. Circ Res 1991;69: 571–81.

111. Venkatesh N, Lamp ST, Weiss J-N. Sulfonylureas, ATP-sensitive K+ channels, and cellular K+ loss during hypoxia, ischemia, and metabolic inhibition in mammalian ventricle. Circ Res 1991;69(3):623–37.

112. McPherson CD, Pierce GN, Cole WC. Ischemic cardioprotection by ATP-sensitive K+ channels involves high-energy phosphate preservation. Am J Physiol 1993;265:H1809–18.

113. Suzuki M, Sasaki N, Miki T, et al. Role of sarcolemmal K(ATP) channels in cardioprotection against ischemia/reperfusion injury in mice. J Clin Invest 2002;109:509–16.

114. Zingman LV, Hodgson DM, Bast PH, et al. Kir6.2 required for adaptation to stress. Proc Natl Acad Sci U S A 2002;99:13278–83.

115. Yamada S, Kane GC, Behfar A, et al. Protection conferred by myocardial ATP-sensitive K+ channels in pressure overload-induced congestive heart failure revealed in KCNJ11 Kir6.2-null mutant. J Physiol 2006;577:1053–65.

116. Hu X, Xu X, Huang Y, et al. Disruption of sarcolemmal ATP-sensitive potassium channel activity impairs the cardiac response to systolic overload. Circ Res 2008;103:1009–17.

117. Kane GC, Behfar A, Dyer RB, et al. KCNJ11 gene knockout of the Kir6.2 K$_{ATP}$ channel causes maladaptive remodeling and heart failure in hypertension. Hum Mol Genet 2006;15:2285–97.

118. Stoller D, Kakkar R, Smelley M, et al. Mice lacking sulfonylurea receptor 2 (SUR2) ATP-sensitive potassium channels are resistant to acute cardiovascular stress. J Mol Cell Cardiol 2007;43: 445–54.

119. Elrod JW, Harrell M, Flagg TP, et al. Role of sulfonylurea receptor type 1 subunits of ATP-sensitive potassium channels in myocardial

ischemia/reperfusion injury. Circulation 2008;117: 1405–13.

120. Schramm TK, Gislason GH, Vaag A, et al. Mortality and cardiovascular risk associated with different insulin secretagogues compared with metformin in type 2 diabetes, with or without a previous myocardial infarction: a nationwide study. Eur Heart J 2011;32:1900–8.

121. Gore MO, McGuire DK. Resolving drug effects from class effects among drugs for type 2 diabetes mellitus: more support for cardiovascular outcome assessments. Eur Heart J 2011;32:1832–4.

122. Zhang HX, Akrouh A, Kurata HT, et al. HMR 1098 is not an SUR isotype specific inhibitor of heterologous or sarcolemmal K ATP channels. J Mol Cell Cardiol 2010;50:552–60.

123. Flagg TP, Nichols CG. "Cardiac K$_{ATP}$": a family of ion channels. Circ Arrhythm Electrophysiol 2011;4:796–8.

124. Flanagan SE, Clauin S, Bellanne-Chantelot C, et al. Update of mutations in the genes encoding the pancreatic beta-cell K(ATP) channel subunits Kir6.2 (KCNJ11) and sulfonylurea receptor 1 (ABCC8) in diabetes mellitus and hyperinsulinism. Hum Mutat 2009;30:170–80.

Potassium Channel Remodeling in Heart Disease

Vincent Algalarrondo, MD, PhD[a,b,c], Stanley Nattel, MD[a,b,c],*

KEYWORDS

- Cardiac repolarization • Heart disease • Potassium • Potassium channel • Arrhythmia
- Atrial Fibrillation

KEY POINTS

- Cardiac repolarization and underlying ionic mechanisms are substantially altered by heart disease.
- In hypertrophy, myocardial infarction, and heart failure, potassium channels and currents are downregulated and repolarization is delayed, creating a substrate for ventricular tachyarrhythmia.
- Mechanisms leading to arrhythmia with potassium channel downregulation include early afterdepolarizations, reduced cardiomyocyte resting membrane resistance, and increased repolarization heterogeneity.
- A variety of extracardiac conditions (eg, hypokalemia, class III antiarrhythmic drugs) further reduce repolarization reserve and increase the arrhythmic risk in patients with heart disease.
- In atrial fibrillation, the combined effects of reduced calcium current and increased potassium current reduce action potential duration and refractory period and promote reentry, while hyperpolarizing the resting membrane potential, stabilizing reentrant rotors.

INTRODUCTION

Potassium channels are substantially altered in cardiovascular diseases (for an overview, see **Table1**). Teleologically, the types of potassium channel remodeling could be classified into 2 general secondary categories. The first type of remodeling, occurring in the ventricles with heart failure (HF), aims to prolong the action potential (AP) to increase calcium entry into the cytoplasm and compensate cardiomyocyte contraction. The second type of remodeling process, typically occurring in atria during atrial fibrillation (AF), aims to shorten the cardiomyocyte refractory period to allow cardiomyocytes to sustain very high activation rates. These pathophysiologic processes are complex and include redundancy and negative feedback. Although apparently designed to maintain cardiac homeostasis, they also induce electrophysiologic alterations that lead to potentially serious arrhythmias. Therefore, understanding them is of value for cardiologists in daily practice. In addition, K^+ channel remodeling can be induced by a host of other cardiac and extracardiac conditions.

Disclosures: V. Algalarrondo received scholarship funding from St. Jude Medical, Biotronik, Boston, Medtronic and Sorin.
Funding Sources: Canadian Institutes of Health Research (6957 and 44365, S. Nattel) and Heart and Stroke Foundation of Canada (S. Nattel). Fédération Française de Cardiologie (V. Algalarrondo).
[a] Department of Medicine, Research Center, Montreal Heart Institute, University of Montreal, 5000 Belanger Street East, Montreal, Quebec H1T 1C8, Canada; [b] Department of Pharmacology and Therapeutics, McGill University, 3655 Promenade Sir-William-Osler, Montréal, Québec H3G 1Y6, Canada; [c] Faculty of Medicine, University Duisburg-Essen, Hufelandstr. 55, Essen 45122, Germany
* Corresponding author. Montreal Heart Institute, University of Montreal, 5000 Belanger Street East, Montreal, Quebec H1T 1C8, Canada.
E-mail address: stanley.nattel@icm-mhi.org

cardiacEP.theclinics.com

Table 1
Main disease-related modifications in K$^+$ currents in pathologic situations

Current Density	Ventricular Hypertrophy		Heart Failure		Myocardial Infarction		Atrial Fibrillation	
	Exercise	Overload	Atria	Ventricle	Border Zone	Normal Zone	Atria	PV[a]
APD	↔	↑	—	↑	↑	↑	↓	↓
I_{to}	↔	↓	↓	↓	↓/↔ [b]	↓	↓	↓
I_{Kur}[c]	—	—	—	—	—	—	↓(?)[d]	—
I_{K1}	↑	↓	↔	↓	↓	↓	↑	↓
I_{Kr}	↔	↓	↔	↔	↓	↓	↔	↑
I_{Ks}	↔	—	↓	↓	↓ [e]	↓	↔	↑
I_{Kss}	↑	↓	—	↔	—	—	—	—
I_f[f]	—	—	↓	—	—	—	—	—
$I_{K(Ach,c)}$[c]	—	—	—	—	—	—	↑	—
$I_{K(ATP)}$	—	—	—	—	—	↑	?[d]	—
I_{SK}	—	—	—	↑	—	↑	↔[d]	↑
I_{K2P}[c]	—	—	—	—	—	—	↑	—

When discrepancies were noted across models, results documented on human samples are reported.

Abbreviations: ↑, current is increased; ↓, current is decreased; ↔, current is unchanged; APD, action potential duration; I_{to}, transient outward K$^+$ current; I_{K1}, inward rectifier K$^+$ current; I_{K2P} 2-pore-domain K$^+$ current; I_{Kur} ultrarapid rectifier K$^+$ current; I_{Kr}, delayed rectifier K$^+$ current; I_{Ks}, slow rectifier K$^+$ current; I_{Kss}, steady-state outward K$^+$ current; $I_{K(ACh)}$, acetylcholine-dependent K$^+$ current; I_{SK}, small calcium-activated K$^+$ current; PV, pulmonary veins.

[a] Compared with the left atrium.
[b] I_{to} is reduced initially then return to normal within 2 months.
[c] Atrial-specific currents.
[d] Conflicting results.
[e] ERG, KvLQT1 and minK are down regulated at day 2 after MI then ERG and KvLQT1 normalized at day 5 after MI, whereas minK remains downregulated.
[f] In sinoatrial node.
Data from Refs.[7,12,30,73,74]

Cardiac repolarization is in itself a complex process. Current state of the art recognizes more than 10 different types of cardiac K$^+$ currents, and more than 20 types of K$^+$ channels are known to be expressed in the heart.[1,2] Herein, we aim to present the K$^+$ channel remodeling processes in 4 common pathologic situations: cardiac hypertrophy, HF, myocardial infarction (MI), and AF. Specific regional remodeling profiles such as the border zone of the MI scar and the pulmonary veins (PVs) are also detailed.

OVERVIEW OF THE REMODELING PROCESSES OF POTASSIUM CHANNELS IN PATHOLOGIC SITUATIONS
Remodeling of K$^+$ Currents Associated with Hypertrophy

Hypertrophy
Cardiac hypertrophy is an adaptive response to volume or pressure overload that occurs in various pathologic situations (hypertension,

valvular ischemic or congenital heart diseases). In hypertensive patients, there is a weak but significant correlation between QTc interval and blood pressure and hypertrophic indices like the Cornell voltage indices.[3] It is also known that hypertensive patients with prolonged QTc intervals are at increased risk of cardiovascular morbidity and mortality.[4] In patients with successful antihypertensive therapy, left ventricular mass reduction is correlated with a decrease in the QTc interval[5]; for a review, see Ref.[6] In experimental models of cardiac hypertrophy, prolongation of repolarization has been documented by longer QTc intervals and AP durations (APDs). In patch clamp analysis, total K$^+$ current amplitudes are similar in cardiac hypertrophy subjects and controls, but because the membrane capacitance is larger in hypertrophy, the resulting K$^+$ current densities are reduced in cardiac hypertrophy.[7] This phenomenon has been documented for transient outward K$^+$ current (I_{to}), I_{K1} and slow rectifier K$^+$ current (I_{Ks}): compared with control, proteins and transcripts are unchanged in cardiac hypertrophy but current densities are lower because the cells are larger (for I_{to}: Kv4.2, Kv4.3 and KChIP2; for I_{K1}: Kir2.1 and Kir2.2).[7] For I_{Ks}, downregulation is observed at the transcript and the protein levels, especially in the epicardium. Finally, I_{ss} amplitude (noninactivating current) is increased in cardiac hypertrophy but not enough to restore a normal I_{ss} current density.[7] Together, these results suggest downregulation of repolarizing K^+ current densities in cardiac hypertrophy owing to pressure overload. This downregulation prolongs the APD; this could be proarrhythmic and may explain, at least in part, the correlation between hypertrophy, QT_c interval, and cardiovascular events.

Exercise-induced hypertrophy

In contrast with hypertrophy owing to chronic pressure overload, exercise-induced hypertrophy does not modify corrected QT_c interval and QT_c interval dispersion in professional athletes.[8] However, T wave morphology is commonly altered in trained athletes, suggesting that repolarization is remodeled in cardiac hypertrophy owing to exercise. In 2010, Yang and colleagues[9] reported an extensive study of cardiac repolarization in a swim training mouse model. Although myocytes had a 17% increase in membrane capacitance with exercise training, most of the electrical parameters were similar between trained mice and controls: ECG intervals were similar and APDs were unchanged. Using patch clamp methods, the authors documented that K^+ and Ca^{2+} currents increased in parallel with each other, resulting in unchanged AP shapes in exercise. The increased current densities were due to increased transcription and translation of channel subunits. The voltage-gated properties were unaltered. In contrast with hypertrophy caused by pressure overload, the repolarization remodeling in exercise parallels cardiac hypertrophy and returns to normal if training is stopped.

Remodeling of K^+ Currents Associated with Congestive Heart Failure

Between one-third and one-half of HF-related deaths are caused by ventricular tachyarrhythmias, and sudden death prevention is crucial in HF. QT_c prolongation occurs in HF[10] and is associated with an increased sudden death rate in ischemic cardiomyopathy.[11] In experimental HF models, the APs are prolonged and early afterdepolarization have been reproducibly documented (**Figs. 1A and 3A**; for a review, see Ref.[12]). APD prolongation is induced by downregulation of the main "classical" cardiac K^+ currents: I_{to}, slow (I_{KS}) and rapid delayed rectifier K^+ current (I_{Kr}),

and I_{K1}, although there are some discrepancies among studies. These discrepancies could be caused by differences in the HF models or to time-course differences in electrophysiologic remodeling after the onset of HF.[13] **Table 2** summarizes the changes in messenger RNA (mRNA) and protein expression in various models. Because the classical K^+ currents are downregulated, other K^+ currents could play an important role in the repolarization of remodeled myocytes. For instance, inhibition of the small conductance Ca^{2+}-activated K^+ current small calcium-activated K^+ current (I_{SK}) has been recently reported to prolong APD by 9% in failing human hearts, suggesting a compensatory role.[14] This report supports previous results in HF rabbits, in which increased cytosolic Ca^{2+} in HF seems to activate I_{SK}, thus reducing APD and compensating for the HF-induced reduction in repolarization reserve (**Fig. 2**).[14–16]

Reduced repolarizing currents induce proarrhythmic consequences in several ways. First, increased duration of repolarization may induce early afterdepolarizations (see **Fig. 1A**). Early afterdepolarizations are triggered if AP is prolonged in the specific voltage and time window that allows either the late Ca^{2+} current I_{CaL} or the Na^+ current I_{Na} to reactivate and generate a new AP.[12] In HF patients, repolarization reserve is reduced and the addition of class III antiarrhythmic drugs or hypokalemia may trigger early afterdepolarizations and ventricular tachyarrhythmias more easily. The downregulation of inward rectifying I_{K1} current increases the membrane resistance in the phase 4 of the AP, increasing the risk that a delayed afterdepolarization will generate an arrhythmia (see **Fig. 1B**).

Remodeling of K^+ Currents Associated with Myocardial Infarction

MI causes changes in K^+ current expression, density and function. In most cases, the proarrhythmic substrate in ischemic cardiomyopathy results from a heterogeneous scar where islands of living cells, called the border zone, are partially surrounded by fibrotic tissue.

Remodeling in the myocardial infarction border zone

Post MI border zone remodeling is characterized by prolonged repolarization owing to global downregulation of K^+ currents that promotes early afterdepolarizations (**Fig. 3B**; see **Table 1**). Remodeling begins within the first days after MI and is observed in both Purkinje cells and cardiomyocytes. It tends to recover after the MI episode for I_{to}, I_{Kr}, and I_{Ks}. The α-subunit expression for these 3 currents normalizes after the acute episode.

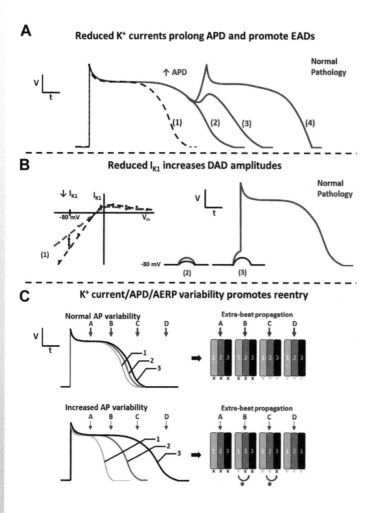

Fig. 1. (*A*) Compared with normal action potential (AP) (1), the reduced K⁺ currents in ventricular pathology prolong the action potential duration (APD) (2); this may induce early afterdepolarizations (3) that can trigger an ectopic AP (4). (*B*) Reduced I_{K1} (1) reduces resting membrane conductance, which increases membrane resistance R. Since the voltage change (V) induced by any membrane current (I) is influenced by the membrane resistance (V = IR), any given depolarizing current during a delayed afterdepolarization will induce a stronger depolarization in pathologic condition than in normal (2), thus more easily reaching the threshold potential of the myocyte to trigger an ectopic AP (3). (*C*) Propagation of ectopic activations according to timing and APD variability. APDs in 3 cells (from 1 to 3) at 4 different ectopic beat coupling intervals (from A to D) are represented. If AP variability is high as often occurs in disease states (*lower panel*), premature beats with coupling conditions B and C arrive when some cell(s) are refractory whereas other(s) are available for activation, which may induce unidirectional block and reentry (*asterisk*). AERP, atrial effective refractory period; DAD, delayed afterdepolarization; EAD, early afterdepolarization.

Table 2
Changes reported in mRNA and protein expression of K⁺ currents in heart failure

Reference	Subunit mRNA Changes	Model/Remarks
Kääb et al,[75] 1998	Kv4.3 ↓; HERG, Kv1.4, Kir2.1 ↔	Human heart
Wang et al,[76] 1998	Kir2.1, Kir2.2, Kir2.3 ↔	Human heart
Borlak and Thum,[77] 2003	Kv4.3, Kv1.5, K2P 1.1, Kir2.1, Kir3.4, Kir6.2 ↓; ERG ↔; KvLQT1, Mink ↑	Human heart
Zicha et al,[78] 2004	Kv4.3 ↓; KChIP2 ↔	Human and dog hearts, proteins correspond with mRNA
Akar et al,[79] 2005	Kv4.3 ↓; KChIP2, KvLQT1, Mink, Kir2.1 ↔; Kv1.4, ERG ↑	Dog heart; proteins correspond with mRNA but not to current
Rose et al,[80] 2005	Kv1.4, Kv4.2, KChIP2, Kir2.1 ↓; Kv4.3, ERG, KvLQT1, Mink ↔	Tachypacing in rabbit; proteins: Kv1.4, Kv4.2, Kv4.3, KChIP2, Kir2.1 KvLQT1 ↔
Tsuji et al,[41] 2006	Kv1.4, Kv4.3, KvLQT1, minK ↓; ERG ↔	AVB in rabbit; proteins correspond with mRNA
Yang et al,[81] 2015	—	Rat with AVF. proteins: SK3 ↑ SK2 ↔

Abbreviations: ↓, decrease; ↑, increase; ↔, no change; AVB, atrioventricular block; AVF, arteriovenous fistula; mRNA, messenger RNA.
Data from Refs.[41,75–81]

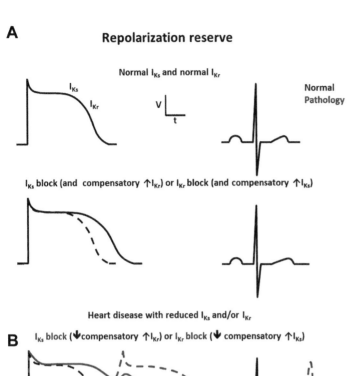

Fig. 2. Consequences of repolarization reserve on action potentials (APs) and the associated surface electrocardiograph (ECG). Under normal conditions (*A*), individual reductions of I_{Kr} or I_{Ks} induce only a minor prolongation of AP duration (APD) and QT interval because of repolarization reserve. (*B*) When this compensatory effect is impaired (eg, in heart disease with reduced I_{Kr} and/or I_{Ks}) (*C*), the APD prolongation is enhanced, as is as the risk of early after depolarizations (*dashed red line*).

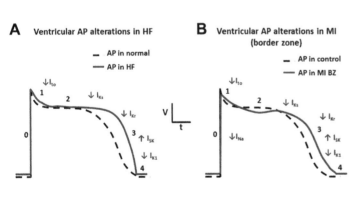

Fig. 3. Schematic summarizing the principal alterations in the action potential (AP) and corresponding K⁺ currents alterations in 4 situations: heart failure (HF; *A*), border zone of the myocardial infarction (MI; *B*), atrial fibrillation (AF; *C*) and pulmonary veins (*D*). Blue numbers indicate AP phases. Red are changes in pathology (*A–C*) or differences in pulmonary vein versus atrium (*D*).

However, this recovery is incomplete and the β-subunit minK remains downregulated in the longer term, which would accelerate I_{Ks} inactivation and decrease its amplitude (for a review see Ref.[12]).

Remodeling in the normal zones of hearts with prior myocardial infarction

Studies of zones remote from the MI scar zone have been performed in small animal models (rabbit and rat). APD prolongation leads to triggered activity and spatial refractoriness heterogeneity. As in the border zone, APD prolongation is caused by downregulation of the main K^+ currents. Mathematical modeling of border and normal zones in MI ventricles highlights the interplay between the 2 zones and the crucial role of refractoriness heterogeneity in generating a substrate for arrhythmia (**Fig. 1C**).[17]

Remodeling of K^+ Currents Associated with Atrial Fibrillation

Remodeling of K^+ currents in atrial fibrillation

AF, the most common sustained cardiac arrhythmia, results from a variety of conditions, like ectopic activity in the PVs and atrial remodeling in HF and hypertension. By itself, AF induces electrical remodeling that shortens atrial refractory periods and promotes AF ("AF begets AF"[18]). This remodeling has been reproduced in experimental models by performing high-rate atrial pacing. It has been shown that K^+ current changes play a key role in the pathogenesis of AF. The remodeling process begins within the first day after the onset of AF and results in complex modifications of the atrial AP (see **Fig. 3C**). During the initial phase of repolarization (phase 1), APD is prolonged because of the downregulation of I_{to}; ultrarapid rectifier K^+ current (I_{Kur}) was documented as reduced or unchanged.[12] Thereafter, the combining effects of stable I_{Kr}/I_{Ks}, decreased I_{CaL} and increased I_{K1}/acetylcholine-dependent K^+ current [$I_{K(Ach)}$]/2-pore-domain K^+ current (I_{K2P}) induce a shortening of phases 2 and 3 of the AP.

I_{K1} increases also occur, paralleling upregulation of Kir2.1 (KCNJ2) mRNA and protein. This upregulation is associated with a decreased expression of microRNAs 1 and 26 (miR-1 and miR-26) both in humans and in experimental models.[19,20] Similarly, decreases in I_{to} density parallel the downregulation of Kv4.3 mRNA and protein. Several reports in experimental models suggest that reduced miR-1 and increased miR-301a may decrease the expression of KCND2 (Kv4.2), and that increased miR-133 may reduce the expression of KChIP2 (for further reviews, see Refs.[2,21]).

The upregulation of $I_{K(Ach)}$ has been documented both in experimental models and in AF

patients.[22] This increased $I_{K(Ach)}$ is caused by activation of the basal current (with downregulation of the carbachol-induced current); Kv3.1 mRNA and protein remain stable. Functional upregulation of constitutive $I_{K(Ach)}$ seems to be caused by changes in regulation by protein kinase C isoforms.[23]

Two-pore domain K^+ channels (K_{2P}) have been recently identified as potential contributors to AF pathophysiology. Expressed mostly in the atria, these channels are regulated by various factors, including lipids, pH, temperature, or membrane stretch (but not voltage) and thus they conduct a background current throughout the AP. The electrophysiologic role of the cardiac K_{2P} channel $K_{2P}3.1$ was first characterized in mice.[24] Recently, Schmidt and colleagues[25] documented that $K_{2P}3.1$ transcripts, protein, and the corresponding I_{K2P} current are upregulated in the atria of patients with chronic AF, contributing to AP abbreviation.

The contribution of small conductance calcium-activated potassium channels in AF is still controversial. It was first documented that increased I_{SK} was associated with arrhythmia and that pharmacologic inhibition of I_{SK} was antiarrhythmic in experimental models.[26,27] In subsequent reports, however, I_{SK} inhibition did not modify AP shape and the expression of SK2 and SK3 subunits was reduced in human AF atria.[27] Therefore, the precise role of I_{SK} in human AF remains to be clarified.

Remodeling of K^+ currents in pulmonary veins

Following the observations from Haïssaguerre and colleagues[28] of the crucial role of PVs in the initiation of AF, basic research characterized further the electrophysiology of the myocardial sleeves in PVs.[29,30] Anatomically, myocardial fibers extend from left atria to PVs for 1 to 3 cm, with a specific structure that transits from a linear to a circular organization. At the cellular level, PV cardiomyocytes have distinct properties, including decreased phase 0 upstroke velocity and short APD, and the fibers have a specific organization (**Fig. 3D**).[29–32] PV sleeve cardiomyocytes also have small background I_{K1} that could lead to depolarization and spontaneous activity.[30,33] Furthermore, as compared with the left atrium, PVs show lower expression of Kir3.1 and Kir3.4 that underlie $I_{K(Ach)}$. This K^+ channel subunit profile is associated with lower resting vagal tone at baseline, greater response to vagal stimulation, and shorter refractory periods in PVs than in left atrium.[34] The intrinsic ion channel and AP properties of PVs make them more susceptible to reentrant arrhythmias. With remodeling, the short PV AP becomes even shorter; however, remodeling-induced increases in I_{K1} should restore the intrinsically smaller resting potential in PV cells. Overall, AF-related tachycardia remodeling decreases the AP differences between PV and left atrial cardiomyocytes and in the absence of other cardiac pathology the PVs do not play a central role in the AF promotion caused by atrial tachycardia remodeling.[35]

K+ CHANNEL REMODELING: TRANSLATIONAL INTEREST AND CLINICAL IMPORTANCE
Hypokalemia and K+ Currents in Heart Disease Patients

Hypokalemia ($[K^+]<3.6$ mmol/L) is a common situation in daily clinical practice that is associated with increased morbidity and mortality in patients with heart diseases like hypertension, MI, resuscitation from out-of-hospital cardiac arrest, and HF.[36,37] Whereas low $[K^+]$ should enhance extracellular/intracellular K^+ gradient, thus increasing K^+ currents, the main effect of hypokalemia's is to prolong the QTc interval and APD. This prolongation is caused by hypokalemia-induced reductions in multiple K^+ currents including I_{Kr}, I_{K1}, and I_{to}. Recently, it was demonstrated that downregulation of I_{Kr} in hypokalemia is caused, at least in part, by accelerated internalization and degradation of hERG channels.[38] Furthermore, hypokalemia downregulates the Na^+–K^+ ATPase pump and increases $[Na^+]_i$, which leads to increased $[Ca^{2+}]_i$ via activation of the Na^+/Ca^{2+} exchanger. Low $[K^+]_e$ correspondingly increases the effects of class III antiarrhythmic drugs by reducing repolarization reserve; conversely, high $[K^+]_e$ protects against drug-induced torsades de pointes. The combined proarrhythmic effects of electrolyte imbalance and/or class III antiarrhythmic agents multiply the risk of life-threatening arrhythmia if they occur on top of a predisposed substrate with reduced repolarization reserve.

Repolarization Reserve

The term "repolarization reserve" refers to the ability of cardiomyocytes to compensate for the loss of a repolarizing current by recruiting another one and thus to minimize the APD prolongation induced by this loss.[39] Repolarization reserve may result in limited alterations in the AP with K^+ channel block, and the surface ECG could be unchanged compared with normal. However, if this compensatory mechanism is lost or overridden by additional repolarization abnormalities, the resulting effect on the AP, the ECG, and finally the cardiac arrhythmic risk could be exaggerated (see **Fig. 2**). Downregulation of K^+ currents and associated repolarization reserve has been documented in HF,[40,41] consistent with the deleterious effect of the I_{Kr} blocker sotalol in patients with HF in the Survival With ORal D-sotalol (SWORD) trial[42] and the increased proarrhythmic risk with sotalol in HF.[43] The increased predisposition to excess APD prolongation with class III agents may occur without any APD prolongation at baseline.[36] Practically, loss of repolarization reserve could be detected by recording ECGs and measuring QTc intervals after the initiation of class III antiarrhythmic drugs, possibly within a few hours of the first oral dose. Another phenomenon that should be considered in the adverse event risk of class III antiarrhythmic drugs is their "reverse use dependency." This "reverse use dependency" means that the APD prolonging effect is greater for low cardiac frequencies, which increases the risk of EAD-triggered arrhythmia with bradycardia (for a review see Ref.[44]).

Specific Targets in Atrial Fibrillation

The upregulation of K^+ currents in AF promotes the arrhythmia and may contribute to its increasing resistance to drug therapy over time, but may also create opportunities for new pharmacologic approaches. In particular, drugs that inhibit inward-rectifier K^+ currents may be particularly interesting in view of their role in AF perpetuation.[45] On the other hand, downregulation of ionic currents like I_{Kur} may limit the value of targeting them in AF.[45]

PHARMACOLOGIC MODULATION OF K+ CHANNELS IN HEART DISEASE PATIENTS

Reentry is a crucial arrhythmic mechanism. Because short refractory periods increase the likelihood of reentry, it has long been recognized that drugs that prolong APD and refractory periods by blocking K^+ channels have antiarrhythmic effects against reentry. Such drugs were allocated to class III of the Singh and Vaughan Williams[46] antiarrhythmic drug classification. After the Cardiac Arrhythmia Suppression Trial (CAST), class III agents were widely studied to treat patients with significant heart diseases. Great successes, but also great failures, have been recorded in this field of research.

Amiodarone

Amiodarone blocks I_{Kr} and I_{Ks} to prolong the APD (class III action),[47] but also blocks Na^+ channels to reduce conduction velocities (class I action),[48] has a noncompetitive blocking effect on β receptors (class II effect)[49] and inhibits I_{CaL} (class IV action).[50] These multiple blocking effects likely contribute to its clinical efficacy and safety.

Clinically, cardiac side effects like torsades de pointes or HF worsening are unusual, which has made amiodarone a first-line antiarrhythmic drug to treat HF patients, illustrating the notion that multiple channel blockers may have increased safety in patients with remodeling-related decreases in repolarization reserve. Clinical efficacy was specifically reported in the AF treatment of HF patients.[51] In patients with a high risk of sudden cardiac death, amiodarone does not prevent sudden death per se; however, in implantable cardioverter–defibrillator carriers, amiodarone plus β-blockers prevent shocks with greater efficacy than sotalol or β-blockers alone.

Other Class III Antiarrhythmic Drugs and Heart Disease

Available class III anti arrhythmic agents include ibutilide, dofetilide, and sotalol. All block I_{Kr}, prolonging effective refractory periods with minimal effects on conduction velocity, and thereby suppress reentry.[52–56] They also, however, carry a risk of torsades de pointes (incidence 2.4% for sotalol, 3.6%–8.3% for ibutilide, and 1%–3% for dofetilide), which is increased in the presence of heart disease.[45] Predisposing factors for drug-induced torsades de pointes include female sex, high drug doses, HF, recent cardioversion, hypokalemia, bradycardia, and elevated baseline serum creatinine level.[57]

Sotalol is a mixed class III and class II drug. The class II action is advantageous to allow for rate control in addition to the rhythm control effect owing to class III properties. However, the bradycardic action of sotalol may increase the risk of torsades de pointes. Sotalol may also be useful to reduce the number of shocks in implantable cardioverter–defibrillator carriers. Ibutilide was constructed by comparing sotalol with other β-blockers and with clofilium phosphate, another class III antiarrhythmic agent.[58] Intravenous ibutilide is used to cardiovert AF and atrial flutter; the risk of ibutilide-induced long QT syndrome is enhanced in HF patients.[56] Because of the risk of torsades de pointes with dofetilide, only certified physicians are authorized to prescribe the drug; initiation is usually performed in hospital, which limits its clinical use.

Other Multichannel Blockers and Heart Diseases

Dronedarone

Dronedarone was constructed on the basis of the amiodarone structure, designed to retain similar efficacy while avoiding the leading type of amiodarone side effect (thyroid disorders). Like amiodarone, dronedarone blocks I_{Na}, I_{CaL}, I_{Kr}, I_{Ks}, I_{to}, $I_{K(ACh)}$, and β-adrenergic receptors[59,60] Clinically, the drug has moderate efficacy to maintain sinus rhythm in AF patients and clearly inferior efficacy compared to amiodarone. Clinical studies that included significant numbers of HF patients (European Trial of Dronedarone in Moderate to Severe Congestive Heart Failure [ANDROMEDA] and Permanent Atrial Fibrillation Outcome Study Using Dronedarone on Top of Standard Therapy [PALLAS]) were interrupted early because of excess events in the dronedarone group,[61] again highlighting the risks of reduced repolarization reserve with heart disease. As a consequence, dronedarone should be avoided for patients with significant cardiovascular disease.[62]

Vernakalant

Vernakalant is a multicurrent blocker that was developed as an atrial selective antiarrhythmic agent.[63] The electrophysiologic profile of vernakalant includes inhibition of I_{Kur}, I_{to}, I_{Kr}, $I_{K(ACh)}$, and I_{Na}.[64] Vernakalant modestly increases the QT_c interval and is contraindicated in patients with a long QT_c.[65–67] Current clinical use only involves intravenous administration to convert AF. The only clinical report on patients with heart diseases involved patients undergoing cardiac surgery and vernakalant was safe.[68]

Ranolazine

Ranolazine was initially described as a late Na^+ current blocker and was primarily evaluated to treat chronic angina. However, experimental and clinical studies showed that ranolazine had an interesting electrophysiologic profile and could be potentially helpful to treat AF (for a review see Ref.[69]). Ranolazine prolongs atrial APD and refractory periods but does not prolong ventricular repolarization in experimental models of hypertrophy and CHF.[56] Ranolazine is a multichannel blocker that inhibits (peak and late) I_{Na}, I_{CaL}, Na^+/Ca^{2+} exchanger, I_{Kr}, and stabilizes RyR2.[70,71] Ranolazine was recently tested in a reduced-dose combination with dronedarone; the combination was found to have synergistic efficacy with low toxicity in AF patients.[72]

SUMMARY

Heart disease produces substantial remodeling of K^+ channels that in general promotes arrhythmia occurrence. In the case of ventricular arrhythmias, K^+ channel remodeling contributes to the arrhythmic risk and increases vulnerability to torsades de pointes with K^+ channel inhibiting drugs. Atrial K^+ channel remodeling caused by AF promotes arrhythmia stability and presents opportunities for the development of new drugs targeting atrial inward rectifier K$^+$ currents.

REFERENCES

1. Nerbonne JM, Kass RS. Molecular physiology of cardiac repolarization. Physiol Rev 2005;85:1205–53.
2. Schmitt N, Grunnet M, Olesen S-P. Cardiac potassium channel subtypes: new roles in repolarization and arrhythmia. Physiol Rev 2014;94:609–53.
3. Schillaci G, Pirro M, Ronti T, et al. Prognostic impact of prolonged ventricular repolarization in hypertension. Arch Intern Med 2006;166:909–13.
4. Salles GF, Cardoso CRL, Muxfeldt ES. Prognostic value of ventricular repolarization prolongation in resistant hypertension: a prospective cohort study. J Hypertens 2009;27:1094–101.
5. Karpanou EA, Vyssoulis GP, Psichogios A, et al. Regression of left ventricular hypertrophy results in improvement of QT dispersion in patients with hypertension. Am Heart J 1998;136:765–8.
6. Klimas J, Kruzliak P, Rabkin SW. Modulation of the QT interval duration in hypertension with antihypertensive treatment. Hypertens Res 2015;38:447–54.
7. Marionneau C, Brunet S, Flagg TP, et al. Distinct cellular and molecular mechanisms underlie functional remodeling of repolarizing K+ currents with left ventricular hypertrophy. Circ Res 2008;102:1406–15.
8. Omiya K, Sekizuka H, Kida K, et al. Influence of gender and types of sports training on QT variables in young elite athletes. Eur J Sport Sci 2014;14(Suppl 1):S32–8.
9. Yang K-C, Foeger NC, Marionneau C, et al. Homeostatic regulation of electrical excitability in physiological cardiac hypertrophy. J Physiol 2010;588:5015–32.
10. Davey PP, Barlow C, Hart G. Prolongation of the QT interval in heart failure occurs at low but not at high heart rates. Clin Sci (Lond) 2000;98:603–10.
11. Karwatowska-Prokopczuk E, Wang W, Cheng ML, et al. The risk of sudden cardiac death in patients with non-ST elevation acute coronary syndrome and prolonged QTc interval: effect of ranolazine. Europace 2013;15:429–36.
12. Nattel S, Maguy A, Le Bouter S, et al. Arrhythmogenic ion-channel remodeling in the heart: heart failure, myocardial infarction, and atrial fibrillation. Physiol Rev 2007;87:425–56.
13. Long VP, Bonilla IM, Vargas-Pinto P, et al. Heart failure duration progressively modulates the arrhythmia substrate through structural and electrical remodeling. Life Sci 2015;123:61–71.
14. Yu C-C, Corr C, Shen C, et al. Small conductance calcium-activated potassium current is important in transmural repolarization of failing human ventricles. Circ Arrhythm Electrophysiol 2015;8:667–76.
15. Chua S-K, Chang P-C, Maruyama M, et al. Small-conductance calcium-activated potassium channel and recurrent ventricular fibrillation in failing rabbit ventricles. Circ Res 2011;108:971–9.
16. Hsieh Y-C, Chang P-C, Hsueh C-H, et al. Apamin-sensitive potassium current modulates action potential duration restitution and arrhythmogenesis of failing rabbit ventricles. Circ Arrhythm Electrophysiol 2013;6:410–8.
17. Decker KF, Rudy Y. Ionic mechanisms of electrophysiological heterogeneity and conduction block in the infarct border zone. Am J Physiol Heart Circ Physiol 2010;299:H1588–97.
18. Wijffels MC, Kirchhof CJ, Dorland R, et al. Atrial fibrillation begets atrial fibrillation. A study in awake chronically instrumented goats. Circulation 1995;92:1954–68.
19. Girmatsion Z, Biliczki P, Bonauer A, et al. Changes in microRNA-1 expression and IK1 up-regulation in human atrial fibrillation. Heart Rhythm 2009;6:1802–9.
20. Luo X, Pan Z, Shan H, et al. MicroRNA-26 governs profibrillatory inward-rectifier potassium current changes in atrial fibrillation. J Clin Invest 2013;123:1939–51.
21. Luo X, Yang B, Nattel S. MicroRNAs and atrial fibrillation: mechanisms and translational potential. Nat Rev Cardiol 2015;12:80–90.
22. Voigt N, Trausch A, Knaut M, et al. Left-to-right atrial inward rectifier potassium current gradients in patients with paroxysmal versus chronic atrial fibrillation. Circ Arrhythm Electrophysiol 2010;3:472–80.
23. Makary S, Voigt N, Maguy A, et al. Differential protein kinase C isoform regulation and increased constitutive activity of acetylcholine-regulated potassium channels in atrial remodeling. Circ Res 2011;109:1031–43.
24. Donner BC, Schullenberg M, Geduldig N, et al. Functional role of TASK-1 in the heart: studies in TASK-1-deficient mice show prolonged cardiac repolarization and reduced heart rate variability. Basic Res Cardiol 2011;106:75–87.
25. Schmidt C, Wiedmann F, Voigt N, et al. Upregulation of K(2P)3.1 K+ Current causes action potential shortening in patients with chronic atrial fibrillation. Circulation 2015;132:82–92.
26. Ozgen N, Dun W, Sosunov EA, et al. Early electrical remodeling in rabbit pulmonary vein results from trafficking of intracellular SK2 channels to membrane sites. Cardiovasc Res 2007;75:758–69.
27. Skibsbye L, Poulet C, Diness JG, et al. Small-conductance calcium-activated potassium (SK) channels contribute to action potential repolarization in human atria. Cardiovasc Res 2014;103:156–67.
28. Haïssaguerre M, Jaïs P, Shah DC, et al. Spontaneous initiation of atrial fibrillation by ectopic beats

originating in the pulmonary veins. N Engl J Med 1998;339(10):659–66.

29. Ehrlich JR, Cha T-J, Zhang L, et al. Characterization of a hyperpolarization-activated time-dependent potassium current in canine cardiomyocytes from pulmonary vein myocardial sleeves and left atrium. J Physiol 2004;557:583–97.

30. Ehrlich JR, Cha T-J, Zhang L, et al. Cellular electrophysiology of canine pulmonary vein cardiomyocytes: action potential and ionic current properties. J Physiol 2003;551:801–13.

31. Jaïs P, Hocini M, Macle L, et al. Distinctive electrophysiological properties of pulmonary veins in patients with atrial fibrillation. Circulation 2002;106: 2479–85.

32. Chen Y-C, Pan N-H, Cheng C-C, et al. Heterogeneous expression of potassium currents and pacemaker currents potentially regulates arrhythmogenesis of pulmonary vein cardiomyocytes. J Cardiovasc Electrophysiol 2009;20:1039–45.

33. Nattel S. Paroxysmal atrial fibrillation and pulmonary veins: relationships between clinical forms and automatic versus re-entrant mechanisms. Can J Cardiol 2013;29:1147–9.

34. Arora R, Ng J, Ulphani J, et al. Unique autonomic profile of the pulmonary veins and posterior left atrium. J Am Coll Cardiol 2007;49:1340–8.

35. Cha T-J, Ehrlich JR, Zhang L, et al. Atrial ionic remodeling induced by atrial tachycardia in the presence of congestive heart failure. Circulation 2004; 110:1520–6.

36. Gennari FJ. Hypokalemia. N Engl J Med 1998;339: 451–8.

37. Osadchii OE. Mechanisms of hypokalemia-induced ventricular arrhythmogenicity. Fundam Clin Pharmacol 2010;24:547–59.

38. Guo J, Massaeli H, Xu J, et al. Extracellular K+ concentration controls cell surface density of IKr in rabbit hearts and of the HERG channel in human cell lines. J Clin Invest 2009;119:2745–57.

39. Roden DM. Taking the "idio" out of "idiosyncratic": predicting torsades de pointes. Pacing Clin Electrophysiol 1998;21:1029–34.

40. Han W, Chartier D, Li D, et al. Ionic remodeling of cardiac Purkinje cells by congestive heart failure. Circulation 2001;104:2095–100.

41. Tsuji Y, Zicha S, Qi X-Y, et al. Potassium channel subunit remodeling in rabbits exposed to long-term bradycardia or tachycardia: discrete arrhythmogenic consequences related to differential delayed-rectifier changes. Circulation 2006;113: 345–55.

42. Waldo AL, Camm AJ, deRuyter H, et al. Effect of d-sotalol on mortality in patients with left ventricular dysfunction after recent and remote myocardial infarction. The SWORD Investigators. Survival with Oral d-Sotalol. Lancet 1996;348:7–12.

43. Lehmann MH, Hardy S, Archibald D, et al. Sex difference in risk of torsade de pointes with d,l-sotalol. Circulation 1996;94:2535–41.

44. Dorian P. Mechanisms of action of class III agents and their clinical relevance. Europace 2000; 1(Suppl C):C6–9.

45. Dobrev D, Carlsson L, Nattel S. Novel molecular targets for atrial fibrillation therapy. Nat Rev Drug Discov 2012;11:275–91.

46. Singh BN, Vaughan Williams EM. A third class of anti-arrhythmic action. Effects on atrial and ventricular intracellular potentials, and other pharmacological actions on cardiac muscle, of MJ 1999 and AH 3474. Br J Pharmacol 1970;39:675–87.

47. Kodama I, Kamiya K, Toyama J. Cellular electropharmacology of amiodarone. Cardiovasc Res 1997;35: 13–29.

48. Mason JW, Hondeghem LM, Katzung BG. Block of inactivated sodium channels and of depolarization-induced automaticity in guinea pig papillary muscle by amiodarone. Circ Res 1984;55:278–85.

49. Kadoya M, Konishi T, Tamamura T, et al. Electrophysiological effects of amiodarone on isolated rabbit heart muscles. J Cardiovasc Pharmacol 1985;7: 643–8.

50. Nattel S, Talajic M, Quantz M, et al. Frequency-dependent effects of amiodarone on atrioventricular nodal function and slow-channel action potentials: evidence for calcium channel-blocking activity. Circulation 1987;76:442–9.

51. Deedwania PC, Singh BN, Ellenbogen K, et al. Spontaneous conversion and maintenance of sinus rhythm by amiodarone in patients with heart failure and atrial fibrillation: observations from the veterans affairs congestive heart failure survival trial of antiarrhythmic therapy (CHF-STAT). The Department of Veterans Affairs CHF-STAT Investigators. Circulation 1998;98:2574–9.

52. Sanguinetti MC, Jurkiewicz NK. Two components of cardiac delayed rectifier K+ current. Differential sensitivity to block by class III antiarrhythmic agents. J Gen Physiol 1990;96:195–215.

53. Jurkiewicz NK, Sanguinetti MC. Rate-dependent prolongation of cardiac action potentials by a methanesulfonanilide class III antiarrhythmic agent. Specific block of rapidly activating delayed rectifier K+ current by dofetilide. Circ Res 1993;72:75–83.

54. Yang T, Snyders DJ, Roden DM. Ibutilide, a methanesulfonanilide antiarrhythmic, is a potent blocker of the rapidly activating delayed rectifier K+ current (IKr) in AT-1 cells. Concentration-, time-, voltage-, and use-dependent effects. Circulation 1995;91: 1799–806.

55. Tai CT, Chen SA, Feng AN, et al. Electropharmacologic effects of class I and class III antiarrhythmia drugs on typical atrial flutter: insights into the mechanism of termination. Circulation 1998;97:1935–45.

56. Kowey PR, VanderLugt JT, Luderer JR. Safety and risk/benefit analysis of ibutilide for acute conversion of atrial fibrillation/flutter. Am J Cardiol 1996;78:46–52.

57. Kannankeril P, Roden DM, Darbar D. Drug-induced long QT syndrome. Pharmacol Rev 2010;62:760–81.

58. Hester JB, Gibson JK, Cimini MG, et al. N-[(omega-amino-1-hydroxyalkyl)phenyl]methanesulfonamide derivatives with class III antiarrhythmic activity. J Med Chem 1991;34:308–15.

59. Varró A, Takács J, Németh M, et al. Electrophysiological effects of dronedarone (SR 33589), a noniodinated amiodarone derivative in the canine heart: comparison with amiodarone. Br J Pharmacol 2001;133:625–34.

60. Gautier P, Guillemare E, Marion A, et al. Electrophysiologic characterization of dronedarone in guinea pig ventricular cells. J Cardiovasc Pharmacol 2003;41:191–202.

61. Nattel S. Dronedarone in atrial fibrillation–Jekyll and Hyde? N Engl J Med 2011;365:2321–2.

62. Camm AJ, Lip GYH, De Caterina R, et al. ESC Committee for Practice Guidelines-CPG, Document Reviewers. 2012 focused update of the ESC Guidelines for the management of atrial fibrillation: an update of the 2010 ESC Guidelines for the management of atrial fibrillation–developed with the special contribution of the European Heart Rhythm Association. Europace 2012;14:1385–413.

63. Nattel S, De Blasio E, Beatch GN, et al. RSD1235: a novel antiarrhythmic agent with a unique electrophysiological profile that terminates AF in dogs. Eur Heart J 2001;22(Suppl):448.

64. Fedida D, Orth PMR, Chen JYC, et al. The mechanism of atrial antiarrhythmic action of RSD1235. J Cardiovasc Electrophysiol 2005;16:1227–38.

65. Dorian P, Pinter A, Mangat I, et al. The effect of vernakalant (RSD1235), an investigational antiarrhythmic agent, on atrial electrophysiology in humans. J Cardiovasc Pharmacol 2007;50:35–40.

66. Roy D, Pratt CM, Torp-Pedersen C, et al, Atrial Arrhythmia Conversion Trial Investigators. Vernakalant hydrochloride for rapid conversion of atrial fibrillation: a phase 3, randomized, placebo-controlled trial. Circulation 2008;117:1518–25.

67. Camm AJ, Capucci A, Hohnloser SH, et al. A randomized active-controlled study comparing the efficacy and safety of vernakalant to amiodarone in recent-onset atrial fibrillation. J Am Coll Cardiol 2011;57:313–21.

68. Kowey PR, Dorian P, Mitchell LB, et al, Atrial Arrhythmia Conversion Trial Investigators. Vernakalant hydrochloride for the rapid conversion of atrial fibrillation after cardiac surgery: a randomized, double-blind, placebo-controlled trial. Circ Arrhythm Electrophysiol 2009;2:652–9.

69. Gupta T, Khera S, Kolte D, et al. Antiarrhythmic properties of ranolazine: a review of the current evidence. Int J Cardiol 2015;187:66–74.

70. Antzelevitch C, Belardinelli L, Zygmunt AC, et al. Electrophysiological effects of ranolazine, a novel antianginal agent with antiarrhythmic properties. Circulation 2004;110:904–10.

71. Parikh A, Mantravadi R, Kozhevnikov D, et al. Ranolazine stabilizes cardiac ryanodine receptors: a novel mechanism for the suppression of early afterdepolarization and torsades de pointes in long QT type 2. Heart Rhythm 2012;9:953–60.

72. Reiffel JA, Camm AJ, Belardinelli L, et al, HARMONY Investigators. The HARMONY trial: combined ranolazine and dronedarone in the management of paroxysmal atrial fibrillation: mechanistic and therapeutic synergism. Circ Arrhythm Electrophysiol 2015;8:1048–56.

73. Volk T, Nguyen TH, Schultz JH, et al. Regional alterations of repolarizing K+ currents among the left ventricular free wall of rats with ascending aortic stenosis. J Physiol 2001;530:443–55.

74. Yang K-C, Nerbonne JM. Mechanisms contributing to myocardial potassium channel diversity, regulation and remodeling. Trends Cardiovasc Med 2015;15:S1050–738.

75. Kääb S, Dixon J, Duc J, et al. Molecular basis of transient outward potassium current downregulation in human heart failure: a decrease in Kv4.3 mRNA correlates with a reduction in current density. Circulation 1998;98:1383–93.

76. Wang Z, Yue L, White M, et al. Differential distribution of inward rectifier potassium channel transcripts in human atrium versus ventricle. Circulation 1998;98:2422–8.

77. Borlak J, Thum T. Hallmarks of ion channel gene expression in end-stage heart failure. FASEB J 2003;17:1592–608.

78. Zicha S, Xiao L, Stafford S, et al. Transmural expression of transient outward potassium current subunits in normal and failing canine and human hearts. J Physiol 2004;561:735–48.

79. Akar FG, Wu RC, Juang GJ, et al. Molecular mechanisms underlying K+ current downregulation in canine tachycardia-induced heart failure. Am J Physiol Heart Circ Physiol 2005;288:H2887–96.

80. Rose J, Armoundas AA, Tian Y, et al. Molecular correlates of altered expression of potassium currents in failing rabbit myocardium. Am J Physiol Heart Circ Physiol 2005;288:H2077–87.

81. Yang D, Wang T, Ni Y, et al. Apamin-Sensitive K(+) current upregulation in volume-overload heart failure is associated with the decreased interaction of CK2 with SK2. J Membr Biol 2015;248:1181–9.

Modulation of Cardiac Potassium Current by Neural Tone and Ischemia

Todd T. Tomson, MD, Rishi Arora, MD*

KEYWORDS

- Autonomic nervous system • Cardiac arrhythmias • Potassium channels
- Acetylcholine-activated potassium channel • ATP-sensitive potassium channel • Atrial fibrillation

KEY POINTS

- Modulation of the flow of potassium across myocyte cell membranes results in changes to the cardiac action potential, and abnormalities of potassium current can result cardiac arrhythmias.
- The autonomic nervous system (ANS) has a role in regulation of cardiac potassium currents, and abnormalities in autonomic regulation of cardiac potassium currents can result in arrhythmias, including atrial fibrillation (AF), that may result from abnormal modulation of acetylcholine (ACh)-activated potassium channels.
- Ischemia is another important modulator of cardiac cellular electrophysiology that alters cardiac potassium current through effects on ATP-sensitive potassium channels in ways that may result in cardiac arrhythmias, in particular ventricular fibrillation.

INTRODUCTION

The cardiac action potential is generated by intricate flows of ions across myocyte cell membranes in a coordinated fashion that ultimately results in myocyte depolarization and then repolarization, which on a myocardial tissue level coordinates myocardial contraction and the heart rhythm. Modulation of the flow of these ions (primarily sodium, calcium, and potassium) in response to a variety of stimuli results in changes to the action potential. Although inward sodium and calcium currents are primarily responsible for the depolarization and plateau phases of the cardiac action potential, potassium currents contribute to the plateau phase but are primarily responsible for the repolarization phase of the cardiac action potential. Modulation of the potassium current results in alterations in cardiac action potential duration and repolarization, and abnormalities of the

potassium current can result in cardiac arrhythmias. The ANS plays an important role in the modulation of cardiac electrophysiology as a whole and has a particularly important role in modulation of the potassium current in particular. The role of the ANS in modulation of the cardiac potassium current is discussed in this review. In addition, the effect of ischemia, another modulator of cardiac cellular electrophysiology, on potassium current is also discussed.

OVERVIEW OF THE CARDIAC AUTONOMIC NERVOUS SYSTEM

The heart is richly innervated by autonomic nerves. A general understanding of the anatomy of the cardiac ANS is useful in understanding the effects of the autonomic system in normal and diseased states. The cardiac ANS can be divided into extrinsic and intrinsic systems, with the extrinsic

Disclosures: No disclosures (T.T. Tomson); Rhythm Therapeutics, Inc (R. Arora).
Bluhm Cardiovascular Institute, Northwestern University Feinberg School of Medicine, Chicago, IL, USA
* Corresponding author. Northwestern University-Feinberg School of Medicine, 251 East Huron, Feinberg 8-503, Chicago, IL 60611.
E-mail address: r-arora@northwestern.edu

Card Electrophysiol Clin 8 (2016) 349–360
http://dx.doi.org/10.1016/j.ccep.2016.01.007

ANS comprising nerves outside the heart and the intrinsic ANS made up of nerves and ganglia within the pericardium and on the epicardial surface[1,2] (**Fig. 1**).

The extrinsic cardiac ANS consists of sympathetic and parasympathetic nerves. Preganglionic sympathetic neurons originate in the spinal cord and travel to the prevertebral autonomic ganglia, including the superior cervical ganglia, the stellate ganglia, and the thoracic ganglia.[3,4] The cell bodies of the postganglionic sympathetic neurons reside in these ganglia, and postganglionic sympathetic neurons travel from these ganglia to innervate both the atrial and ventricular surfaces of the heart via the superior, middle, and inferior cardiac nerves. Preganglionic parasympathetic neurons originate in the medulla oblongata. Parasympathetic neurons travel to the heart in the vagus nerve where they terminate primarily in fats pads in the atria and superior vena cava.

The intrinsic cardiac ANS consists of sympathetic and parasympathetic neurons after they enter the pericardial sac.[5] After entering the pericardial sac, sympathetic neurons either directly innervate the myocardium or form synapses within cardiac ganglia. All parasympathetic fibers, in contrast, form synapses within the cardiac ganglia. They are concentrated within the fat pads on the epicardial surface of the atria and ventricle and generally form groups of ganglionated plexi. Within the atria, the ganglionated plexi have been located in several areas, including the superior right atrium, the posterior right atrium, the superior left atrium (LA), the posteromedial LA, and the inferolateral LA, and they have been noted to be close to the PV ostia. Ventricular ganglionated plexi primarily localize to fat pads around the aortic root and the origins of the major coronary arteries.

CELLULAR MECHANISMS OF CARDIAC AUTONOMIC SIGNALING

Several reviews have discussed the cellular mechanisms of autonomic signaling in detail and are summarized in brief.[6–8] In response to stimulation, postganglionic sympathetic neurons release norepinephrine, which exerts its effects on cardiac myocytes primarily by activating β-receptors on the myocyte cell surface. β-Receptors are one of the numerous types of 7 transmembrane domain G protein–coupled receptors. Three subtypes of β-receptors exist, with the β_1-receptors the most common on cardiac cells, accounting for approximately 80% of cardiac β-receptors.[7] The G protein–coupled receptors are associated with G proteins that consist of 3 subunits, Gα, Gβ, and Gγ. When simulated by norepinephrine, the β_1-receptor triggers conversion of guanosine triphosphate (GTP) to guanosine diphosphate (GDP) on the Gα subunit of the G protein, causing Gα to dissociate from Gβ and Gγ. The primary Gα subunit associated with β-receptors is the stimulatory $G\alpha_s$ subunit. The dissociated $G\alpha_s$ subunit is then free to activate adenylyl cyclase, which converts ATP to cyclic adenosine monophosphate

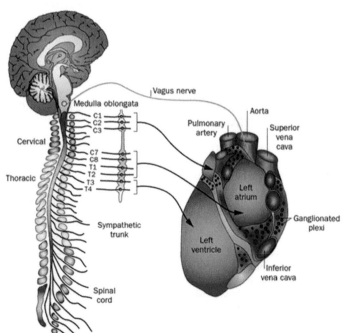

Fig. 1. Autonomic innervations of the heart. The extrinsic ANS comprises nerves outside the heart. The sympathetic ganglia include the cervical ganglia, the stellate ganglia, and the thoracic ganglia. The parasympathetic innervations of the heart arises from the vagus nerve. The intrinsic ANS is made up of nerves and ganglionated plexi within the pericardium and on the epicardial surface of the heart. (*From* Shen MJ, Choi EK, Tan AY, et al. Neural mechanisms of atrial arrhythmias. Nat Rev Cardiol 2011;9:30–9; with permission.)

(cAMP), the primary second messenger for the β-receptors. cAMP then activates protein kinase A (PKA), which phosphorylates a variety of proteins involved in calcium handling, including the L-type calcium channel (I_{CaL}), the ryanodine receptor, and phospholamban, resulting in enhanced calcium cycling. In addition, sympathetic stimulation also affects several potassium channels, in particular activation of the slow and rapid delayed rectifier potassium currents (I_{Ks} and I_{Kr}, respectively), which offsets the inward current that results from enhanced calcium inflow[9–12] (**Fig. 2**).

The parasympathetic neurons exert their influence on cardiac myocytes through the release of ACh. ACh binds to the M_2 muscarinic receptor on the myocyte surface. The M_2-receptor is another G protein–coupled receptor.[6] The Gα subunit associated with the muscarinic receptor is the inhibitor $G\alpha_i$ subunit. When ACh binds to the M_2-receptor, the receptor catalyzes the conversion of GTP to GDP on the $G\alpha_i$ subunit of the G protein coupled to the receptor. Conversion of GTP to GDP causes release of the $G\alpha_i$ subunit from the Gβγ subunit, freeing the Gβγ subunit. In the case of parasympathetic stimulation, the Gβγ subunits are the active subunits and are responsible primarily for activation of the ACh-gated potassium channel I_{K-ACh}. I_{K-ACh} is the predominant ion channel responsible for parasympathetic

effects on the action potential duration and effective refractory period (ERP) of the atrium.[13] I_{K-ACh} activation leads to action potential duration shortening that may be necessary for promoting abnormal atrial rhythms, such as AF and atrial tachycardias.

AUTONOMIC EFFECTS ON ATRIAL POTASSIUM CURRENTS: SINOATRIAL NODE AND HEART RATE

The ANS is the primary system responsible for modulating cardiac pacemaker cell automaticity and thus heart rate.[14] With brief reference to potassium currents, activation of I_{K-ACh} channels in the sinoatrial (SA) nodal and atrioventricular (AV) nodal tissue in response to parasympathetic stimulation is a major mechanism by which parasympathetic stimulation reduces heart rate and slows conduction in the AV node. Activation of I_{K-ACh} in the pacemaker cells of the SA node leads to cell membrane hyperpolarization, which decreases spontaneous firing of the SA node and reduces heart rate.[15] In addition to the effects on I_{K-ACh}, parasympathetic stimulation more directly opposes sympathetic stimulation by causing a decrease in the funny current (I_f) and I_{CaL}.[16,17] The combination of these effects results in hyperpolarization and a slower automatic depolarization

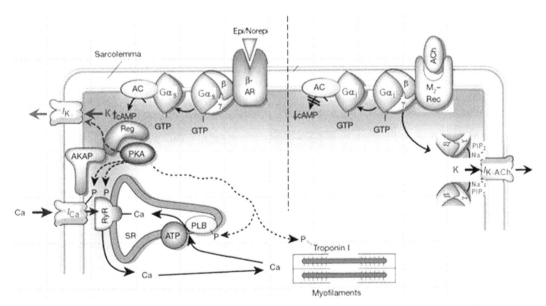

Fig. 2. Sympathetic and parasympathetic signaling pathways. AC, adenylyl cyclase; ACh, acetylcholine; AKAP, A-kinase-anchoring-proteins; ATP, adenosine triphosphate; β-AR, β-adrenergic receptor; Ca, calcium; cAMP, cyclic adenosine monophosphate; Epi, epinephrine; GTP, guanosine triphosphate; M2-Rec, M_2-receptor; Na, sodium; Norepi, norepinephrine; P, phosphate; PIP, phosphatidyl inositol bisphosphate; PKA, protein kinase A; PLB, phospholamban; reg, regulatory; RyR, ryanodine receptor; SR, sarcoplasmic reticulum. (*Adapted from* Arora R. Recent insights into the role of the autonomic nervous system in the creation of substrate for atrial fibrillation – implications for therapies targeting the atrial autonomic nervous system. Circ Arrhythm Electrophysiol 2012;5:850–59; with permission.)

of the SA nodal cells, resulting in a reduced heart rate. Although parasympathetic stimulation exerts its influence on heart rate in a large part through activation of I_{K-ACh} channels, the effect of sympathetic stimulation is driven primarily by effects on If and I_{CaL}, with sympathetic stimulation resulting in an increased heart rate by enhancing the activity of both I_f and I_{CaL}.[14,18] Sympathetic stimulation, however, also effects the activity of I_{Ks} and I_{Kr} currents, which also play a part in regulating automaticity and in leading to the action potential shortening necessary at more rapid heart rates.

ATRIAL MYOCARDIUM AND ATRIAL ARRHYTHMIAS

Autonomic effects on myocardial potassium currents are most prominent in the atria, and imbalances in the ANS and the subsequent effects on potassium currents may play a role in the genesis of diseases, such as AF, the most common sustained arrhythmia in clinical practice. Several studies have demonstrated an association between autonomic effects and AF. For example, exercise-induced AF may be sympathetically driven,[19] whereas the parasympathetic nervous system may play a role in AF in young patients with no structural heart disease.[20] The unique autonomic innervations of the LA and the autonomic effects on potassium currents, in particular I_{K-ACh}, may be a key contributor to AF. Although there are autonomic nerves throughout the atria, this innervation is heterogeneous. The PVs and posterior LA (PLA) have a unique autonomic profile in comparison to the rest of the atria, and these differences in autonomic innervations and the subsequent electrophysiologic effects on potassium

currents may play an important contributing role in the genesis of arrhythmias like AF.

The unique distribution of autonomic innervation of the PVs and PLA was demonstrated in a canine study by Arora and colleagues.[21] In this study, the distribution and physiology of sympathetic and parasympathetic nerves in various parts of the LA were investigated. The study found that both parasympathetic and sympathetic fibers most richly innervated the PLA, with nerve bundles colocalized mainly in fibrofatty tissue but also in the surrounding myocardium (**Fig. 3**). In the PLA, parasympathetic nerves were more numerous than sympathetic nerves. Not only did autonomic nerves localize to the PLA, with a predominance of parasympathetic fibers, but also M_2-receptor density was significantly more pronounced in the PLA than in the rest of the LA. Finally, the study showed that because a majority of parasympathetic fibers and M_2-receptors in the LA are located in the PLA, selective parasympathetic blockade in the PLA significantly altered vagal responsiveness in the entire LA. These findings were applied to the effects on AF inducibility. Selective blockade of the parasympathetic effects in the PLA resulted in attenuation of parasympathetic effects in the entire LA and resulted in near complete elimination of vagal-induced AF in this model, demonstrating the importance of the PLA and parasympathetic activity in the induction of AF.

Another canine study by Arora and colleagues[22] specifically investigated the electrophysiologic profile of the PVs and LA and found heterogeneous electrophysiologic responses in the LA (**Fig. 4**). In this study, the effect of modulating autonomic tone on ERPs in various part of the LA was investigated. In addition, these findings were correlated with I_{K-ACh} distribution within the LA. The study

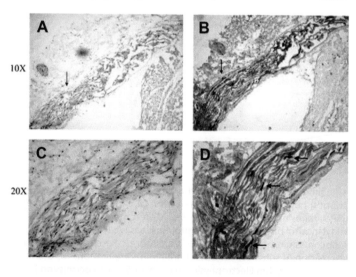

Fig. 3. Colocalization of sympathetic and parasympathetic nerves in a PV. (A) Hematoxylin stain of a single large nerve fiber (arrow) at ×10 magnification. (B) Double-staining of a nerve fiber (arrow) with sympathetic elements in blue and parasympathetic elements in brown at ×10 magnification. (C) Hematoxylin stain of a single large nerve fiber at ×20 magnification. (D) Double-staining of a nerve fiber with sympathetic elements in blue (arrows) and parasympathetic elements in brown at ×20 magnification. (Adapted from Arora R, Ulphani JS, Villuendas R, et al. Neural substrate for atrial fibrillation: implications for targeted parasympathetic blockade in the posterior left atrium. Am J Physiol Heart Circ Physiol 2008;294:H134–44; with permission.)

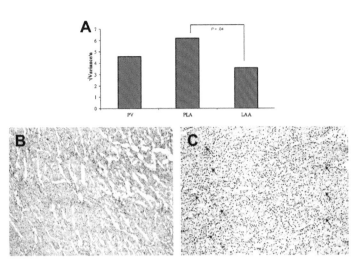

Fig. 4. Differences in heterogeneity of parasympathetic-induced ERP shortening correspond with differences in heterogeneity of I_{K-ACh} distribution in the PLA and left atrial appendage (LAA). (A) Heterogeneity in ERP shortening (measured as $\sqrt{Variance/N}$) is greater in the PLA than the LAA. (B) Immunohistochemical staining for I_{K-ACh} in the LAA is very homogeneous (magnification 10×). (C) Immunohistochemical staining for I_{K-ACh} in the PLA is significantly more heterogeneous, with arrows indicating areas of heterogeneous staining (magnification 10×). (Adapted from Arora R, Ng J, Ulphani J, et al. Unique autonomic profile of the pulmonary veins and posterior left atrium. J Am Coll Cardiol 2007;49:1340–48; with permission.)

showed autonomic stimulation resulted in a greater degree of ERP change in the LAA compared with the PV and PLA. These findings correlated with a greater concentration of I_{K-ACh} channels expressed in the LAA compared with the rest of the LA. Although the cumulative effect of changes in autonomic tone was greatest in the LAA, the heterogeneity of changes in ERP (measured by the variance of changes in ERP within the different areas of the LA) was significantly greater in the PLA than the LAA. This increased heterogeneity in ERP changes in response to autonomic tone within the PLA correlated with a more heterogeneous distribution of I_{K-ACh} channel concentration within the PLA, as identified by immunohistochemical staining. Other studies have shown that I_{K-ACh} concentrations are higher in the LA than the RA,[23] but this study highlights the heterogeneity of I_{K-ACh} distribution within the tissue of the LA. Because heterogeneity of ERP shortening within the LA is thought to be a major contributor to the induction and maintenance of AF, allowing for re-entry within the atrium to occur,[24] the unique electrophysiologic properties of the PLA, with heterogeneous I_{K-ACh} distribution and ERP changes in response to changes in autonomic tone, in combination with the previous study's finding of increased parasympathetic nerve innervations and M_2-receptor concentration in the PLA, suggest the importance of the PLA as a contributor to AF induction. These data also support the idea that I_{K-ACh} plays an important role in vagal influence on AF.[25]

Human studies have also confirmed the heterogeneous distribution of autonomic nerves in the atria. In a human study by Chevalier and colleagues,[26] heterogeneous nerve distribution was described in the region of the PV and surrounding LA. The study showed higher concentrations of epicardial nerve fibers and ganglia at the ostia of the 4 PVs and in the PLA. Tan and colleagues[27] also demonstrated that the highest concentrations of autonomic nerves were at the junction of the PVs and the LA and that sympathetic and parasympathetic nerves were colocalized in the human LA. A human study by Deneke and colleagues[28] again showed that nerve density was higher in the region of the PV ostia and antrum compared with other areas of the atria. The study also demonstrated a high degree of colocalization of sympathetic and parasympathetic nerves within the atria. These findings in humans seem consistent with the findings of animal studies.

Although the studies discussed previously investigated the heterogeneous autonomic innervations of the LA and the heterogeneous effects of modulation of autonomic tone in the LA potassium channels and currents in normal subjects, studies have also investigated changes in autonomic innervations of the atria and subsequent effects on potassium current seen in the setting of structural heart disease and showed that these autonomic alterations may play a role in the genesis of AF. Ng and colleagues[29] studied the effects of congestive heart failure (CHF) on autonomic remodeling in the atria and subsequent changes in the electrophysiologic properties of the atria in a canine model of CHF. In this study, CHF was induced by rapid ventricular pacing over a period of weeks. CHF dogs demonstrated remodeling of both the sympathetic and parasympathetic innervations of the LA. In both normal and CHF dogs, autonomic nerves were located in the fibrofatty tissue overlaying the epicardium, with colocalization of both sympathetic and parasympathetic nerves. In CHF, autonomic innervation was increased in the LA, as noted by increases in nerve bundle size and density of cardiac ganglia. Neural remodeling was most prominent in the PVs and PLA, which correlates with the baseline increased innervations of the PLA, discussed previously. Sympathetic remodeling was suggested by both an increase in sympathetic nerve fiber density and an increase in β_1-receptor density, which was accompanied by an increased effect of sympathetic stimulation on atrial ERPs, particularly in the PLA and PVs. The increased parasympathetic innervation, on the other hand, was not associated with any change in the M_2-receptor activity, which remained unchanged compared with control dogs. This observation was accounted for by an increase in acetylcholinesterase activity, which caused a reduction in synaptic ACh and thus a reduction in M_2-receptor stimulation. These changes led to a decreased effect of parasympathetic stimulation on atrial ERP, likely through altered effects on I_{K-ACh} potassium current. Despite the decreased parasympathetic responsiveness of the LA, some effect of parasympathetic tone was maintained in the LA. The continued effect of parasympathetic tone was demonstrated most importantly by the fact that parasympathetic blockade led to a significant decrease in the duration of induced AF, which also suggests that parasympathetic activity is an important contributor to AF substrate in CHF and that parasympathetic blockade may be a potential target for AF treatment. Both sympathetic and parasympathetic blockade together did not result in a further decreased in AF duration, although it did decrease AF dominant frequency. This finding suggests that the sympathetic innervation may play a more modulatory role in AF induction and that parasympathetic innervation and its downstream effects on potassium current is the dominant autonomic limb affecting the atrium in CHF.

Canine models of AF induced by rapid atrial pacing (RAP) have also been used to study the effects of AF on autonomic innervation and atrial electrophysiology. A study by Jayachandran and colleagues[30] showed that RAP-induced AF in dogs resulted in both autonomic and electrophysiologic remodeling of the atria. After 4 weeks of RAP, all paced dogs developed sustained AF. PET of the atria was performed using carbon-11 hydroxyephedrine (HED) to label sympathetic nerve terminals. HED activity in the atria was significantly greater in the atria of paced dogs, and these findings correlated with increased norepinephrine levels in atrial tissue samples of paced dog, suggesting an increased sympathetic innervation in paced dogs with AF. HED retention

was also noted to be significantly more heterogeneous in the atria of paced dogs compared with controls, which correlates with the findings in CHF models of AF. Another study by Chang and colleagues[31] looked at histologic evidence for autonomic changes in a canine models of RAP-induced AF. Dogs that had sustained AF induced by RAP had a significantly higher density of atrial sympathetic innervation compared with control animals. In addition, the histologic data showed a heterogeneous distribution of nerves within the atria, correlating with the imaging data from the previous study. These findings suggest the importance of autonomic changes in AF and likely underlie some of the changes in potassium current seen in AF. In another study, Nishida and colleagues[32] investigated the effects of PV encircling ablation and linear left atrial roof lines on AF induced by RAP in a canine model. PV encircling ablation, which can affect autonomic ganglia near the PVs and result in autonomic denervation, suppressed AF initiation in this canine model by prolonging left atrial ERPs.

Similar changes in autonomic innervation in subjects with AF have been observed in human subjects. Gould and colleagues[33] investigated atrial sympathetic innervation in patients with and without AF undergoing cardiac surgery. The right atrial appendage of 24 patients (half in sinus rhythm and half in persistent AF) were collected during surgery, and the degree of sympathetic innervation was examined by immunostaining for sympathetic nerves. Sympathetic innervation was significantly higher in the atrial tissue of the AF cohort compared with the patients in sinus rhythm. In addition, right atrial tissue was more densely innervated than left atrial tissue in patients with AF. The heterogeneously increased sympathetic innervation seen in patients with persistent AF corresponds to that seen in the animal models. Sympathetic innervation seems to increase the most in the right atrium, whereas changes in parasympathetic innervation seem greatest in the LA. This heterogeneity of autonomic innervation and its subsequent effects on potassium currents and atrial ERPs may play a role in the initiation and maintenance of clinical AF.

These studies demonstrating the heterogeneous effects of autonomic innervation in both normal hearts and in the setting of structural heart disease highlight the importance of the ANS as a contributing factor to atrial arrhythmias. These data also underscore the potential importance of the ANS as a suitable therapeutic target in AF in both normal and diseased hearts.

A final potassium current in the atria that is at least indirectly modulated by the autonomic system is the small conductance calcium-activated potassium (SK) current. SK channels also likely may play a role in the cardiac arrhythmias. They are sensitive to intracellular calcium levels and link intracellular calcium concentrations and cellular membrane potentials at the myocyte level and are important in modulation of action potential duration and repolarization, particularly of atrial myocytes.[34,35] SK channels have been found up-regulated in heart failure in both animal models and in humans.[36–39] Although a specific modulation of the SK channel by the ANS has not been clearly shown, some studies suggest that SK channels play a role in AF,[40,41] possibly by modulating the membrane potentials in response to different calcium loading situations that result from different degrees of sympathetic stimulation. As such, SK current may represent a therapeutic target for AF treatment.

MODULATION OF AUTONOMIC EFFECTS ON ATRIAL POTASSIUM CURRENT AS A POSSIBLE THERAPEUTIC TARGET FOR ATRIAL FIBRILLATION

The observations that the ANS modulates atrial myocardial electrophysiologic properties, particularly through parasympathetic alterations in I_{K-ACh}, have led to the idea that modulation of the intrinsic cardiac nervous system may be one therapeutic avenue for the treatment of atrial arrhythmias, in particular AF. At a gross anatomic level, ganglionated plexi ablation has been attempted as a way of reducing autonomic innervation of the LA, thus reducing AF burden by limiting the effects of the ANS on the atria. One method of ablating ganglionated plexi is to use high-frequency stimulation to identify ganglionated plexi at the time of ablation, and use of this method to identify ganglionated plexi for ablation in addition to standard PV isolation has shown promising results in treating AF.[42] Another approach to autonomic denervation is an anatomically based approach to ablation. A randomized controlled trial performed by Katritsis and colleagues[43] showed the benefit of anatomically based GP ablation for AF. In this trial, 242 patients with paroxysmal AF were randomized to either standard PV isolation, anatomic ablation of left atrial GP, or standard PV isolation plus left atrial GP ablation. At 2 years of follow-up, patients who received standard PV isolation plus left atrial GP ablation had a significantly higher freedom from recurrent AF (74%) compared with either PV isolation alone (56%) or left atrial GP ablation alone (48%). A recent meta-analysis of cardiac autonomic denervation in addition to standard PV ablation for AF also suggests improved freedom from

recurrent AF with cardiac autonomic denervation.[44] This strategy of treating AF may be effective because cardiac autonomic denervation reduces the heterogeneity of ERP changes in the LA seen as a result of the ANS's effect on heterogeneously distributed potassium channels, particularly in the PLA where much of the ablation is performed.

In addition to modification of the gross anatomy of the LA by ablation, more targeted approaches of modulating the potassium currents in the atria through alteration in cell signaling at a cellular level may also be a target for AF treatment. A targeted approach to modulating the effects of the ANS on potassium current is of interest because there are several drawbacks to the current strategy of GP ablation. First, because sympathetic and parasympathetic fibers are colocalized, ablation nonselectively destroys both limbs of the ANS. Second, ablation carries other risks, such as damage to the atrial myocardium or other structures surrounding the LA. Third, because ablation targets only specific areas, some nerves could be left unaffected by ablation, limiting the overall effect of ablation. Given these drawbacks, a more targeted approach to modulation of the ANS using molecular or biologic approaches to target ANS cell signaling has been investigated.

One biologic approach to treating AF is to modulate I_{K-ACh} activity and potassium current by targeting the parasympathetic G protein–coupled receptor signaling mechanism. As discussed previously, M_2-receptor stimulation by the parasympathetic nervous system leads to activation of the I_{K-ACh} through a G protein–coupled mechanism, leading to increased potassium current and atrial ERP shortening that promotes initiation and maintenance of AF. Aistrup and colleagues[45,46] have shown in 2 studies that inhibition of G-protein signaling in the atrium can lead to attenuated parasympathetic effects in the atrium. In a proof-of-concept animal study, G protein–inhibitory peptides targeting the C-terminus of the $G\alpha_{i/o}$ subunit, the subunit associated with parasympathetic M_2-receptors, were used to inhibit parasympathetic signaling in the atrium.[46] Peptides targeting the C-terminal portion of $G\alpha_i$ were selectively delivered to the PLA by direct injection into the myocardium with associated electroporation. These $G\alpha_i$ C-terminal peptides ($G\alpha_i$ctp) selectively inhibited parasympathetic signaling by disrupting binding of the native $G\alpha_i$ to the G-protein complex associated with the M_2-receptor and reducing signal transduction. Injection of these inhibitory peptides into the PLA resulted in prolongation of the atrial ERP both at baseline and during parasympathetic stimulation, demonstrating the effects of reduced activation of I_{K-ACh}. A second animal study tested the ability of minigene plasmids expressing inhibitory Gα C-terminal peptides to modulate parasympathetic stimulation and downstream potassium current.[45] In this gene-based approach, plasmid DNA expressing either inhibitory Gα$_i$ctp alone or in combination with inhibitory Gα$_o$ctp (Gα$_o$ C-terminal peptide) were injected into the PLA of canines and incorporated into the cells via electroporation. Effects on atrial ERPs and AF inducibility were investigated under conditions of parasympathetic stimulation. When both inhibitory Gα$_i$ctp and Gα$_o$ctp were expressed in the PLA, parasympathetic-induced atrial ERP shortening as well as AF inducibility were almost entirely eliminated (**Fig. 5**). Both of these studies showed that parasympathetic denervation, resulting in decreased I$_{K-ACh}$ activity, can be achieved on a selective basis by introduction of small inhibitory peptides in a targeted fashion into the LA.

AUTONOMIC CONTROL OF POTASSIUM CURRENT IN THE VENTRICLE

Although AF seems to be promoted by parasympathetic stimulation, parasympathetic stimulation may be protective against ventricular arrhythmias, such as ventricular fibrillation.[47] The difference in parasympathetic effect between the atrium and ventricle may be explained by differences in I$_{K-ACh}$ distribution between the atria and ventricles and thus the effect of parasympathetic stimulation on potassium current and refractory periods in each chamber. Whereas, I$_{K-ACh}$ is abundant in most

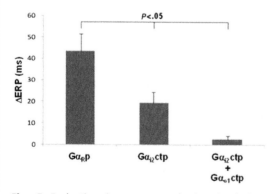

Fig. 5. Reduction in parasympathetic stimulation-induced ERP shortening in the canine PLA by plasmid DNA vectors (minigenes) expressing Gα$_i$ctp injected in the PLA either alone or in combination with a minigene expressing Gα$_o$ctp compared with injection of a control minigene expressing scrambled peptide (Gα$_R$p). (*Adapted from* Aistrup GL, Cokic I, Ng J, et al. Targeted nonviral gene-based inhibition of Galpha(i/o)-mediated vagal signaling in the posterior left atrium decreases vagal-induced atrial fibrillation. Heart Rhythm 2011;8(11):1722–9; with permission.)

atrial tissue,[46] I$_{K-ACh}$ is expressed to a much lower degree in the ventricle, with ventricular myocytes having little or no I$_{K-ACh}$.[48] This finding may be responsible for the observed fact that, although parasympathetic stimulation significantly shortens the action potential duration in the atria, it either lengthens the action potential duration[49] or shortens it by a significantly smaller amount in the ventricle.[50,51]

Although there is little I$_{K-ACh}$ in ventricular myocardium, the ANS may exert effects on ventricular potassium currents through effects on the I$_{Ks}$ and I$_{Kr}$, which are largely responsible for the repolarization phase of the cardiac action potential. In normal hearts, effects on these currents in response to autonomic inputs allows for dynamic control of the cardiac action potential to match diastolic filling with changes in heart rate caused by changes in autonomic tone.

I$_{Ks}$ may be the potassium current in the ventricle that is most affected by the changes in sympathetic stimulation.[52] Sympathetic stimulation through the β-receptor results in an increased I$_{Ks}$ current, through PKA-mediated phosphorylation of the *KCNQ1* subunit, and shortens the action potential duration and thus myocardial repolarization, which is necessary to ensure diastolic filling time during higher heart rates that also result from sympathetic stimulation. Loss-of-function mutations in the *KCNQ1* subunit of the I$_{Ks}$ channel are linked to the most common long QT syndrome (LQTS), LQTS type 1 (LQTS1), which is associated with prolongation of the cardiac action potential and sudden death.[53] Adverse events and cardiac arrhythmias in patients with LQTS1 are particularly associated with activities, such as exercise or swimming, in which sympathetic stimulation would normally result in increased I$_{Ks}$ current.[54] In patients with LQTS1 and mutations in the I$_{Ks}$ channel subunit, however, sympathetic stimulation paradoxically tends to cause APD prolongation, presumably because of an imbalance in the repolarizing I$_{Ks}$ current and other ion currents. Modulation of the ANS with β-blocking drugs that reduce sympathetic stimulation on the heart has been shown to reduce the risk of adverse events in patients with LQTS1.[55]

The other main delayed rectifier potassium current, I$_{Kr}$, may also be regulated by the ANS in the ventricle. Like I$_{Ks}$, I$_{Kr}$ is involved in the repolarization phase of the cardiac action potential. Mutations in the *KCNH2* subunit of I$_{Kr}$ are associated with the second most common form of LQTS, LQTS2.[56] Sympathetic stimulation modulates I$_{Kr}$ current in a variety of ways. Sympathetic stimulation, through the activation of Gα$_s$, results in an increase in intracellular cAMP concentration, which can directly interact with the I_{Kr} channel, and in PKA-dependent phosphorylation of the I_{Kr} channel.[9,10]

MODULATION OF VENTRICULAR AUTONOMIC TONE AS A TREATMENT OF VENTRICULAR ARRHYTHMIAS

As in the atrium, where ablation of autonomic ganglia may serve as a method of reducing atrial arrhythmias, modulation of autonomic input to the ventricle may reduce the risk of ventricular arrhythmias. Autonomic denervation of the ventricle by cervical sympathectomy alters sympathetic stimulation of the ventricle and can reduce the risk of ventricular arrhythmias in some patients, particularly in patients with syndromes associated with congenital sudden cardiac death, such as LQTS and catecholaminergic polymorphic ventricular tachycardia.[57–59] Another method of modulating autonomic input to the ventricle, which may be effective in reducing ventricular arrhythmias, is spinal cord stimulation, which may result in parasympathetic stimulation and sympathetic inhibition.[60,61] These therapeutic treatments of ventricular arrhythmias almost certainly exert their antiarrhythmic effect, at least in part, by reducing the modulation of autonomic stimulation-associated changes in potassium current in the myocardium. Further elucidation of the exact mechanism by which modulation of the extrinsic autonomic system leads to antiarrhythmic effects, particularly on potassium current modulation, may lead to the identification of more specific targets for treatments of ventricular arrhythmias.

EFFECTS OF ISCHEMIA ON POTASSIUM CURRENTS

In addition to autonomic stimulation, other factors, such as ischemia, can modulate the cardiac potassium current. The ATP-sensitive inwardly rectifying potassium channel (I_{K-ATP}), which is inhibited by ATP, modulates potassium current as a function of the metabolic state of the heart.[62] Under normal conditions with a normal intracellular ATP/ADP ratio, I_{K-ATP} remains closed. During states of ischemia or hypoxia, the relative concentration of ATP to ADP decreases. The decreased ATP/ADP ratio that results from ischemia leads to activation of I_{K-ATP}, helping to preserve the resting membrane potential and to reduce the cardiac action potential duration, cardiac contraction, and thus energy/ATP usage during times of stress on the myocardium. In this way, I_{K-ATP} may function to protect the myocardium from the effects of ischemia. Knockout mice lacking Kir6.2, a the

pore-forming subunit of I_{K-ATP}, have a reduced ability to perform exercise, a compromised cardiac performance in response to sympathetic stimulation, and an increased susceptibility to arrhythmias and sudden death as a response to sympathetic stimulation.[63] I_{K-ATP} may also play a role in ischemic preconditioning, the phenomenon whereby brief periods of ischemia followed by reperfusion can result in reduced myocardial injury to an ischemic insult. Animal studies have shown not only that agonists of the I_{K-ATP} channel reproduce the effects of preconditioning but also that I_{K-ATP} blockers prevent the protective effects of ischemic preconditioning.[64–66] Although the initial activation of I_{K-ATP} in response to ischemia may be protective, prolonged I_{K-ATP} activation may actually lead to early repolarization and thus may be proarrhythmic.[67] Early repolarization syndromes associated with ventricular fibrillation have been associated with gain of function mutations in the I_{K-ATP} channel.[68,69]

Modulators of I_{K-ATP} channel activity may be a potential target for antiarrhythmic and anti-ischemic mediations. I_{K-ATP} activators and inhibitors generally act on the sulfonylureas subunit of the channel. I_{K-ATP} channels are present in many tissues, including cardiac myocytes, insulin-secreting pancreatic cells where they regulate insulin secretion, and vascular smooth muscle where they regulate muscle constriction. Nonselective I_{K-ATP} blockers or activators may, therefore, cause abnormalities in regulation of blood glucose levels or blood pressure through their effects on other tissue. Cardiac-specific I_{K-ATP} blockers have the potential to reduce the effects of ischemia on cardiac action potential shortening without the sided effects of nonselective agents.[70,71] On the other hand, I_{K-ATP} channel openers may be useful in simulating ischemic preconditioning and may be protective in the setting of acute ischemia.[71] Again, selective activators of I_{K-ATP} are needed to avoid the unwanted side effects, such as unwanted changes in blood pressure, from changes in activation of I_{K-ATP} in vascular smooth muscle. Focus has been placed on evaluating the properties of drugs that have specificity for either the sarcolemmal or the mitochondrial I_{K-ATP} channels. Mitochondrial I_{K-ATP} activators, in particular, have shown promising anti-ischemic properties with minimal side effects on vascular tone.[72]

SUMMARY

Modulation of the potassium current in the heart plays an important part in cardiac electrophysiology by altering the cardiac action potential duration. The ANS is one major modulator of the cardiac potassium current. Changes in autonomic tone in response to changes in physiologic states lead to physiologic alterations in potassium current, affecting cardiac action potential duration and repolarization. Abnormalities of autonomic regulation, such as those seen in heart failure, may contribute to cardiac arrhythmias. Understanding the mechanisms by which the ANS alters potassium current to cause diseases, such as AF, can potentially lead to more targeted treatments of these conditions. The same holds true for understanding other modulators of potassium currents, such as the effect of ischemia on ATP-sensitive potassium currents, a better understanding of which could lead to improved management of cardiac arrhythmias.

REFERENCES

1. Kapa S, Venkatachalam KL, Asirvatham SJ. The autonomic nervous system in cardiac electrophysiology: an elegant interaction and emerging concepts. Cardiol Rev 2010;18(6):275–84.
2. Kapa S, DeSimone CV, Asirvatham SJ. Innervation of the heart: an invisible grid within a black box. Trends Cardiovasc Med 2016;26(3):245–57.
3. Smith DC. Synaptic sites in sympathetic and vagal cardioaccelerator nerves of the dog. Am J Physiol 1970;218(6):1618–23.
4. Randall WC, Armour JA, Geis WP, et al. Regional cardiac distribution of the sympathetic nerves. Fed Proc 1972;31(4):1199–208.
5. Armour JA, Murphy DA, Yuan BX, et al. Gross and microscopic anatomy of the human intrinsic cardiac nervous system. Anat Rec 1997;247(2):289–98.
6. Kurachi Y. G protein regulation of cardiac muscarinic potassium channel. Am J Physiol 1995;269(4 Pt 1):C821–30.
7. Salazar NC, Chen J, Rockman HA. Cardiac GPCRs: GPCR signaling in healthy and failing hearts. Biochim Biophys Acta 2007;1768(4):1006–18.
8. Wess J. G-protein-coupled receptors: molecular mechanisms involved in receptor activation and selectivity of G-protein recognition. FASEB J 1997;11(5):346–54.
9. Thomas D, Zhang W, Karle CA, et al. Deletion of protein kinase A phosphorylation sites in the HERG potassium channel inhibits activation shift by protein kinase A. J Biol Chem 1999;274(39):27457–62.
10. Cui J, Melman Y, Palma E, et al. Cyclic AMP regulates the HERG K(+) channel by dual pathways. Curr Biol 2000;10(11):671–4.
11. Marx SO, Kurokawa J, Reiken S, et al. Requirement of a macromolecular signaling complex for beta adrenergic receptor modulation of the KCNQ1-KCNE1 potassium channel. Science 2002;295(5554):496–9.
12. Terrenoire C, Houslay MD, Baillie GS, et al. The cardiac IKs potassium channel macromolecular complex includes the phosphodiesterase PDE4D3. J Biol Chem 2009;284(14):9140–6.
13. Lomax AE, Rose RA, Giles WR. Electrophysiological evidence for a gradient of G protein-gated K+ current in adult mouse atria. Br J Pharmacol 2003;140(3):576–84.
14. Mangoni ME, Nargeot J. Genesis and regulation of the heart automaticity. Physiol Rev 2008;88(3):919–82.
15. Noma A, Trautwein W. Relaxation of the ACh-induced potassium current in the rabbit sinoatrial node cell. Pflugers Arch 1978;377(3):193–200.
16. DiFrancesco D, Ducouret P, Robinson RB. Muscarinic modulation of cardiac rate at low acetylcholine concentrations. Science 1989;243(4891):669–71.
17. Fischmeister R, Hartzell HC. Mechanism of action of acetylcholine on calcium current in single cells from frog ventricle. J Physiol 1986;376:183–202.
18. Brown HF, DiFrancesco D, Noble SJ. How does adrenaline accelerate the heart? Nature 1979;280(5719):235–6.
19. Chen PS, Tan AY. Autonomic nerve activity and atrial fibrillation. Heart Rhythm 2007;4(3 Suppl):S61–4.
20. Coumel P. Paroxysmal atrial fibrillation: a disorder of autonomic tone? Eur Heart J 1994;15(Suppl A):9–16.
21. Arora R, Ulphani JS, Villuendas R, et al. Neural substrate for atrial fibrillation: implications for targeted parasympathetic blockade in the posterior left atrium. Am J Physiol Heart Circ Physiol 2008;294(1):H134–44.
22. Arora R, Ng J, Ulphani J, et al. Unique autonomic profile of the pulmonary veins and posterior left atrium. J Am Coll Cardiol 2007;49(12):1340–8.
23. Sarmast F, Kolli A, Zaitsev A, et al. Cholinergic atrial fibrillation: I(K,ACh) gradients determine unequal left/right atrial frequencies and rotor dynamics. Cardiovasc Res 2003;59(4):863–73.
24. Liu L, Nattel S. Differing sympathetic and vagal effects on atrial fibrillation in dogs: role of refractoriness heterogeneity. Am J Physiol 1997;273(2 Pt 2):H805–16.
25. Dobrev D, Friedrich A, Voigt N, et al. The G protein-gated potassium current I(K,ACh) is constitutively active in patients with chronic atrial fibrillation. Circulation 2005;112(24):3697–706.
26. Chevalier P, Tabib A, Meyronnet D, et al. Quantitative study of nerves of the human left atrium. Heart Rhythm 2005;2(5):518–22.
27. Tan AY, Li H, Wachsmann-Hogiu S, et al. Autonomic innervation and segmental muscular disconnections at the human pulmonary vein-atrial junction: implications for catheter ablation of atrial-pulmonary vein junction. J Am Coll Cardiol 2006;48(1):132–43.
28. Deneke T, Chaar H, de Groot JR, et al. Shift in the pattern of autonomic atrial innervation in subjects

with persistent atrial fibrillation. Heart Rhythm 2011; 8(9):1357–63.

29. Ng J, Villuendas R, Cokic I, et al. Autonomic remodeling in the left atrium and pulmonary veins in heart failure: creation of a dynamic substrate for atrial fibrillation. Circ Arrhythm Electrophysiol 2011;4(3): 388–96.

30. Jayachandran JV, Sih HJ, Winkle W, et al. Atrial fibrillation produced by prolonged rapid atrial pacing is associated with heterogeneous changes in atrial sympathetic innervation. Circulation 2000;101(10): 1185–91.

31. Chang CM, Wu TJ, Zhou S, et al. Nerve sprouting and sympathetic hyperinnervation in a canine model of atrial fibrillation produced by prolonged right atrial pacing. Circulation 2001;103(1):22–5.

32. Nishida K, Sarrazin JF, Fujiki A, et al. Roles of the left atrial roof and pulmonary veins in the anatomic substrate for persistent atrial fibrillation and ablation in a canine model. J Am Coll Cardiol 2010;56(21): 1728–36.

33. Gould PA, Yii M, McLean C, et al. Evidence for increased atrial sympathetic innervation in persistent human atrial fibrillation. Pacing Clin Electrophysiol 2006;29(8):821–9.

34. Zhang XD, Lieu DK, Chiamvimonvat N. Small-conductance Ca2+ -activated K+ channels and cardiac arrhythmias. Heart Rhythm 2015;12(8): 1845–51.

35. Skibsbye L, Poulet C, Diness JG, et al. Small-conductance calcium-activated potassium (SK) channels contribute to action potential repolarization in human atria. Cardiovasc Res 2014;103(1): 156–67.

36. Chua SK, Chang PC, Maruyama M, et al. Small-conductance calcium-activated potassium channel and recurrent ventricular fibrillation in failing rabbit ventricles. Circ Res 2011;108(8):971–9.

37. Hsieh YC, Chang PC, Hsueh CH, et al. Apamin-sensitive potassium current modulates action potential duration restitution and arrhythmogenesis of failing rabbit ventricles. Circ Arrhythm Electrophysiol 2013;6(2):410–8.

38. Chang PC, Turker I, Lopshire JC, et al. Heterogeneous upregulation of apamin-sensitive potassium currents in failing human ventricles. J Am Heart Assoc 2013;2(1):e004713.

39. Qi XY, Diness JG, Brundel BJ, et al. Role of small-conductance calcium-activated potassium channels in atrial electrophysiology and fibrillation in the dog. Circulation 2014;129(4):430–40.

40. Ellinor PT, Lunetta KL, Glazer NL, et al. Common variants in KCNN3 are associated with lone atrial fibrillation. Nat Genet 2010;42(3):240–4.

41. Ellinor PT, Lunetta KL, Albert CM, et al. Meta-analysis identifies six new susceptibility loci for atrial fibrillation. Nat Genet 2012;44(6):670–5.

42. Po SS, Nakagawa H, Jackman WM. Localization of left atrial ganglionated plexi in patients with atrial fibrillation. J Cardiovasc Electrophysiol 2009; 20(10):1186–9.

43. Katritsis DG, Pokushalov E, Romanov A, et al. Autonomic denervation added to pulmonary vein isolation for paroxysmal atrial fibrillation: a randomized clinical trial. J Am Coll Cardiol 2013;62(24):2318–25.

44. Zhang Y, Wang Z, Zhang Y, et al. Efficacy of cardiac autonomic denervation for atrial fibrillation: a meta-analysis. J Cardiovasc Electrophysiol 2012;23(6): 592–600.

45. Aistrup GL, Cokic I, Ng J, et al. Targeted nonviral gene-based inhibition of Galpha(i/o)-mediated vagal signaling in the posterior left atrium decreases vagal-induced atrial fibrillation. Heart Rhythm 2011; 8(11):1722–9.

46. Aistrup GL, Villuendas R, Ng J, et al. Targeted G-protein inhibition as a novel approach to decrease vagal atrial fibrillation by selective parasympathetic attenuation. Cardiovasc Res 2009;83(3):481–92.

47. Ando M, Katare RG, Kakinuma Y, et al. Efferent vagal nerve stimulation protects heart against ischemia-induced arrhythmias by preserving connexin43 protein. Circulation 2005;112(2):164–70.

48. Dobrzynski H, Marples DD, Musa H, et al. Distribution of the muscarinic K+ channel proteins Kir3.1 and Kir3.4 in the ventricle, atrium, and sinoatrial node of heart. J Histochem Cytochem 2001;49(10): 1221–34.

49. Hoffman BF, Suckling EE. Cardiac cellular potentials; effect of vagal stimulation and acetylcholine. Am J Physiol 1953;173(2):312–20.

50. Zhang Y, Mazgalev TN. Arrhythmias and vagus nerve stimulation. Heart Fail Rev 2011;16(2):147–61.

51. Zang WJ, Chen LN, Yu XJ. Progress in the study of vagal control of cardiac ventricles. Sheng Li Xue Bao 2005;57(6):659–72.

52. Lo CF, Numann R. Independent and exclusive modulation of cardiac delayed rectifying K+ current by protein kinase C and protein kinase A. Circ Res 1998;83(10):995–1002.

53. Wang Q, Curran ME, Splawski I, et al. Positional cloning of a novel potassium channel gene: KVLQT1 mutations cause cardiac arrhythmias. Nat Genet 1996;12(1):17–23.

54. Schwartz PJ, Priori SG, Spazzolini C, et al. Genotype-phenotype correlation in the long-QT syndrome: gene-specific triggers for life-threatening arrhythmias. Circulation 2001;103(1):89–95.

55. Moss AJ, Zareba W, Hall WJ, et al. Effectiveness and limitations of beta-blocker therapy in congenital long-QT syndrome. Circulation 2000;101(6):616–23.

56. Curran ME, Splawski I, Timothy KW, et al. A molecular basis for cardiac arrhythmia: HERG mutations cause long QT syndrome. Cell 1995; 80(5):795–803.

57. Scott PA, Sandilands AJ, Morris GE, et al. Successful treatment of catecholaminergic polymorphic ventricular tachycardia with bilateral thoracoscopic sympathectomy. Heart Rhythm 2008;5(10):1461–3.

58. Schwartz PJ, Priori SG, Cerrone M, et al. Left cardiac sympathetic denervation in the management of high-risk patients affected by the long-QT syndrome. Circulation 2004;109(15):1826–33.

59. Wilde AA, Bhuiyan ZA, Crotti L, et al. Left cardiac sympathetic denervation for catecholaminergic polymorphic ventricular tachycardia. N Engl J Med 2008;358(19):2024–9.

60. Issa ZF, Zhou X, Ujhelyi MR, et al. Thoracic spinal cord stimulation reduces the risk of ischemic ventricular arrhythmias in a postinfarction heart failure canine model. Circulation 2005;111(24):3217–20.

61. Lopshire JC, Zhou X, Dusa C, et al. Spinal cord stimulation improves ventricular function and reduces ventricular arrhythmias in a canine postinfarction heart failure model. Circulation 2009;120(4):286–94.

62. Noma A. ATP-regulated K+ channels in cardiac muscle. Nature 1983;305(5930):147–8.

63. Zingman LV, Hodgson DM, Bast PH, et al. Kir6.2 is required for adaptation to stress. Proc Natl Acad Sci U S A 2002;99(20):13278–83.

64. Gross GJ, Auchampach JA. Blockade of ATP-sensitive potassium channels prevents myocardial preconditioning in dogs. Circ Res 1992;70(2): 223–33.

65. D'Alonzo AJ, Darbenzio RB, Parham CS, et al. Effects of intracoronary cromakalim on postischaemic contractile function and action potential duration. Cardiovasc Res 1992;26(11):1046–53.

66. Schulz R, Rose J, Heusch G. Involvement of activation of ATP-dependent potassium channels in ischemic preconditioning in swine. Am J Physiol 1994;267(4 Pt 2):H1341–52.

67. Tinker A, Aziz Q, Thomas A. The role of ATP-sensitive potassium channels in cellular function and protection in the cardiovascular system. Br J Pharmacol 2014;171(1):12–23.

68. Haissaguerre M, Chatel S, Sacher F, et al. Ventricular fibrillation with prominent early repolarization associated with a rare variant of KCNJ8/KATP channel. J Cardiovasc Electrophysiol 2009;20(1):93–8.

69. Barajas-Martinez H, Hu D, Ferrer T, et al. Molecular genetic and functional association of Brugada and early repolarization syndromes with S422L missense mutation in KCNJ8. Heart Rhythm 2012;9(4):548–55.

70. Liu Y, Ren G, O'Rourke B, et al. Pharmacological comparison of native mitochondrial K(ATP) channels with molecularly defined surface K(ATP) channels. Mol Pharmacol 2001;59(2):225–30.

71. Grover GJ, Garlid KD. ATP-Sensitive potassium channels: a review of their cardioprotective pharmacology. J Mol Cell Cardiol 2000;32(4):677–95.

72. Grover GJ, D'Alonzo AJ, Garlid KD, et al. Pharmacologic characterization of BMS-191095, a mitochondrial K(ATP) opener with no peripheral vasodilator or cardiac action potential shortening activity. J Pharmacol Exp Ther 2001;297(3):1184–92.

Clinical Features of Genetic Cardiac Diseases Related to Potassium Channelopathies

Arnon Adler, MD, Sami Viskin, MD*

KEYWORDS

- Potassium channels • Inherited arrhythmias • Sudden cardiac death • Long QT syndrome
- Brugada syndrome • Short QT syndrome • Early repolarization syndrome • Familial atrial fibrillation

KEY POINTS

- With the exception of familial atrial fibrillation, symptoms are related to the development of ventricular arrhythmias. Extracardiac manifestations are extremely rare.
- Personal and family history and typical electrocardiographic findings are instrumental for the diagnosis of these syndromes with most auxiliary tests being used to uncover latent electrocardiographic patterns.
- Genetic testing has a high yield in long QT syndrome but a low to very low yield in all other syndromes.
- With few exceptions, implantable cardioverter-defibrillators are recommended for secondary prevention and for primary prevention in certain high-risk patients.
- The mainstay of pharmacologic therapy includes β-blockers for almost all patients with long QT syndrome and quinidine for some patients with short QT, Brugada, and early repolarization syndromes.

Potassium channels are the most diverse ion channels in the human heart and contribute to all phases of the action potential. Most importantly, their function is key to the normal repolarization of the cardiomyocyte.[1] It should, therefore, come as no surprise that dysfunction of these channels, whether inherited or acquired, results in a variety of arrhythmogenic syndromes. These syndromes include long QT syndrome (LQTS), short QT syndrome (SQTS), Brugada syndrome (BrS), early repolarization syndrome (ERS), and familial atrial fibrillation (AF). In some of these syndromes (eg, LQTS) mutations in genes encoding for cardiac potassium channels or their subunits play a central role in the pathophysiology. In other syndromes (eg, BrS) the association with disease of rare genetic variants in these genes is less robust. In the case of familial AF the inherited syndrome represents a small fraction of a common and multifactorial condition. This article discusses the clinical manifestation of these syndromes and delineates the approach to their diagnosis and management.

CONGENITAL LONG QT SYNDROME

The first genes underlying the pathophysiology of any inherited arrhythmia syndrome were

Conflicts of Interests: None.
Financial Support and Sponsorship: None.
Department of Cardiology, Tel Aviv Sourasky Medical Center, Sackler School of Medicine, Tel Aviv University, 6 Weizmann Street, Tel Aviv 64239, Israel
* Corresponding author.
E-mail address: saviskin@tasmc.health.gov.il

Card Electrophysiol Clin 8 (2016) 361–372
http://dx.doi.org/10.1016/j.ccep.2016.02.001
1877-9182/16/$ – see front matter © 2016 Elsevier Inc. All rights reserved.

discovered in 1995.[2,3] These genes, KCNQ1 and KCNH2, encode for the potassium channels KvLQT1 and hERG and are responsible for LQTS type 1 and 2 (LQT1 and LQT2), respectively. Since then several other genes encoding for potassium channels or their accessory subunits have been associated with LQTS (**Table 1**).

Clinical Presentation

As with all channelopathies the main symptoms (syncope, cardiac arrest [CA], and sudden cardiac death [SCD]) are the result of ventricular arrhythmias (torsades de pointes in the case of LQTS). In most patients with LQT1 and LQT2 the first symptom is syncope, which may facilitate diagnosis before CA.[4] In LQT3 (which is the result of sodium-channel and not potassium-channel dysfunction) there is a greater risk of SCD as the presenting symptom.[4] Triggers associated with an increased risk of arrhythmias include exercise (especially swimming) in LQT1 and sudden auditory stimulus and the postpartum period in LQT2.[5]

Age at time of first symptom varies widely and ranges from infancy to old age; however, the risk of cardiac events changes with puberty and aging. Gender and LQT type have also been associated with risk of cardiac events. In males with LQTS the risk is mitigated after adolescence, whereas in women such a trend is not observed.[4,6] This is especially true in LQT1 in which males have an increased risk during childhood but a lower one after puberty.[4]

Extracardiac manifestations are rare in LQTS. Jervell and Lange-Nielsen syndrome is an autosomal-recessive disease caused by mutations in KCNQ1 or KCNE1 and manifests as severe QT prolongation and sensorineural deafness.[7] Andersen-Tawil syndrome is caused by mutations in KCNJ2 and is regarded as LQT7.[8] This syndrome is characterized by periodic paralysis, dysmorphic features, and moderate QT prolongation

Table 1
Genes encoding for potassium channels and their subunits associated with cardiac arrhythmia syndromes

Gene	Protein	Effect on Ionic Current	OMIM Entry
Long QT syndrome			
KCNQ1	Kv7.1/KvLQT1	$I_{Ks}\downarrow$	607542
KCNH2	Kv11.1/hERG	$I_{Kr}\downarrow$	152427
KCNE1	minK	$I_{Ks}\downarrow$	613695
KCNE2	MiRP1	$I_{Kr}\downarrow$	603796
KCNJ2	Kir2.1/IRK1	$I_{K1}\downarrow$	600681
AKAP9	AKAP9/Yotiao	$I_{Ks}\downarrow$	604001
KCNJ5	Kir3.4/GIRK4	$I_{K-ACh}\downarrow$	600734
Short QT syndrome			
KCNH2	Kv11.1/hERG	$I_{Kr}\uparrow$	152427
KCNQ1	Kv7.1/KvLQT1	$I_{Ks}\uparrow$	607542
KCNJ2	Kir2.1/IRK1	$I_{K1}\uparrow$	600681
Brugada syndrome			
KCNE3	MiRP2	$I_{to}\uparrow$	604433
KCND3	Kv4.3	$I_{to}\uparrow$	616399
KCNJ8	Kir6.1	$I_{K-ATP}\uparrow$	600935
ABCC9	SUR2A	$I_{K-ATP}\uparrow$	601439
Early repolarization syndrome			
KCNJ8	Kir6.1	$I_{K-ATP}\uparrow$	600935
ABCC9	SUR2A	$I_{K-ATP}\uparrow$	601439

For details regarding genes associated with familial atrial fibrillation see review by Tucker and Ellinor.[84]

(but very prolonged QU intervals). Furthermore, although arrhythmias are frequent in these patients typical torsades de pointes is not, leading some experts to exclude Andersen-Tawil from the typical LQTS family.

Diagnosis

Diagnosis of LQTS is primarily based on measurement of the QT interval on the electrocardiogram (ECG). Corrected QT (QTc) intervals longer than 450 ms in men and 460 ms in women are regarded as abnormal; nevertheless, a large overlap between patients and healthy individuals exists.[9] Therefore, most individuals with an abnormal QTc according to these definitions do not have LQTS. QTc intervals longer than 480 ms, however, are very rarely normal and those longer than 500 ms invariably represent LQTS in the absence of QT prolonging factors (**Table 2**). Importantly, about half of patients with LQTS have a QTc shorter than 480 ms or even in the normal range, and therefore a normal QTc does not exclude LQTS.

One tool that may aid in the diagnosis is the Schwartz score,[10] which incorporates ECG and clinical data (**Table 3**). Furthermore, several tests have been developed to uncover repolarization abnormalities in suspected patients without overt QTc prolongation. These tests include the epinephrine test,[11,12] adenosine test,[13] exercise test,[14] and stand-up test.[15,16] On top of the QT interval duration, the T-wave morphology is also beneficial for diagnosis of LQTS. Patients with

LQT1 typically have a broad-based T wave and those with LQT2 a bifid T wave (**Fig. 1**),[17] which may be apparent at rest or be uncovered by one of the aforementioned tests.[18,19]

Finally, genetic testing is beneficial in confirming the diagnosis, identifying the type of LQTS, and facilitating family screening. The yield of genetic testing in LQTS is about 80%. Mutations in KCNQ1 and KCNH2 are found in 30% to 35% and 25% to 40% of patients tested, respectively.[20]

Management

All patients with LQTS should receive recommendation regarding lifestyle precautions including avoidance of QT-prolonging drugs,[21] auditory stimulus (in LQT2), and competitive sports. In certain low-risk cases (eg, asymptomatic non-LQT1 patients with a normal QTc) participation in sports may be considered after a detailed discussion with the patient and his or her family.[22,23]

The first line of medical therapy for patients with LQTS is β-blockers. Long-acting propranolol and nadolol have been advocated as the most protective with metoprolol regarded as less effective, although this issue is a matter of debate.[24–26] Patients with LQT1 have an especially low event rate on β-blockers, whereas those with LQT2 have a higher arrhythmic breakthrough on this therapy.[27] Although the yield of β-blockers for low-risk patients (eg, asymptomatic patients >40 years of age with QTc <470 ms) is probably low, it should be considered in absence of contraindications.[22]

Table 2
Causes of secondary electrocardiographic patterns

LQTS	SQTS	BrS	ERS
Hypokalemia, hypomagnesemia, and hypocalcemia	Hyperkalemia and hypercalcemia	Hyperkalemia and hypercalcemia	Hypokalemia and hypocalcemia
Hypothermia	Hyperthermia	Hypothermia	Hypothermia
Early postmyocardial infarction period	Ischemia	Acute myocardial ischemia or myocarditis	Ischemia
QT prolonging drugs	Digitalis	Acute pericarditis	
Bradycardia/AV block	Acidosis	Atypical right bundle branch block	
Stroke	Central and autonomic nervous system abnormalities	Central and autonomic nervous system abnormalities	
Structural heart disease		Left ventricular hypertrophy	
Stress-induced cardiomyopathy		Arrhythmogenic right ventricular cardiomyopathy	
S/P cardioversion		Muscular dystrophies	
		Pectus excavatum	
		RVOT compression (eg, mediastinal tumor, hemopericardium)	
		Thiamine deficiency	
		S/P cardioversion	

These causes should be excluded before diagnosis of a specific syndrome.
Abbreviations: AV block, atrioventricular block; RVOT, right ventricular outflow tract; S/P, status/post.

Table 3
Schwartz score for diagnosis of long QT syndrome

ECG findings[a]	
(A) QTc[b]	
≥480 ms	3 points
460–479 ms	2 points
450–459 ms (in males)	1 point
(B) QTc[b] 4th minute of recovery form exercise test ≥ 480 ms	
(C) Torsade de pointes[c]	2 points
(D) T wave alternans	1 point
(E) Notched T wave in three leads	1 point
(F) Low heart rate for age[d]	0.5 point
Clinical history	
(A) Syncope[c]	
With stress	2 points
Without stress	1 point
(B) Congenital deafness	0.5 point
Family history[e]	
(A) Family members with definite LQTS[f]	1 point
(B) Unexplained sudden cardiac death below age 30 among immediate family members	0.5 point

Scoring: ≤1 point, low probability of LQTS; 1.5–3 points, intermediate probability of LQTS; ≥5 points, high probability of LQTS.
  [a] In the absence of medications or disorders known to affect these ECG features.
  [b] Calculated by Bazett's formula, where QTc = QT/√RR.
  [c] Mutually exclusive.
  [d] Resting heart rate below the second percentile for age.
  [e] The same family member cannot be counted in A and B.
  [f] Definite LQTS is defined by an LQTS score ≥4.
From Schwartz PJ, Crotti L. QTc Behavior During Exercise and Genetic Testing for the Long-QT Syndrome. Circulation 2011;124:2182; with permission.

Survivors of CA and patients with syncope while taking β-blockers have an indication for an implantable cardioverter-defibrillator (ICD).[22] This may also be considered in patients at very high risk (eg, patients with Jervell and Lange-Nielsen syndrome). In those with a contraindication for ICD implantation or those who refuse such a device, left cardiac sympathetic denervation is recommended.[22,28] It may also be considered in those with repeated ICD shocks or a contraindication for β-blockers.

SHORT QT SYNDROME

SQTS is a rare disease described for the first time in 2000 by Gussak and colleagues.[29] It is characterized by a short QT interval and a propensity for development of atrial and ventricular arrhythmias. Gain of function mutations in three genes encoding for potassium channels (*KCNH2*,[30] *KCNQ1*,[31] and *KCNJ2*[32]) have been associated with SQTS types 1 to 3, respectively (see **Table 1**).

Interestingly, loss of function mutations in these genes is responsible for LQT2, LQT1, and LQT7.

Clinical Presentation

Knowledge of SQTS is limited by the paucity of patients diagnosed. Data from the two largest series including 53 and 73 patients demonstrates that most are male (75%–84%).[33,34] In one-quarter to one-third of cases the clinical presentation was CA and in 15% syncope. Although age at time of first symptom ranged between infancy and old age, most patients presenting with syncope, CA, or SCD were young men in their second to fourth decades.[33] Most ventricular arrhythmias occurred during sleep or rest.[34]

Diagnosis

As with LQTS the diagnosis of SQTS relies heavily on the ECG and is encumbered by the problem of overlap between patients and healthy subjects. Population studies have demonstrated

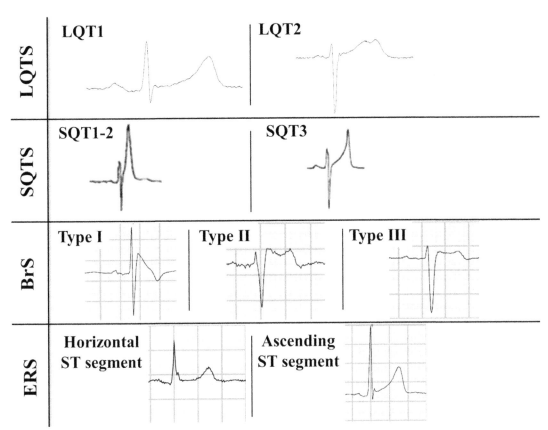

Fig. 1. Typical electrocardiographic patterns. BrS: only type I (2-mm coved ST-segment elevation in one of right precordial leads) is considered diagnostic; ERS: J-point elevation of at least 1 mm followed by a horizontal ST segment has been associated with higher risk (see text); LQTS: typical T wave in LQT1 is normal or broad-based; LQT2: typical T wave is bifid; SQTS: typical T-wave morphology in SQT1 and SQT2 is symmetric, pointed, tall, and with no ST segment; SQT3: T wave is asymmetrical with a rapid descending limb. (*Adapted from* [*SQT1 & SQT2*] Brugada R, Hong K, Dumaine R, et al. Sudden death associated with short-QT syndrome linked to mutations in HERG. Circulation 2004;109:31 and; [*SQT3*] Priori SG, Pandit SV, Rivolta I, et al. A novel form of short QT syndrome (SQT3) is caused by a mutation in the KCNJ2 gene. Circ Res 2005;96:802.)

that a QTc of 350 for men and 360 for women represents two standard deviations from the mean.[35] In the large SQTS series the mean QTc was 314 to 329 ms but QTc intervals as short as 220 ms have been reported.[33,34] For diagnosis of asymptomatic patients, cutoff values of 330 to 340 have been recommended.[22,33,34] A value of 360 ms has been recommended for diagnosis of patients with one of the following: history of CA, documented ventricular arrhythmias, positive family history of SQTS/SCD at a young age (≤40), or presence of a disease-causing mutation. A scoring system incorporating these parameters, similar to the Schwartz score in LQTS, has been proposed by Gollob and colleagues[36] (**Table 4**).

Importantly, the QT adaptation to heart rate in SQTS is abnormal with blunted prolongation of the QT during bradycardia.[37] Consequently, the

short QT is more pronounced at slow heart rates. Furthermore, the commonly used Bazett formula is notorious for undercorrection of the QT interval during tachycardia and may result in pseudonormal QTc intervals if measured at fast heart rates. Accordingly, it is recommended that for diagnosis of SQTS the QT interval be measured at heart rates lower than 80 beats per minute.

T-wave morphology may raise the suspicion of SQTS in certain cases. Typically, it is tall, symmetric, peaked, and follows the QRS immediately with no ST segment (see **Fig. 1**). In SQT3 the T wave may be asymmetrical with a rapidly descending downslope (see **Fig. 1**).[32]

The yield of genetic testing in SQTS is relatively low (≈20%). Nevertheless, it may be considered in patients with strong clinical evidence of SQTS and in family members of a proband found to harbor a disease-causing mutation.[20]

Table 4
Gollob score for diagnosis of short QT syndrome

ECG findings[a]	
(A) QTc[b]	
<370 ms	1 point
<300 ms	2 points
<350 ms	3 points
(B) J point–T peak interval[c] <120 ms	1 point
Clinical history[d]	
(A) History of sudden cardiac arrest	2 points
(B) Documented polymorphic VT or VF	2 points
(C) Unexplained syncope	1 point
(D) Atrial fibrillation	1 point
Family history[e]	
(A) First- or second-degree relative with high-probability SQTS	2 points
(B) First- or second-degree relative with autopsy-negative sudden cardiac death	1 point
(C) Sudden infant death syndrome	1 point
Genotype	
(A) Genotype positive	2 points
(A) Mutation of undetermined significance in a culprit gene	1 point

Abbreviations: VF, ventricular fibrillation; VT, ventricular tachycardiaa.

High-probability SQTS, ≥4 points; intermediate-probability SQTS, 3 points; low-probability SQTS, ≤2 points.

[a] A minimum of 1 point must be obtained in the electrocardiographic section to obtain additional.

[b] Electrocardiogram must be recorded in the absence of modifiers known to shorten the QT.

[c] J point–T peak interval must be measured in the precordial lead with the greatest amplitude T wave.

[d] Clinical history: events must occur in the absence of an identifiable cause, including structural heart disease. Points can only be received for one of cardiac arrest, documented polymorphic VT, or unexplained syncope.

[e] Family history: points can only be received once in this section.

From Gollob MH, Redpath CJ, Roberts JD. The short QT syndrome: proposed diagnostic criteria. J Am Coll Cardiol 2011;57:809; with permission.

Electrophysiologic studies (EPS) are of limited value for diagnosis of SQTS. However, studies in a small group of patients demonstrated short effective refractory periods (140–200 ms).[33]

Finally, as is the case in other inherited arrhythmia syndromes, structural heart disease and QT shortening secondary to other conditions needs to be ruled out before diagnosis (see **Table 2**).

Management

The mainstay of treatment in SQTS is ICD implantation for prevention of SCD. In patients with history of CA or documented ventricular arrhythmias this is clearly indicated because they have a high risk of recurrent events (10% per year).[34] In patients with syncope thought to be of arrhythmic origin such treatment can also be considered although very little evidence supporting this approach is available. Indications for ICD implantation as a primary prevention measure are less clear because of limited knowledge regarding risk stratification in asymptomatic patients. Surprisingly, a shorter QT interval has not been associated with higher risk of cardiac events.[33,34] EPS has also been disappointing as a risk-stratifier.[33] Nevertheless, in patients with family history of SCD an ICD may be considered after discussing the possible complications. In this regard, inappropriate shocks are a particular problem in SQTS because of the propensity for supraventricular arrhythmias and higher risk of T-wave oversensing as a result of the tall T waves. This latter problem is overcome in many cases by appropriate ICD programming.

Several antiarrhythmic drugs have been used in patients with SQTS; however, available data suggest quinidine to be the most effective in prolonging the QT interval and preventing arrhythmias.[33,37] Sotalol has also been suggested as a treatment option.[22] Isoproterenol was shown to be effective in controlling an arrhythmic storm in one case report[38]; however, studies on canine cardiac-wedge models have demonstrated that this drug may exacerbate the underlying pathophysiologic process.[39] Accordingly, the role of isoproterenol in SQTS is yet to be elucidated. Antiarrhythmic therapy (usually quinidine) may be considered in the following cases: (1) patients with an indication for an ICD who refuse implantation or have a contraindication for such a procedure, (2) patients with recurrent appropriate ICD shocks or arrhythmic storms, and (3) patients with SCD at a young age in their family.

BRUGADA SYNDROME

BrS was described for the first time in 1992[40] but despite more than two decades of study the underlying pathophysiology is still not entirely clear. The main gene associated with BrS is the sodium-channel encoding SCN5A. Several potassium channels have also been implicated (see **Table 1**) but their association with the disease is less robust.

Population studies have demonstrated that a type I Brugada pattern can be found in 0% to 0.3% depending on the population studied (the prevalence is higher in East Asia).[41] There is a clear male predominance with 70% to 95% of patients in large cohorts being men.[42–44]

Clinical Presentation

Arrhythmias (almost always ventricular fibrillation [VF] or polymorphic ventricular tachycardia [VT]) typically occur during rest or sleep with a peak between midnight and 6 AM.[45,46] Accordingly, BrS should be included in the differential diagnosis of patients with nocturnal agonal respiration. Fever has been shown to be a potent arrhythmic trigger in BrS[47,48] and increase vagal tone has also been proposed as such.[49]

Most symptomatic patients (with SCD, CA, or syncope) are men in their fourth or fifth decade of life.[42,43,50] Children are rarely symptomatic but VF has been described even in infants.[51–53] Data from recent studies suggest that symptoms are also rare in the elderly with few symptomatic patients beyond the age of 60.[54,55]

Patients with BrS also have an increased risk of AF. This should be kept in mind when evaluating young patients with AF, especially if they also have a history of syncope or SCD in the family.

Diagnosis

The diagnosis of BrS is based on the finding of the typical coved 2-mm ST-segment elevation in one of the right precordial leads (type I Brugada pattern; see **Fig. 1**) and in the absence of conditions known to induce such a pattern (see **Table 2**). Saddle-back type ST-segment elevation or elevation less than 2 mm (type II-III Brugada pattern; see **Fig. 1**) is not regarded as diagnostic. Because a type I pattern is intermittent in most patients,[56] serial ECG recordings or a Holter test[57] may be used to increase the sensitivity. Elevating leads V1 and V2 to the third and second intercostal space also increases the sensitivity of the test[58] and is recommended in any case with suspected BrS. In patients with suspected BrS but no diagnostic ECG findings, infusion of a sodium-channel blocker is useful for uncovering the type I pattern.[59]

In the most recent guidelines addressing the diagnosis of BrS[22] the finding of a type I pattern was deemed sufficient for diagnosis. Nevertheless, according to some experts a definite diagnosis should be made only if clinical features are also present.[41,60] These proposed features include history of CA, agonal nocturnal respiration, documented VT/VF, unexplained syncope, or positive family history (unexplained SCD <45 years or diagnosed BrS in a first-degree relative).

Genetic testing may be used for screening of family members of probands in whom a disease-causing mutation was found.[20] Mutations in SCN5A thought to be disease-causing are uncovered in 25% to 30% of probands[20]; however, mutations in genes encoding for potassium channels are responsible for a small minority of gene-positive patients with BrS (see **Table 1**).

Management

All patients with BrS are recommended to avoid drugs that block the sodium current and may increase the risk of cardiac events. An updated list of such drugs is available at burgadadrugs.org.[61] Excessive alcohol intake and use of cocaine may also be deleterious.[59] Because of the arrhythmogenic effect of fever it is advised that patients with BrS use antipyretics during febrile illness.

Symptomatic patients with BrS have a clear indication for ICD implantation because of their high risk of recurrent events (48% at 10 years).[22,62] Asymptomatic patients with BrS are at a low but not trivial risk of cardiac events (0.5%–1.5% per year).[42,43,63] Unfortunately, their risk stratification remains a challenge and topic of debate. The main controversy centers on the utility of inducible ventricular arrhythmias during EPS as a predictor of future cardiac events.[64,65] Although many other markers have been associated with increased risk,[66] a widely accepted risk stratification strategy useful for clinical decision-making is unavailable.

Several pharmacologic agents have been studied in BrS but most experience is with quinidine. This drug has been shown to be effective in prevention of cardiac events in multiple studies[67,68]; however, its side effects prevent it from being indiscriminately used. The side effects are gastrointestinal but the most feared is its QT-prolonging effect and torsadogenic potential. It is, therefore, recommended for patients with ICDs and arrhythmic storms or multiple appropriate ICD shocks. It may also be considered in patients with an indication for an ICD who cannot or will not undergo implantation. Its role for primary prevention in asymptomatic patients without an ICD is undetermined. Data on other drugs (eg, cilostazol, beperidil) are limited[69] but these may be considered in patients with multiple ICD shocks who cannot tolerate quinidine. Isoproterenol has been demonstrated to be effective for control of arrhythmic storms.[70]

Epicardial ablation of the right ventricular outflow tract has been shown to significantly reduce the number of ICD shocks in patients with BrS[71] and may be considered in patients with recurrent shocks.

EARLY REPOLARIZATION SYNDROME

ERS has been defined as a clinical entity only recently.[22,72] The pathophysiology of ERS is thought to involve dispersion of repolarization as a result of aberration in the transient outward potassium current (I_{to}).[73] Unlike some of the other inherited syndromes discussed previously, very few families with ERS have been described and most cases are sporadic. Accordingly, data regarding putative genetic mutations underlying this syndrome are less than robust (see **Table 1**).

Importantly, early repolarization is a very common electrocardiographic sign (found in 5% of the population)[74] but ERS is very rare. It, therefore, should be emphasized that most asymptomatic patients with an early repolarization pattern are at very low risk of CA or SCD. A discussion regarding risk stratification of asymptomatic patients with early repolarization is beyond the scope of this article and may found elsewhere.[75,76]

Clinical Presentation

Patients with ERS are most commonly men (approximately 70%) who present at a young age (mean, 35–37).[77,78] The presenting symptom is most commonly CA and less than 40% have syncope as a warning sign. There are no specific activities that predispose patients to increased risk and no arrhythmic trigger has been identified.

Diagnosis

ERS is diagnosed in patients resuscitated from CA who have an early repolarization pattern on their ECG and after exclusion of all other causes of CA or J-point elevation (see **Table 2**). The exact definition of early repolarization has been fraught with controversy and confusion but recently a consensus statement[72] has defined it as follows: J-point elevation of greater than or equal to 0.1 mV in two or more contiguous leads excluding V1 to 3. The J-point elevation may be either a notch or a slur appearing on the last portion of the QRS (final half of R wave downslope) and in the absence of QRS prolongation ($\geq$120 ms).

Some caution, however, is in place when making the diagnosis of ERS. Because early repolarization is not rare in the general population the appearance of a J wave on the ECG of a CA survivor does not automatically mean it has something to do with the cause of the CA. Therefore, other characteristics supporting the diagnosis should be sought. In an optimal (and rare) scenario, an increase in J-wave amplitude before initiation of VF or polymorphic VT is documented and the diagnosis can be made with a high level of confidence. Documentation of dynamic changes in J-wave amplitude, short-coupled premature ventricular complexes, nonsustained polymorphic VT, or tall J-waves ($\geq$0.2 mV) in inferior leads also support the diagnosis. The ST segment following the J wave is usually horizontal or descending in patients with ERS (see **Fig. 1**); however, this is not invariably true.[78] Therefore, such a finding may support the diagnosis but an ascending ST segment does not exclude it. Finally, family history of ERS or SCD at a young age is not common in patients with ERS but does support the diagnosis of an inherited syndrome rather than an acquired condition.

The use of the Valsalva maneuver has been suggested to uncover J waves or increase their amplitude in patients with ERS and their first-degree relatives[79] but further studies are necessary to define this method's role in the diagnosis of ERS.

Although mutations in several genes (see **Table 1**) have been associated with ERS, the role of genetic testing in this syndrome is still limited because of the paucity of data. Accordingly, such testing is not routinely recommended and, when performed, interpretation of the results should be done with a great deal of caution.

Management

Once more, the mainstay of therapy is implantation of an ICD for secondary prevention.[22] Several lines of evidence suggest that quinidine (an I_{to} blocker) is beneficial in prevention of cardiac events.[80,81] Similar to the recommendations in BrS, it should be considered in patients with arrhythmic storms, recurrent ICD shocks, or those who refuse or have a contraindication for an ICD. Isoproterenol for acute control of arrhythmic storms is advised as in BrS.[81]

In rare cases an asymptomatic patient may present with early repolarization and high-risk features (eg, tall dynamic J waves, short-coupled premature ventricular complexes, nonsustained polymorphic VT, horizontal ST pattern) and/or a strong family history (relative with ERS or ≥ 2 family members with SCD at a young age). In these cases ICD implantation or quinidine for primary prevention may be discussed, although direct data supporting such an approach do not exist.

Ablation of ectopic foci originating from ventricular myocardium or Purkinje fibers has been suggested[77] but evidence supporting this approach is limited.

FAMILIAL ATRIAL FIBRILLATION

AF is a common and multifactorial arrhythmia but in about 15% of patients it is diagnosed in the absence of conventional risk markers.[82] It has been hypothesized that these patients have a genetic background that predisposes them to the development of AF. Studies demonstrating increased risk of AF in first-degree relatives of patients with AF[83] and genome-wide association studies revealing specific risk-loci for AF support this hypothesis.[84] Nevertheless, only in a minority of cases a familial form of the disease is suspected (estimated at 5%–15%).[85] Several putative mutations (mostly gain-of-function) in genes encoding for potassium channels have been described in such families.[84] Furthermore, development of AF at a young age occurs in some patients with LQTS, SQTS, and BrS.

Unfortunately, the use of clinical genetic testing for familial AF is still limited. Patients with familial AF are not known to have a different prognosis than those with nonfamilial AF and no specific screening strategy is recommended for patients carrying a putative AF-associated mutation.

Therefore, genetic testing is not currently recommended for patients with AF.[20]

SUMMARY

With the exception of familial AF, all genetic cardiac diseases related to potassium channel dysfunction share several common characteristics: (1) a normal or near-normal heart structure, (2) a propensity for the development of ventricular arrhythmias (almost invariably polymorphic VT or VF), (3) the main symptoms (SCD, CA, or syncope) are related to ventricular arrhythmias and extracardiac manifestations are extremely rare, (4) typical findings on the ECG are a crucial part of the diagnosis, and (5) an ICD for secondary prevention is recommended for survivors of a CA with few exceptions.

ICD implantation for primary prevention should also be considered in certain high-risk patients, especially in LQTS in which risk-stratification is more accurate. The mainstay of pharmacologic therapy that reduces arrhythmic events includes β-blockers in LQTS and quinidine in SQTS and BrS. Isoproterenol for control of arrhythmic storms is effective in BrS, ERS, and possibly in SQTS.

Familial AF differs from the other syndromes because it is responsible for a small minority of cases of a very common and multifactorial disease. Currently, the management of patients with familial and nonfamilial AF is identical but research in this field holds great promise for future developments.

REFERENCES

1. Grant AO. Cardiac ion channels. Circ Arrhythm Electrophysiol 2009;2:185–94.
2. Curran ME, Splawski I, Timothy KW, et al. A molecular basis for cardiac arrhythmia: HERG mutations cause long QT syndrome. Cell 1995;80:795–803.
3. Wang Q, Curran ME, Splawski I, et al. Positional cloning of a novel potassium channel gene: KVLQT1 mutations cause cardiac arrhythmias. Nat Genet 1996;12:17–23.
4. Zareba W, Moss AJ, Locati EH, et al. Modulating effects of age and gender on the clinical course of long QT syndrome by genotype. J Am Coll Cardiol 2003;42:103–9.
5. Schwartz PJ, Priori SG, Spazzolini C, et al. Genotype-phenotype correlation in the long-QT syndrome: gene-specific triggers for life-threatening arrhythmias. Circulation 2001;103:89–95.
6. Goldenberg I, Moss AJ, Bradley J, et al. Long-QT syndrome after age 40. Circulation 2008;117:2192–201.

7. Jervell A, Lange-Nielsen F. Congenital deaf-mutism, functional heart disease with prolongation of the Q-T interval and sudden death. Am Heart J 1957;54:59–68.

8. Andersen ED, Krasilnikoff PA, Overvad H. Intermittent muscular weakness, extrasystoles, and multiple developmental anomalies. A new syndrome? Acta Paediatr Scand 1971;60:559–64.

9. Taggart NW, Haglund CM, Tester DJ, et al. Diagnostic miscues in congenital long-QT syndrome. Circulation 2007;115:2613–20.

10. Schwartz PJ, Moss AJ, Vincent GM, et al. Diagnostic criteria for the long QT syndrome. An update. Circulation 1993;88:782–4.

11. Ackerman MJ, Khositseth A, Tester DJ, et al. Epinephrine-induced QT interval prolongation: a gene-specific paradoxical response in congenital long QT syndrome. Mayo Clin Proc 2002;77:413–21.

12. Shimizu W, Noda T, Takaki H, et al. Diagnostic value of epinephrine test for genotyping LQT1, LQT2, and LQT3 forms of congenital long QT syndrome. Heart Rhythm 2004;1:276–83.

13. Viskin S, Rosso R, Rogowski O, et al. Provocation of sudden heart rate oscillation with adenosine exposes abnormal QT responses in patients with long QT syndrome: a bedside test for diagnosing long QT syndrome. Eur Heart J 2006;27:469–75.

14. Sy RW, van der Werf C, Chattha IS, et al. Derivation and validation of a simple exercise-based algorithm for prediction of genetic testing in relatives of LQTS probands. Circulation 2011;124:2187–94.

15. Viskin S, Postema PG, Bhuiyan ZA, et al. The response of the QT interval to the brief tachycardia provoked by standing: a bedside test for diagnosing long QT syndrome. J Am Coll Cardiol 2010;55:1955–61.

16. Adler A, van der Werf C, Postema PG, et al. The phenomenon of "QT stunning": the abnormal QT prolongation provoked by standing persists even as the heart rate returns to normal in patients with long QT syndrome. Heart Rhythm 2012;9:901–8.

17. Zhang L, Timothy KW, Vincent GM, et al. Spectrum of ST-T-wave patterns and repolarization parameters in congenital long-QT syndrome: ECG findings identify genotypes. Circulation 2000;102:2849–55.

18. Khositseth A, Hejlik J, Shen WK, et al. Epinephrine-induced T-wave notching in congenital long QT syndrome. Heart Rhythm 2005;2:141–6.

19. Chorin E, Havakuk O, Adler A, et al. Diagnostic value of T-wave morphology changes during "QT stretching" in patients with long QT syndrome. Heart Rhythm 2015;12(11):2263–71.

20. Ackerman MJ, Priori SG, Willems S, et al. HRS/EHRA expert consensus statement on the state of genetic testing for the channelopathies and cardiomyopathies this document was developed as a partnership between the Heart Rhythm Society (HRS) and the European Heart Rhythm Association (EHRA). Heart Rhythm 2011;8:1308–39.

21. Woosley RaR, KA. Available at: www.Crediblemeds.org, QT drugs List, Accession Date, AZCERT, Inc. 1822 Innovation Park Dr., Oro Valley, AZ 85755.

22. Priori SG, Wilde AA, Horie M, et al. HRS/EHRA/APHRS expert consensus statement on the diagnosis and management of patients with inherited primary arrhythmia syndromes: document endorsed by HRS, EHRA, and APHRS in May 2013 and by ACCF, AHA, PACES, and AEPC in June 2013. Heart Rhythm 2013;10:1932–63.

23. Schwartz PJ, Ackerman MJ. The long QT syndrome: a transatlantic clinical approach to diagnosis and therapy. Eur Heart J 2013;34:3109–16.

24. Chockalingam P, Crotti L, Girardengo G, et al. Not all beta-blockers are equal in the management of long QT syndrome types 1 and 2: higher recurrence of events under metoprolol. J Am Coll Cardiol 2012;60:2092–9.

25. Abu-Zeitone A, Peterson DR, Polonsky B, et al. Efficacy of different beta-blockers in the treatment of long QT syndrome. J Am Coll Cardiol 2014;64:1352–8.

26. Wilde AA, Ackerman MJ. Beta-blockers in the treatment of congenital long QT syndrome: is one beta-blocker superior to another? J Am Coll Cardiol 2014;64:1359–61.

27. Priori SG, Napolitano C, Schwartz PJ, et al. Association of long QT syndrome loci and cardiac events among patients treated with beta-blockers. JAMA 2004;292:1341–4.

28. Schwartz PJ. Cardiac sympathetic denervation to prevent life-threatening arrhythmias. Nat Rev Cardiol 2014;11:346–53.

29. Gussak I, Brugada P, Brugada J, et al. Idiopathic short QT interval: a new clinical syndrome? Cardiology 2000;94:99–102.

30. Brugada R, Hong K, Dumaine R, et al. Sudden death associated with short-QT syndrome linked to mutations in HERG. Circulation 2004;109:30–5.

31. Bellocq C, van Ginneken AC, Bezzina CR, et al. Mutation in the KCNQ1 gene leading to the short QT-interval syndrome. Circulation 2004;109:2394–7.

32. Priori SG, Pandit SV, Rivolta I, et al. A novel form of short QT syndrome (SQT3) is caused by a mutation in the KCNJ2 gene. Circ Res 2005;96:800–7.

33. Giustetto C, Schimpf R, Mazzanti A, et al. Long-term follow-up of patients with short QT syndrome. J Am Coll Cardiol 2011;58:587–95.

34. Mazzanti A, Kanthan A, Monteforte N, et al. Novel insight into the natural history of short QT syndrome. J Am Coll Cardiol 2014;63:1300–8.

35. Kobza R, Roos M, Niggli B, et al. Prevalence of long and short QT in a young population of 41,767 predominantly male Swiss conscripts. Heart Rhythm 2009;6:652–7.

36. Gollob MH, Redpath CJ, Roberts JD. The short QT syndrome: proposed diagnostic criteria. J Am Coll Cardiol 2011;57:802–12.

37. Wolpert C, Schimpf R, Giustetto C, et al. Further insights into the effect of quinidine in short QT syndrome caused by a mutation in HERG. J Cardiovasc Electrophysiol 2005;16:54–8.

38. Bun SS, Maury P, Giustetto C, et al. Electrical storm in short-QT syndrome successfully treated with Isoproterenol. J Cardiovasc Electrophysiol 2012;23: 1028–30.

39. Extramiana F, Antzelevitch C. Amplified transmural dispersion of repolarization as the basis for arrhythmogenesis in a canine ventricular-wedge model of short-QT syndrome. Circulation 2004; 110:3661–6.

40. Brugada P, Brugada J. Right bundle branch block, persistent ST segment elevation and sudden cardiac death: a distinct clinical and electrocardiographic syndrome. A multicenter report. J Am Coll Cardiol 1992;20:1391–6.

41. Mizusawa Y, Wilde AA. Brugada syndrome. Circ Arrhythm Electrophysiol 2012;5:606–16.

42. Probst V, Veltmann C, Eckardt L, et al. Long-term prognosis of patients diagnosed with Brugada syndrome: results from the FINGER Brugada syndrome registry. Circulation 2010;121:635–43.

43. Kamakura S, Ohe T, Nakazawa K, et al. Long-term prognosis of probands with Brugada-pattern ST-elevation in leads V1-V3. Circ Arrhythm Electrophysiol 2009;2:495–503.

44. Brugada J, Brugada R, Antzelevitch C, et al. Long-term follow-up of individuals with the electrocardiographic pattern of right bundle-branch block and ST-segment elevation in precordial leads V1 to V3. Circulation 2002;105:73–8.

45. Matsuo K, Kurita T, Inagaki M, et al. The circadian pattern of the development of ventricular fibrillation in patients with Brugada syndrome. Eur Heart J 1999;20:465–70.

46. Takigawa M, Noda T, Shimizu W, et al. Seasonal and circadian distributions of ventricular fibrillation in patients with Brugada syndrome. Heart Rhythm 2008;5:1523–7.

47. Junttila MJ, Gonzalez M, Lizotte E, et al. Induced Brugada-type electrocardiogram, a sign for imminent malignant arrhythmias. Circulation 2008;117: 1890–3.

48. Amin AS, Meregalli PG, Bardai A, et al. Fever increases the risk for cardiac arrest in the Brugada syndrome. Ann Intern Med 2008;149:216–8.

49. Miyazaki T, Mitamura H, Miyoshi S, et al. Autonomic and antiarrhythmic drug modulation of ST segment elevation in patients with Brugada syndrome. J Am Coll Cardiol 1996;27:1061–70.

50. Conte G, Sieira J, Ciconte G, et al. Implantable cardioverter-defibrillator therapy in Brugada syndrome: a 20-year single-center experience. J Am Coll Cardiol 2015;65:879–88.

51. Priori SG, Napolitano C, Giordano U, et al. Brugada syndrome and sudden cardiac death in children. Lancet 2000;355:808–9.

52. Probst V, Denjoy I, Meregalli PG, et al. Clinical aspects and prognosis of Brugada syndrome in children. Circulation 2007;115:2042–8.

53. Conte G, de Asmundis C, Ciconte G, et al. Follow-up from childhood to adulthood of individuals with family history of Brugada syndrome and normal electrocardiograms. JAMA 2014;312:2039–41.

54. Conte G, DE Asmundis C, Sieira J, et al. Clinical characteristics, management, and prognosis of elderly patients with Brugada syndrome. J Cardiovasc Electrophysiol 2014;25:514–9.

55. Kamakura T, Wada M, Nakajima I, et al. Evaluation of the necessity for cardioverter-defibrillator implantation in elderly patients with Brugada syndrome. Circ Arrhythm Electrophysiol 2015;8(4): 785–91.

56. Veltmann C, Schimpf R, Echternach C, et al. A prospective study on spontaneous fluctuations between diagnostic and non-diagnostic ECGs in Brugada syndrome: implications for correct phenotyping and risk stratification. Eur Heart J 2006;27: 2544–52.

57. Shimeno K, Takagi M, Maeda K, et al. Usefulness of multichannel Holter ECG recording in the third intercostal space for detecting type 1 Brugada ECG: comparison with repeated 12-lead ECGs. J Cardiovasc Electrophysiol 2009;20:1026–31.

58. Sangwatanaroj S, Prechawat S, Sunsaneewitayakul B, et al. New electrocardiographic leads and the procainamide test for the detection of the Brugada sign in sudden unexplained death syndrome survivors and their relatives. Eur Heart J 2001;22:2290–6.

59. Antzelevitch C, Brugada P, Borggrefe M, et al. Brugada syndrome: report of the second consensus conference: endorsed by the Heart Rhythm Society and the European Heart Rhythm Association. Circulation 2005;111:659–70.

60. Sarquella-Brugada G, Campuzano O, Arbelo E, et al. Brugada syndrome: clinical and genetic findings. Genet Med 2016;18(1):3–12.

61. Postema PG, Wolpert C, Amin AS, et al. Drugs and Brugada syndrome patients: review of the literature, recommendations, and an up-to-date website (www.brugadadrugs.org). Heart Rhythm 2009;6: 1335–41.

62. Sacher F, Probst V, Maury P, et al. Outcome after implantation of a cardioverter-defibrillator in patients with Brugada syndrome: a multicenter study-part 2. Circulation 2013;128:1739–47.

63. Priori SG, Gasparini M, Napolitano C, et al. Risk stratification in Brugada syndrome: results of the PRELUDE (PRogrammed ELectrical stimUlation

preDictive valuE) registry. J Am Coll Cardiol 2012;
59:37–45.

64. Brugada J, Brugada R, Brugada P. Electrophysiologic testing predicts events in Brugada syndrome
patients. Heart Rhythm 2011;8:1595–7.

65. Wilde AA, Viskin S. EP testing does not predict
cardiac events in Brugada syndrome. Heart Rhythm
2011;8:1598–600.

66. Adler A, Rosso R, Chorin E, et al. Risk stratification in
Brugada syndrome: clinical characteristics, electro-
cardiographic parameters, and auxiliary testing.
Heart Rhythm 2016;13(1):299–310.

67. Belhassen B, Glick A, Viskin S. Efficacy of quinidine
in high-risk patients with Brugada syndrome.
Circulation 2004;110:1731–7.

68. Hermida JS, Denjoy I, Clerc J, et al. Hydroquinidine
therapy in Brugada syndrome. J Am Coll Cardiol
2004;43:1853–60.

69. Shinohara T, Ebata Y, Ayabe R, et al. Combination
therapy of cilostazol and bepridil suppresses recurrent ventricular fibrillation related to J-wave
syndromes. Heart Rhythm 2014;11:1441–5.

70. Maury P, Couderc P, Delay M, et al. Electrical storm
in Brugada syndrome successfully treated using
isoprenaline. Europace 2004;6:130–3.

71. Nademanee K, Veerakul G, Chandanamattha P,
et al. Prevention of ventricular fibrillation episodes
in Brugada syndrome by catheter ablation over the
anterior right ventricular outflow tract epicardium.
Circulation 2011;123:1270–9.

72. Macfarlane PW, Antzelevitch C, Haissaguerre M,
et al. The early repolarization pattern: a consensus
paper. J Am Coll Cardiol 2015;66:470–7.

73. Koncz I, Gurabi Z, Patocskai B, et al. Mechanisms
underlying the development of the electrocardiographic and arrhythmic manifestations of early
repolarization syndrome. J Mol Cell Cardiol 2014;
68:20–8.

74. Tikkanen JT, Anttonen O, Junttila MJ, et al. Long-
term outcome associated with early repolarization

on electrocardiography. N Engl J Med 2009;361:
2529–37.

75. Junttila MJ, Sager SJ, Tikkanen JT, et al. Clinical
significance of variants of J-points and J-waves:
early repolarization patterns and risk. Eur Heart J
2012;33:2639–43.

76. Adler A, Rosso R, Viskin D, et al. What do we know
about the "malignant form" of early repolarization?
J Am Coll Cardiol 2013;62:863–8.

77. Haissaguerre M, Derval N, Sacher F, et al. Sudden
cardiac arrest associated with early repolarization.
N Engl J Med 2008;358:2016–23.

78. Rosso R, Kogan E, Belhassen B, et al. J-point elevation in survivors of primary ventricular fibrillation and
matched control subjects: incidence and clinical
significance. J Am Coll Cardiol 2008;52:1231–8.

79. Gourraud JB, Le Scouarnec S, Sacher F, et al.
Identification of large families in early repolarization
syndrome. J Am Coll Cardiol 2013;61:164–72.

80. Antzelevitch CJ. Wave syndromes: molecular
and cellular mechanisms. J Electrocardiol 2013;46:
510–8.

81. Haissaguerre M, Sacher F, Nogami A, et al. Characteristics of recurrent ventricular fibrillation associated with inferolateral early repolarization role of
drug therapy. J Am Coll Cardiol 2009;53:612–9.

82. Kopecky SL, Gersh BJ, McGoon MD, et al. The natural
history of lone atrial fibrillation. A population-based
study over three decades. N Engl J Med 1987;317:
669–74.

83. Lubitz SA, Yin X, Fontes JD, et al. Association
between familial atrial fibrillation and risk of new-
onset atrial fibrillation. JAMA 2010;304:2263–9.

84. Tucker NR, Ellinor PT. Emerging directions in the
genetics of atrial fibrillation. Circ Res 2014;114:
1469–82.

85. Darbar D, Herron KJ, Ballew JD, et al. Familial atrial
fibrillation is a genetically heterogeneous disorder.
J Am Coll Cardiol 2003;41:2185–92.

Potassium Channel Block and Novel Autoimmune-Associated Long QT Syndrome

Mohamed Boutjdir, PhD[a,b,c], Pietro Enea Lazzerini, MD[d],
Pier Leopoldo Capecchi, MD[d], Franco Laghi-Pasini, MD[d],
Nabil El-Sherif, MD[a,b],*

KEYWORDS

- Long QT syndrome • Autoimmune disease • Anti-SSA/Ro antibodies • Potassium channels
- Cardiac arrhythmia

KEY POINTS

- Patients with corrected QT (QTc) prolongation are prone to complex ventricular arrhythmias, including torsades de pointes, syncope, and sudden death.
- Emerging clinical evidence demonstrates high prevalence of QTc prolongation and complex ventricular arrhythmias in patients with anti-SSA/Ro antibodies.
- QTc prolongation associated with anti-SSA/Ro antibodies per se may confer an increased risk for developing ventricular arrhythmias and thus represents an additional risk factor for patients with drug-induced or congenital QTc prolongation.
- The identification of the antibodies binding consensus motifs on the human ether-a-go-go—related gene potassium channel may open new avenues in the development of peptide-based pharmacotherapy for autoimmune-associated long QT syndrome.

INTRODUCTION

Autoimmune diseases and related cardiovascular comorbidities are increasingly recognized as a major health problem associated with significant morbidity and mortality and their prevalence is continuously increasing.[1–3] The National Institutes of Health estimates that up to 23.5 million Americans have autoimmune diseases and up to 24 million have heart diseases. As a result, the National Institutes of Health and the American Heart Association estimate the annual direct health care costs for autoimmune diseases to be in the range of $100 billion and $200 billion for heart diseases and stroke. However, autoimmune-associated cardiac rhythm disturbances have gained more attention in the fetal/neonate conduction system electrocardiographic abnormalities commonly known as congenital heart block, which manifest as complete atrioventricular block (AVB),[4] whereas the adult and associated repolarization abnormalities (QT interval prolongation) are just emerging.

Supported in part by Cardiovascular Research program, the Narrows Institute for Biomedical Research and Education and a MERIT Award Number I01BX007080 from Biomedical Laboratory Research & Development Service of Veterans Affairs Office of Research and Development.

Conflict of Interest: None.

[a] Research and Development Service, VA New York Harbor Healthcare System, 800 Poly Place, Brooklyn, NY 11209, USA; [b] Departments of Medicine, Cell Biology and Pharmacology, SUNY Downstate Medical Center, 450 Clarkson Avenue, Brooklyn, NY 11203, USA; [c] Department of Medicine, NYU School of Medicine, 550, 1st Avenue, New York, NY 10016, USA; [d] Department of Medical Sciences, Surgery and Neurosciences, University of Siena, Policlinico "Le Scotte", Viale Bracci, Siena 53100, Italy

* Corresponding author. Division of Cardiology, VA New York Harbor Healthcare System, 800 Poly Place, Brooklyn, NY 11209.

E-mail address: nelsherif@aol.com

This article focuses on the current knowledge of the pathophysiology of autoimmune-associated long QT syndrome.

Autoantibodies and the Heart

Numerous antibodies targeting cardiac proteins have been reported and their pathogenesis well characterized.[5,6] For example, antibodies targeting β-adrenergic and muscarinic receptors, Na/K-ATPase, cardiac troponin I, cardiac myosin heavy chain, and KCNQ1 (Kv7.1), were detected in patients with dilated cardiomyopathy/heart failure and have been suggested to exert their pathogenic role via an electrophysiologic and/or inflammatory processes.[5,7,8] However, only recently has the pathophysiology of autoimmune-associated anti-SSA/Ro antibodies in the adult heart began to emerge. Anti-SSA/Ro antibodies are among the most frequently detected autoantibodies in several autoimmune diseases, particularly connective tissue diseases (CTDs), but also in the general, otherwise healthy, population[9–13] (Table 1).

Autoimmune Anti-SSA/Ro–associated Long QT Syndrome

Clinical aspects

Anti-SSA/Ro antibodies, almost exclusively belonging to the immunoglobulin (Ig) G class and consisting of 2 subtypes (ie, anti–SSA/52kD-Ro and anti–SSA/60kD-Ro), result from an autoimmune response against the intracellular ribonucleoproteins, SSA/Ro (Ro) antigen, which is not accessible to the circulating anti-SSA/Ro antibodies under physiologic conditions.[4]

In recent years, a growing body of evidence from patients with CTDs indicates that the presence of circulating anti-SSA/Ro antibodies is associated with a clinically significant interference with ventricular repolarization seen as corrected

QT (QTc) prolongation at the surface electrocardiogram (ECG)[8,11] (Table 2).

Fifteen years ago, Cimaz and colleagues[14] for the first time reported a high prevalence (42% of the cases) of prolonged QTc in anti-SSA/Ro antibody–positive infants without congenital AVB. Later, the same group showed a concomitant disappearance of ECG abnormality and acquired maternal autoantibodies in these infants during their first year of life.[15] Moreover, another study by Gordon and colleagues[16] found that the QTc was significantly longer in children of anti-SSA/Ro antibody–positive mothers compared with children of anti-SSA/Ro antibody–negative mothers, with a further increase in those with siblings with congenital AVB.

These findings were confirmed and expanded by several subsequent studies performed in adults. In a cohort of adult patients with CTD, including Sjögren syndrome, systemic lupus erythematosus (SLE), mixed CTDs, undifferentiated CTDs, polymyositis/dermatomyositis, and systemic sclerosis, more than a half (58%) of anti-SSA/Ro antibody–positive subjects showed a prolonged QTc, with mean QTc values significantly longer in positive versus negative patients.[17] Accordingly, a similar prevalence of anti-SSA/Ro–associated QTc prolongation (46%) was shown in a another 24-hour ECG monitoring study of 46 patients with CTD, also showing that this ECG abnormality lasted throughout the day and was associated with the presence of complex ventricular arrhythmias[18] (Fig. 1). More recently, Bourré-Tessier and colleagues[19] performed 2 consecutive large studies on 150 and 278 patients with SLE. Using a multivariate logistic regression analysis, the investigators found a 5.1-times to 12.6-times higher risk of QTc prolongation in anti-SSA/Ro antibody–positive patients than in the anti-SSA/Ro antibody–negative patients, and each increase of 10 U/mL was associated with a parallel increase in the risk of having prolonged QTc. Moreover, the longitudinal follow-up of 118 of these patients for a mean of 17 months showed the strong association over the time between anti-SSA/Ro antibody positivity and QTc prolongation.[19] The association between QTc prolongation and the levels of circulating antibodies, as well as the subtype specificity, was confirmed in a further study on 49 patients with CTD. In this cohort, the authors showed a direct correlation between anti-SSA/Ro antibody concentration and QTc interval, but with the anti–SSA/52kD-Ro subtype only when the 2 subtypes (SSA/60kD-Ro) were considered separately.[20] Very recently, 2 additional studies provided evidence of the association between anti-SSA/Ro antibodies and QTc in

Table 1	
Prevalence of anti-SSA/Ro antibodies in different autoimmune diseases	
Diseases	**Anti-SSA/Ro Antibodies (%)**
Sjögren syndrome	70–100
Systemic lupus erythematosus	30–50
Systemic sclerosis	12
Rheumatoid arthritis	11
Undifferentiated CTD	8–30
Healthy general population	2–6

Data from Refs.[9–13]

adults. In the first study, Pisoni and colleagues[21] reported that, among 73 patients with different CTDs, 20% of anti-SSA/Ro antibody–positive subjects versus 0% of anti-SSA/Ro antibody–negative subjects had QTc prolongation. Notably, in patients with prolonged QTc (in all cases anti-SSA/Ro antibody positive) interleukin-1 beta levels were significantly higher compared with patients with normal QTc, thus suggesting a synergistic interplay between autoantibodies and inflammatory cytokines on QTc interval in these patients. In the second study, Sham and colleagues[22] found that mean QTc interval was significantly longer (with mean values approaching 450 milliseconds) in anti-SSA/Ro antibody–positive patients than in anti-SSA/Ro antibody–negative patients in a study of 100 patients with SLE.

Nakamura and colleagues[23] described the case of an anti-SSA/Ro antibody–positive woman with severe QTc prolongation (700 milliseconds) complicated with torsades de pointes arrhythmia, in which clear evidence of a direct mechanistic link between circulating antibodies and QTc prolongation was provided. No known causes of QT prolongation (drugs, electrolyte and hormone imbalance, structural heart disease, mutations in the genes responsible for the congenital long QT syndrome) were detected, although a polymorphism (D85N) in KCNE1 gene was found. The investigators showed the ability of both serum and purified IgG from the patient to significantly and specifically reduce the rectifier potassium ion current (IKr), in transfected HEK293 cells stably expressing the human ether-a-go-go--related gene (HERG) channel. Note that this patient was totally asymptomatic for autoimmune diseases. Because anti-SSA/Ro antibodies are the most common autoantibody found in the general population, and in most cases (60%–70%) is asymptomatic,[11] an intriguing speculation is that by reducing the repolarization reserve, anti-SSA/Ro antibodies may be silently involved as a predisposing factor in several apparently idiopathic life-threatening arrhythmias, including drug-induced torsades de pointes, and sudden unexpected deaths occurring in apparently healthy people.

In addition, recent preliminary data from single case reports show the effectiveness of immunosuppressive therapy in rapidly reversing QTc prolongation and other anti-SSA/Ro–associated electrocardiographic abnormalities in vivo, at least in adults.[24] These findings provide further indirect evidence that the mechanism of anti-SSA/Ro antibody–associated QTc prolongation depends only on the electrophysiologic interference of these autoantibodies with the heart ion channels.

In addition to the supporting data discussed earlier, there are other studies that, although they did not observe significant differences between anti-SSA/Ro antibody–positive and anti-SSA/Ro antibody–negative patients for mean QTc and/or QTc prolongation prevalence, nevertheless found differences in QTc that were close to statistical significance (see **Table 1**). This pattern was the case in the studies in adults by Gordon and colleagues[25] (QTc slightly longer in the anti-SSA/Ro antibody CTD—positive group; $P = .06$), Nomura and colleagues[26] (anti-SSA/Ro antibody positivity slightly more frequent among patients with SLE with QTc prolongation; $P = .08$), and Bourré-Tessier and colleagues[27] (proportion of patients with SLE with prolonged QTc slightly higher [up to about 3-fold] in the anti–SSA/52kD-Ro antibody–positive group, although it did not reach statistical significance for wide confidence intervals; odds ratio, 3.33, 95% confidence interval, −1.35 to 8.00). Similar findings were reported in children by Motta and colleagues.[28]

Although most of the data point to an association between anti-SSA/Ro antibody positivity and QTc prolongation, there are conflicting results from other studies, both in children[29,30] and adults[31–33] (see **Table 1**). However, one of these studies[33] was performed in a cohort of patients with systemic sclerosis who frequently display anti-SSA/Ro antibody positivity but at a low levels,[34] thus possibly not high enough for the threshold required for the manifestation of QTc prolongation.[20,35] In another study[32] involving patients with SLE, the investigators used a cutoff for QTc prolongation (>500 milliseconds), thus excluding a large range of what may be considered abnormal QTc (values between 440 milliseconds and 500 milliseconds).

Collectively, the data discussed above strongly suggest that the electrophysiologic effects of anti-SSA/Ro antibodies in experimental studies have a significant clinical impact in patients with autoimmune diseases despite some discrepancies. Variability of QTc prolongation has been also reported even within patients with CTD from the studies showing a significant association between QTc and anti-SSA/Ro antibodies, ranging from about 10% to 60%.[20] This QTc variability[19,20] can be attributed, at least in part, to the differences among CTD cohorts in terms of autoantibody concentration and specificity (high levels of anti-SSA/52kD-Ro are particularly frequent in Sjögren syndrome, much less in SLE and systemic sclerosis[36]). In contrast, the electrophysiologic

Table 2
Clinical studies on anti-Ro/SSA antibodies and QTc interval

Author, Year	Study Population	Anti-Ro/SSA–positive Patients (n)	Anti-Ro/SSA–negative Patients (n)	Main Findings
Cimaz et al,[14] 2000	Children of mothers with CTD	21	7	Mean QTc significantly longer in anti-Ro/SSA–positive subjects
Gordon et al,[16] 2001	Children of mothers with CTD	38	7	Mean QTc significantly longer in children of anti-Ro/SSA–positive mothers
Gordon et al,[25] 2001	Adult patients with AD	49 (SLE, 29; SS, 11; other ADs, 9)	62 (SLE, 48; SS, 2; other ADs, 12)	Mean QTc slightly longer in anti-Ro/SSA–positive patients ($P = .06$)
Cimaz et al,[15] 2003	Children of mothers with CTD	21	—	Concomitant disappearance of QTc prolongation and acquired maternal antibodies at 1-year follow-up
Lazzerini et al,[17] 2004	Adult patients with CTD	31 (SLE, 6; SS, 14; SSc, 4; UCTD, 5; MCTD, 1)	26 (SLE, 4; SS, 1; SSc, 17; UCTD, 3; MCTD, 1)	Mean QTc significantly longer and prevalence of QTc prolongation significantly higher in anti-Ro/SSA–positive subjects
Costedoat-Chalumeau et al,[29] 2004	Children of mothers with CTD	58	85	No differences in mean QTc duration or in QTc prolongation prevalence between groups
Costedoat-Chalumeau et al,[31] 2005	Adult patients with CTD	32 (SLE, 28; SS, 4)	57 (SLE, 49; UCTD, 4; MCTD, 4)	No differences in mean QTc duration or in QTc prolongation prevalence between groups
Lazzerini et al,[18] 2007	Adult patients with CTD	26 (SLE, 4; SS, 9; SSc, 2; UCTD, 8; MCTD, 2; PM/DM, 1)	20 (SLE, 9; SS, 3; SSc, 4; UCTD, 1; MCTD, 2; PM/DM, 1)	Mean QTc significantly longer and prevalence of QTc prolongation significantly higher in anti-Ro/SSA–positive subjects; QTc prolongation significantly associated with the presence of complex ventricular arrhythmias
Motta et al,[28] 2007	Children of mothers with CTD	51	50	Mean QTc slightly longer in children of anti-Ro/SSA–positive mothers ($P = .06$)

Study	Population			Findings
Gerosa et al,[30] 2007	Children of mothers with AD	60	30	No difference in the prevalence of QTc prolongation between the groups
Bourrè-Tessier et al,[19] 2011	Adult patients with SLE (2 studies)	57 / 113	93 / 165	5.1–12.6-times higher risk of QTc prolongation in anti-Ro/SSA–positive vs anti-Ro/SSA–negative group
Lazzerini et al,[20] 2011	Adult patients with CTD	25 (SLE, 9; SS, 13; UCTD, 2; MCTD, 1)	24 (SLE, 13; SS, 3; UCTD, 6; MCTD, 2)	Mean QTc significantly longer and prevalence of QTc prolongation significantly higher in anti-Ro/SSA–positive subjects; significant correlation between anti-Ro/SSA–52kD concentration and QTc duration
Nomoura et al,[26] 2014	Adult patients with SLE	43	47	Anti-Ro/SSA positivity slightly more frequent among patients with SLE with QTc prolongation (P = .08)
Teixera et al,[32] 2014	Adult patients with SLE	111	206	No difference in the prevalence of marked QTc prolongation (>500 ms) between groups
Massie et al,[33] 2014	Adult patients with SSc	148	541	No difference in the prevalence of QTc prolongation between groups
Bourrè-Tessier et al,[27] 2015	Adult patients with SLE	283	314	Prevalence of QTc prolongation slightly higher in anti-Ro/SSA–positive subjects, but not significant enough for wide confidence intervals
Pisoni et al,[21] 2015	Adult patients with AD	55 (SLE, 16; SS, 20; SSc, 3; UCTD, 11; MCTD, 1; PM/DM, 2; other ADs, 2)	18 (SLE, 14; SS, 1; UCTD, 1; other ADs, 1)	Anti-Ro/SSA positivity significantly more frequent among patients with CTD with QTc prolongation (all patients with QTc prolongation were anti-Ro/SSA positive)
Sham et al,[22] 2015	Adult patients with SLE	47	53	Mean QTc significantly longer in anti-Ro/SSA–positive subjects

Abbreviations: AD, autoimmune disease; MCTD, mixed connective tissue disease; PM/DM, polymyositis/dermatomyositis; SLE, systemic lupus erythematosus; SS, Sjögren syndrome; SSc, systemic sclerosis; UCTD, undifferentiated connective tissue disease.

Data from Refs.[14–22,25–32]; *adapted from* Lazzerini PE, Cappechi PL, Laghi Pasini F. Long QT syndrome: an emerging role for inflammation and immunity. Front Cardiovasc Med 2015;2:26.

A

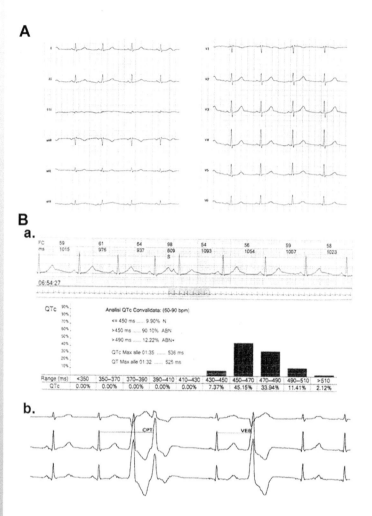

Fig. 1. Anti-SSA/Ro antibody–associated QTc prolongation in a patient with CTD. Examples of ECG tracings from a 35-year-old woman with Sjögren syndrome. (*A*) Resting ECG showed QTc prolongation (480 milliseconds). (*B*) Twenty-four-hour ambulatory ECG findings: (*a*) QTc prolongation lasted for all the 24-hour period, with a significant percentage of values greater than 500 milliseconds (QTc maximum: 535 milliseconds); (*b*) frequent and complex ventricular arrhythmias were recorded throughout the day.

aspects of the autoantibodies on the cardiac myocyte provide a plausible mechanistic explanation that could account for the QTc variability in the clinical studies. Specifically, a large body of experimental data[37–43] clearly show that, despite blocking the HERG potassium currents, anti-SSA/Ro antibodies are able to bind to calcium channels (L and T type) and inhibit its related currents. It is well recognized that calcium and potassium channels have opposing effects on action potential duration, and thus on QT interval. A block of the inward L-type calcium current during the plateau phase shortens the action potential duration, whereas an inhibition of outward IKr current during repolarization prolongs the action potential duration.[44] With this in mind, it is conceivable that a concomitant inhibitory effect of anti-SSA/Ro antibodies on calcium channels is able to partially counteract the IKr inhibition–dependent action potential prolongation in vivo, thus reducing the extent of QTc

prolongation observed.[35] Intrinsic (inherited or acquired) differences in potassium and calcium channel expression on patients' cardiomyocytes may also contribute to the QTc variability observed. In conclusion, evidence as detailed later indicates that anti-SSA/Ro antibodies inhibit IKr, but the clinical QT interval phenotype may not be the same for each patient as a result of the influence of several modifying factors, including the anti- SSA/Ro antibody subtypes and circulating levels, and the cardiomyocyte ion channels' gene expression profiles.

Autoimmune Anti-SSA/Ro–associated Long QT Syndrome

Functional and molecular aspects

The long QT syndrome is one of the most studied channelopathies, in which abnormal prolongation of ventricular repolarization predisposes to life-threatening ventricular arrhythmia or torsades de pointes.[45–47] The long QT syndrome can be congenital or acquired. Although the congenital long QT syndrome is rare and is caused by mutations in ion channel protein–coding genes, the acquired long QT syndrome is more prevalent and often associated with drugs.[48,49] In virtually all cases of drug-induced complex ventricular arrhythmias, the target ion channel is the HERG (also termed KCNH2) encoding the pore-forming subunits (Kv11.1) of the rapidly activating delayed potassium channel conducting IKr current.[49] IKr plays a major role during the repolarization of the cardiac action potential. Its blockade by drugs or genetic defects causes delayed repolarization of the action potential, which manifests as prolongation of the QT interval on the surface ECG.[49] As discussed earlier, a novel acquired form of long QT syndrome, termed autoimmune-associated long QT

syndrome, has been reported in clinical settings and its pathogenesis has recently been characterized.[50]

To demonstrate the pathogenic role of anti-SSA/Ro antibodies in the development of QTc prolongation, an animal model capitulating the clinical ECG phenotype was necessary for proof of concept. Adult guinea pigs were immunized with the SSA/Ro antigen and ECGs were measured after the animals developed significant anti-SSA/Ro antibodies. Significant QTc prolongation (**Fig. 2**A and B) was documented in immunized guinea pigs compared with controls (before immunization). No significant differences in heart rate, PR intervals, or QRS durations were observed before and after immunization.[50] This QTc prolongation was explained by the anti-SSA/Ro antibodies lengthening the guinea pig ventricular action potential (**Fig. 2**C) resulting

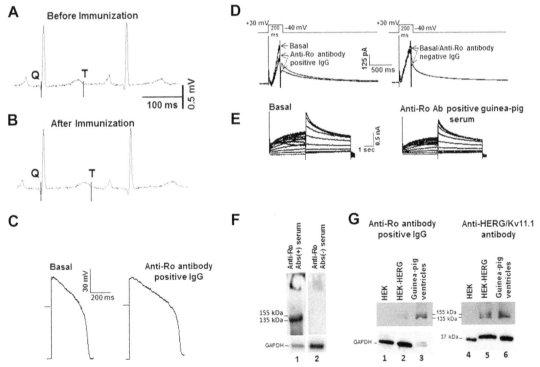

Fig. 2. Representative ECGs from a guinea pig (A) before immunization and (B) after immunization with SSA/52kD-Ro antigen. Vertical lines indicate QT interval. (C) Effects of anti-SSA/Ro antibody–positive IgG from the serum of a patient with connective tissue disease and QTc prolongation on action potential duration and (D) on IKr current recorded from guinea pig ventricular myocytes. (E) Representative IKr tracings from HEK293 cells stably expressing the HERG channel, at basal (*left*) and after (*right*) the application of anti-SSA/Ro antibody–positive serum from an immunized guinea pig. (F) Western blot of guinea pig ventricles probed with anti-SSA/Ro antibody–positive (lane 1) and anti-SSA/Ro antibodies–negative (lane 2) guinea pig sera. (G) Western blots of anti-SSA/Ro antibody–positive IgG (*left panel*) on untransfected HEK293 cells (lane 1), HEK293 cells expressing HERG channel (lane 2), and guinea pig ventricular tissue (lane 3). Additional positive controls with HEK293 cells expressing HERG channel and guinea pig ventricular tissue are shown respectively in lanes 5 and 6, and a negative control with untransfected HEH293 cells (lane 4). Ab, antibody. (*Adapted from* Yue Y, Castrichini M, Srivastava U, et al. Pathogenesis of the novel autoimmune-associated long-QT syndrome. Circulation 2015;132(4):237–8; with permission.)

from the inhibition of the native IKr (**Fig. 2**D) as well as IKr recorded from HEK293 cells stably expressing the HERG channel (**Fig. 2**E). This inhibition probably occurred by direct binding of anti-SSA/Ro antibodies from immunized guinea pig sera (**Fig. 2**F) and from anti-SSA/Ro antibodies from patients with CTD with guinea pig ERG (Ether-a-go-go Related Gene) channel proteins (**Fig. 2**G) as well as HEK293 cells expressing the HERG channel, respectively (see **Fig. 2**G).

Together, these findings are consistent and support the clinical observation that the sole presence of anti-SSA/Ro antibodies is associated with QTc prolongation.

At the patient level, sera, purified IgG, and affinity purified anti-SSA/Ro antibodies from patients with CTD and long QTc also significantly inhibited IKr in a time-dependent and dose-dependent manner in HEK293 cells expressing HERG channels (**Fig. 3**A–I). These effects were not seen with

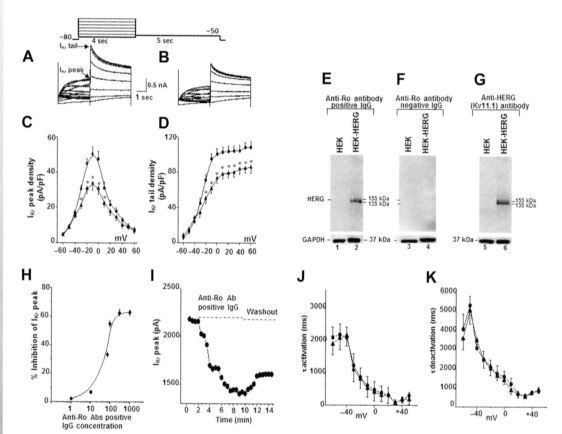

Fig. 3. (*A*) Representative currents were recorded from HEK293 cells stably expressing HERG channels using the protocol shown in the top sections of panels (*A*) under basal conditions and (*B*) in the presence of 75 μg/mL anti-SSA/Ro antibody–positive IgG from a patient with connective tissue disease and QTc prolongation. I-V relationships of IKr peak (*C*) and tail (*D*) current densities during basal (*circles*) and anti-SSA/Ro antibody–positive IgG application (*triangles*). (*H*) Dose-response curve of anti-SSA/Ro antibody–positive IgG resulted in an EC$_{50}$ (half maximal effective concentration) of 87.3 μg/mL. (*I*) Time course of anti-SSA/Ro antibody–positive IgG (75 μg/mL) on IKr peak. (*E*) Proteins from untransfected (lane 1) and transfected HEK293 cells with HERG channels (lane 2) were probed with anti-SSA/Ro antibody–positive IgG from a patient with connective tissue disease and QTc prolongation. Bands at 155 kDa and 135 kDa correspond with glycosylated and endoplasmic reticulum–retained HERG channels in lane 2 only. (*F*) Proteins from untransfected (lane 3) and transfected HEK293 cells with HERG channels (lane 4) were probed with anti-SSA/Ro antibody–negative IgG from a control patient with connective tissue disease but normal QTc. (*G*) Proteins from untransfected (lane 5) and transfected HEK293 cells with HERG channels (lane 6) were probed with commercial anti–HERG channel antibodies. Bands at 155 kDa and 135 kDa were seen in lane 6 only as in lane 2 with anti-SSA/Ro antibody–positive IgG. The 37-kDa bands represent GAPDH (Glyceraldehyde-3-Phosphate Dehydrogenase). (*J*) and (*K*) Boltzmann fit of IKr activation and deactivation respectively, before (*circle*) and after anti-Ro Ab–positive IgG application (*triangle*). The asterisk indicates statistical significance at $P<.05$. (*Adapted from* Yue, Y, Castrichini M, Srivastava U, et al. Pathogenesis of the novel autoimmune-associated long-QT syndrome. Circulation 2015;132(4):234–6; with permission.)

anti-SSA/Ro antibody–negative control patients with CTD and normal QTc.[50] These anti-SSA/Ro antibodies from patients with CTD directly interacted with the HERG channel proteins by Western blots (see **Fig. 3**). Note that the biophysical properties of the IKr were not altered by the antibodies (see **Fig. 3**J and K), suggesting a direct channel block. Nakamura and colleagues,[23] in an elegant study, also showed that anti-SSA/Ro antibodies from serum and purified IgG from the female patient discussed earlier whose QTc was very prolonged (700 milliseconds) with episodes of torsades de pointes, functionally inhibited and biochemically interacted with the HERG channel proteins in a dose-dependent manner. These effects were observed only when HEK293 cells in culture were incubated with anti-SSA/Ro antibodies for 1 to 5 days, but no acute effects (5 minutes) were observed. It is possible that longer periods of time than the 5-minute exposure were

necessary to see an acute effect similar to the one reported recently in the same HEK293 cells stably expressing the HERG channel.[50] Regardless, both studies agree that anti-SSA/Ro antibodies are pathogenic.

As mentioned earlier, and because the antigen SSA/Ro is not accessible to the circulating antibodies, the authors hypothesized that anti-SSA/Ro antibodies must recognize an epitope mimic on the extracellular side of the HERG channel homologous to SSA/52kD-Ro antigen. In this regard, linear homology analysis revealed 44% homology between SSA/52kD-Ro antigen (aa302–aa321) and the HERG alpha-1 subunit (aa574–aa598) at the pore region of which 25% are identical.[50] The presence of this homology at the pore region may be sufficient for anti–SSA/52kD-Ro antibody binding to the HERG channel at this epitope mimic, especially in the tetrameric conformation of the channel where the 4-pore

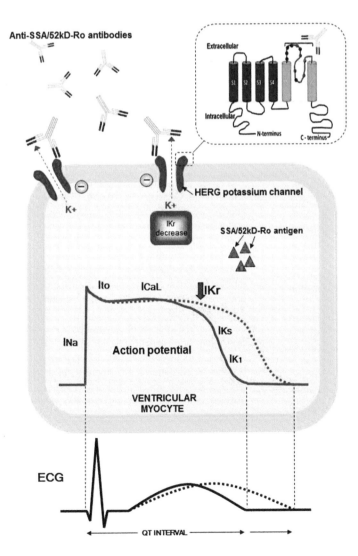

Fig. 4. The molecular and electrophysiologic basis of anti-SSA/Ro–associated QTc prolongation, from the cell to the surface ECG. Circulating anti-SSA/52kD-Ro antibodies cross react with the extracellular loop of the pore-forming region of the HERG potassium channel (*inset*) as a result of a molecular mimicry mechanism with anti-SSA/52kD-Ro antigens (*blue triangles*) that are located inside the cardiac myocyte but are not accessible to autoantibodies. The autoantibody–HERG channel interaction results in the inhibition of the related IKr current, thus leading to an increase in the cardiomyocyte action potential duration (*dotted lines*). The clinical correlate of these electrophysiologic changes is a prolongation of the QT interval on the surface ECG (*dotted lines*).

extracellular loops come together and are accessible to the antibodies. To test this hypothesis, a 31 aa peptide corresponding with a portion of the HERG extracellular loop at the pore region between S5 and S6 was designed and tested against sera from anti–SSA/Ro antibody–positive and anti–SSA/Ro antibody–negative patients with CTD. Significant reactivity to the peptide was observed only in anti–SSA/Ro antibody–positive patients' sera,[50] thus implicating this pore region as a potential binding epitope for the autoantibodies.

Proposed Pathogenic Mechanism for Anti-SSA/Ro Antibodies in the Development of QTc Prolongation

The proposed mechanism by which anti-SSA/Ro antibodies cause QTc prolongation in patients with CTD is summarized in **Fig. 4**: anti-SSA/Ro antibodies directly recognize specific epitope mimics to anti-SSA/52kD-Ro antigen on the HERG channels (see **Fig. 4**, inset) resulting in the inhibition of the repolarizing current, IKr. The IKr inhibition leads to action potential prolongation (see **Fig. 4**, center), which per se translates to a QT interval prolongation on the surface ECG (see **Fig. 4**, lower panel). It is generally accepted that QT interval is a function of ventricular action potential duration and that the two variables are very closely correlated in humans[51,52] and animals.[53] Experimental evidence supports this proposed mechanism: (1) the sole presence of anti-Ro antibodies induced by immunization of guinea pigs resulted in QTc prolongation on the surface ECG; (2) only sera, IgG, and affinity purified anti-Ro antibodies from anti-Ro antibody–positive patients, but not anti-Ro–negative patients, inhibited IKr and directly interacted with HERG channel proteins both in expression systems and in native ventricular myocytes; (3) anti-Ro antibodies did not affect IKr kinetics and their effect was observed within minutes, suggesting a direct block of the HERG channel; (3) the homology between SSA/52kD-Ro antigen and HERG channel at the pore-forming region; (4) the reactivity of anti-Ro antibody–positive sera, but not anti-Ro antibody–negative sera, with the peptide corresponding with the pore-forming region of HERG; (5) anti-Ro antibodies do not affect other currents, such as the delayed rectifier potassium current, IKs, the transient outward current, Ito, the inward rectifier potassium current, IK1, and the Na current, INa.[54,55]

CLINICAL SIGNIFICANCE AND SUMMARY

Patients with QTc prolongation are prone to complex ventricular arrhythmias, including torsades de pointes, syncope, and sudden death.[46,56] QTc prolongation associated with anti–SSA-Ro antibodies per se may confer an increased risk for developing ventricular arrhythmias and thus represents an additional risk factor for patients with drug-induced or congenital QTc prolongation. The identification of the antibodies binding consensus motifs on the HERG channel may open new avenues in the development of peptide-based pharmacotherapy for autoimmune-associated long QT syndrome.

REFERENCES

1. Turesson C, Jacobsson LT, Matteson EL. Cardiovascular co-morbidity in rheumatic diseases. Vasc Health Risk Manag 2008;4(3):605–14.
2. Symmons DP, Gabriel SE. Epidemiology of CVD in rheumatic disease, with a focus on RA and SLE. Nat Rev Rheumatol 2011;7(7):399–408.
3. Lee HC, Huang KT, Wang XL, et al. Autoantibodies and cardiac arrhythmias. Heart Rhythm 2011;8(11): 1788–95.
4. Qu Y, Boutjdir M. Pathophysiology of autoimmune associated congenital heart block. In: Conrad K, Chan KL, Fritzler MJ, et al, editors. From prediction to prevention of autoimmune diseases. vol. 17. Lengerich, Germany: Pabst-Science Publishers; 2011. p. 289–310.
5. Kaya Z, Leib C, Katus HA. Autoantibodies in heart failure and cardiac dysfunction. Circ Res 2012; 110(1):145–58.
6. Lazzerini PE, Capecchi PL, Guideri F, et al. Autoantibody-mediated cardiac arrhythmias: mechanisms and clinical implications. Basic Res Cardiol 2008; 103(1):1–11.
7. Li J, Maguy A, Duverger JE, et al. Induced KCNQ1 autoimmunity accelerates cardiac repolarization in rabbits: potential significance in arrhythmogenesis and antiarrhythmic therapy. Heart Rhythm 2014; 11(11):2092–100.
8. Lazzerini PE, Capecchi PL, Laghi-Pasini F. Long QT Syndrome: an emerging role for inflammation and immunity. Front Cardiovasc Med 2015;2:26.
9. Hayashi N, Koshiba M, Nishimura K, et al. Prevalence of disease-specific antinuclear antibodies in general population: estimates from annual physical examinations of residents of a small town over a 5-year period. Mod Rheumatol 2008;18(2):153–60.
10. Yoshimi R, Ueda A, Ozato K, et al. Clinical and pathological roles of Ro/SSA autoantibody system. Clin Dev Immunol 2012;2012:606195.
11. Lazzerini PE, Capecchi PL, Laghi-Pasini F. Anti-Ro/SSA antibodies and cardiac arrhythmias in the adult: facts and hypotheses. Scand J Immunol 2010;72(3): 213–22.

12. Satoh M, Chan EK, Ho LA, et al. Prevalence and sociodemographic correlates of antinuclear antibodies in the United States. Arthritis Rheum 2012; 64(7):2319–27.

13. Guo YP, Wang CG, Liu X, et al. The prevalence of antinuclear antibodies in the general population of china: a cross-sectional study. Curr Ther Res Clin Exp 2014;76:116–9.

14. Cimaz R, Stramba-Badiale M, Brucato A, et al. QT interval prolongation in asymptomatic anti-SSA/Ro-positive infants without congenital heart block. Arthritis Rheum 2000;43(5):1049–53.

15. Cimaz R, Meroni PL, Brucato A, et al. Concomitant disappearance of electrocardiographic abnormalities and of acquired maternal autoantibodies during the first year of life in infants who had QT interval prolongation and anti-SSA/Ro positivity without congenital heart block at birth. Arthritis Rheum 2003;48(1):266–8.

16. Gordon PA, Khamashta MA, Hughes GR, et al. Increase in the heart rate-corrected QT interval in children of anti-Ro- positive mothers, with a further increase in those with siblings with congenital heart block: comment on the article by Cimaz, et al. Arthritis Rheum 2001;44(1):242–3.

17. Lazzerini PE, Acampa M, Guideri F, et al. Prolongation of the corrected QT interval in adult patients with anti-Ro/SSA-positive connective tissue diseases. Arthritis Rheum 2004;50(4):1248–52.

18. Lazzerini PE, Capecchi PL, Guideri F, et al. Comparison of frequency of complex ventricular arrhythmias in patients with positive versus negative anti-Ro/SSA and connective tissue disease. Am J Cardiol 2007; 100(6):1029–34.

19. Bourré-Tessier J, Clarke AE, Huynh T, et al. Prolonged corrected QT interval in anti-Ro/SSA-positive adults with systemic lupus erythematosus. Arthritis Care Res (Hoboken) 2011;63(7):1031–7.

20. Lazzerini PE, Capecchi PL, Acampa M, et al. Anti-Ro/SSA-associated corrected QT interval prolongation in adults: the role of antibody level and specificity. Arthritis Care Res (Hoboken) 2011; 63(10):1463–70.

21. Pisoni CN, Reina S, Arakaki D, et al. Elevated IL-1beta levels in anti-Ro/SSA connective tissue diseases patients with prolonged corrected QTc interval. Clin Exp Rheumatol 2015;33(5):715–20.

22. Sham S, Medheshwaran M, Tamilselvam T, et al. Correlation of QT interval with disease activity in newly detected SLE patients at baseline and during flare. Indian J Rheumatol 2015;10:121–4.

23. Nakamura K, Katayama Y, Kusano KF, et al. Anti-KCNH2 antibody-induced long QT syndrome: novel acquired form of long QT syndrome. J Am Coll Cardiol 2007;50(18):1808–9.

24. Lazzerini PE, Brucato A, Capecchi PL, et al. Isolated atrioventricular block of unknown origin in the adult

and autoimmunity: diagnostic and therapeutic considerations exemplified by three anti-Ro/SSA-associated cases. HeartRhythm Case Rep 2015;1:293–9.

25. Gordon PA, Rosenthal E, Khamashta MA, et al. Absence of conduction defects in the electrocardiograms [correction of echocardiograms] of mothers with children with congenital complete heart block. J Rheumatol 2001;28(2):366–9.

26. Nomura A, Kishimoto M, Takahashi O, et al. Prolongation of heart rate-corrected QT interval is a predictor of cardiac autonomic dysfunction in patients with systemic lupus erythematosus. Rheumatol Int 2014; 34(5):643–7.

27. Bourré-Tessier J, Urowitz MB, Clarke AE, et al. Electrocardiographic findings in systemic lupus erythematosus: data from an international inception cohort. Arthritis Care Res (Hoboken) 2015;67(1): 128–35.

28. Motta M, Rodriguez-Perez C, Tincani A, et al. Outcome of infants from mothers with anti-SSA/Roantibodies. J Perinatol 2007;27:278–83.

29. Costedoat-Chalumeau N, Amoura Z, Lupoglazoff JM, et al. Outcome of pregnancies in patients with anti-SSA/Ro antibodies: a study of 165 pregnancies, with special focus on electrocardiographic variations in the children and comparison with a control group. Arthritis Rheum 2004; 50(10):3187–94.

30. Gerosa M, Cimaz R, Stramba-Badiale M, et al. Electrocardiographic abnormalities in infants born from mothers with autoimmune diseases–a multicentre prospective study. Rheumatology (Oxford) 2007;46(8):1285–9.

31. Costedoat-Chalumeau N, Amoura Z, Hulot JS, et al. Corrected QT interval in anti-SSA-positive adults with connective tissue disease: comment on the article by Lazzerini, et al. Arthritis Rheum 2005; 52(2):676–7 [author reply: 677–8].

32. Teixeira RA, Borba EF, Pedrosa A, et al. Evidence for cardiac safety and antiarrhythmic potential of chloroquine in systemic lupus erythematosus. Europace 2014;16(6):887–92.

33. Massie C, Hudson M, Tatibouet S, et al. Absence of an association between anti-Ro antibodies and prolonged QTc interval in systemic sclerosis: a multicenter study of 689 patients. Semin Arthritis Rheum 2014;44(3):338–44.

34. Parker JC, Burlingame RW, Bunn CC. Prevalence of antibodies to Ro-52 in a serologically defined population of patients with systemic sclerosis. J Autoimmune Dis 2009;6:2.

35. Lazzerini PE, Capecchi PL, Boutjdir M, et al. Comment on "absence of an association between anti-Ro antibodies and prolonged QTc interval in systemic sclerosis: a multicenter study of 689 patients." Semin Arthritis Rheum 2015;44(5): e16–7.

36. Dugar M, Cox S, Limaye V, et al. Diagnostic utility of anti-Ro52 detection in systemic autoimmunity. Postgrad Med J 2010;86(1012):79–82.

37. Karnabi E, Boutjdir M. Role of calcium channels in congenital heart block. Scand J Immunol 2010; 72(3):226–34.

38. Qu Y, Xiao GQ, Chen L, et al. Autoantibodies from mothers of children with congenital heart block downregulate cardiac L-type Ca channels. J Mol Cell Cardiol 2001;33(6):1153–63.

39. Qu Y, Baroudi G, Yue Y, et al. Novel molecular mechanism involving alpha1D (Cav1.3) L-type calcium channel in autoimmune-associated sinus bradycardia. Circulation 2005;111(23):3034–41.

40. Karnabi E, Qu Y, Wadgaonkar R, et al. Congenital heart block: identification of autoantibody binding site on the extracellular loop (domain I, S5-S6) of alpha(1D) L-type Ca channel. J Autoimmun 2010; 34(2):80–6.

41. Strandberg LS, Cui X, Rath A, et al. Congenital heart block maternal sera autoantibodies target an extracellular epitope on the alpha1G T-type calcium channel in human fetal hearts. PLoS One 2013; 8(9):e72668.

42. Boutjdir M, Chen L, Zhang ZH, et al. Arrhythmogenicity of IgG and anti-52-kD SSA/Ro affinity-purified antibodies from mothers of children with congenital heart block. Circ Res 1997;80(3):354–62.

43. Xiao GQ, Qu Y, Hu K, et al. Down-regulation of L-type calcium channel in pups born to 52 kDa SSA/Ro immunized rabbits. FASEB J 2001;15(9):1539–45.

44. Patel C, Antzelevitch C. Pharmacological approach to the treatment of long and short QT syndromes. Pharmacol Ther 2008;118(1):138–51.

45. Schwartz PJ, Periti M, Malliani A. The long Q-T syndrome. Am Heart J 1975;89(3):378–90.

46. Keating MT, Sanguinetti MC. Molecular and cellular mechanisms of cardiac arrhythmias. Cell 2001; 104(4):569–80.

47. Schwartz PJ, Ackerman MJ. The long QT syndrome: a transatlantic clinical approach to diagnosis and therapy. Eur Heart J 2013;34(40):3109–16.

48. Roden DM. Cellular basis of drug-induced torsades de pointes. Br J Pharmacol 2008;154(7):1502–7.

49. Kannankeril P, Roden DM, Darbar D. Drug-induced long QT syndrome. Pharmacol Rev 2010;62(4):760–81.

50. Yue Y, Castrichini M, Srivastava U, et al. Pathogenesis of the novel autoimmune-associated long-QT syndrome. Circulation 2015;132(4):230–40.

51. Seed WA, Noble MI, Oldershaw P, et al. Relation of human cardiac action potential duration to the interval between beats: implications for the validity of rate corrected QT interval (QTc). Br Heart J 1987; 57(1):32–7.

52. Yan GX, Lankipalli RS, Burke JF, et al. Ventricular repolarization components on the electrocardiogram: cellular basis and clinical significance. J Am Coll Cardiol 2003;42(3):401–9.

53. Yan GX, Antzelevitch C. Cellular basis for the normal T wave and the electrocardiographic manifestations of the long-QT syndrome. Circulation 1998;98(18):1928–36.

54. Xiao GQ, Hu K, Boutjdir M. Direct inhibition of expressed cardiac L- and T-type calcium channels by IgG from mothers whose children have congenital heart block. Circulation 2001;103(11):1599–604.

55. Boutjdir M, Chen L, Zhang ZH, et al. Serum and immunoglobulin G from the mother of a child with congenital heart block induce conduction abnormalities and inhibit L-type calcium channels in a rat heart model. Pediatr Res 1998;44(1):11–9.

56. Farkas AS, Nattel S. Minimizing repolarization-related proarrhythmic risk in drug development and clinical practice. Drugs 2010;70(5):573–603.

Pharmacogenetics of Potassium Channel Blockers

Dan M. Roden, MD

KEYWORDS

• Pharmacogenetics • Potassium channel blockers • Ion channels • Cardiac repolarization

KEY POINTS

- The QT interval on the surface electrocardiogram serves as an interesting model of a multicomponent integrated readout of many different biological systems, including ion channels, modulatory subunits, the signaling systems that modulate their activity, and the mechanisms that regulate the expression of their responsible genes.
- A highly integrated system like this behaves in a fairly consistent way in normal humans, and in people harboring congenital long QT syndrome disease mutations; most heart beats do not trigger fatal cardiac arrhythmias.
- The problem of drug exposure causing exaggerated QT interval prolongation and torsades de pointes has evolved from a historical curiosity as an idiosyncratic drug action to a set of genomic and model system experiments that highlight the multicomponent nature of cardiac repolarization and the way in which simple perturbations can, in some patients, yield exaggerated responses.
- Future directions will involve cellular approaches coupled to evolving technologies that can interrogate not just cells but multicellular systems up to and including the whole heart, and provide an increasingly sophisticated view of mechanisms in this previously idiosyncratic drug reaction.

Drugs vary in their effects for many reasons, such as incomplete compliance, the underlying disease being treated, clinical covariates such as age and sex, and interaction with other drugs being prescribed. Work over the past several decades, and accelerating in the last 10 years, has identified an increasingly large set of DNA variants that can modulate drug actions. Thus, a contemporary view includes a consideration of pharmacogenetic factors as a source of variability in drug action in human patients.[1]

This article focuses on genetic factors modulating the effects of potassium channel blockers whose major clinical action is to prolong cardiac repolarization. In the case of potassium channel blocking antiarrhythmic drugs, this effect on repolarization and its surface electrocardiogram (ECG) correlate, QT interval prolongation, is the desired therapeutic effect and is associated with arrhythmia suppression. In other cases, drugs that inhibit cardiac repolarization are used therapeutically for other clinical conditions, such as psychiatric or infectious diseases. In this setting, QT interval prolongation is an off-target effect. A major reason for the interest in QT pharmacogenomics is the problem that marked QT prolongation can generate the morphologically distinctive polymorphic ventricular tachycardia torsades de pointes, the drug-induced long QT syndrome (diLQTS).

Potassium channels are ubiquitous across many cell types, and a wide range of drugs has been

Supported in part by grants from the United States Public Health Service (R01 HL118952, R01 HL049989, U19 HL65962, and P50 GM115305).
Oates Institute for Experimental Therapeutics, Vanderbilt University School of Medicine, 1285 MRB IV, Nashville, TN 37232-0575, USA
E-mail address: dan.roden@vanderbilt.edu

developed to inhibit their function. For example, sulfonylureas interact with ATP-inhibited potassium channels in the pancreas to produce therapeutic effects in diabetes,[2] and the broad-spectrum potassium channel blocker 4-aminopyridine has been used therapeutically for multiple sclerosis.[3] These drugs do not produce major effects on the QT interval on the surface ECG and are not discussed further here.

Some potassium channel blocking antiarrhythmics produce little or no other cardiac ion channel electrophysiologic effect and are termed pure potassium channel blockers. Sotalol, dofetilide, and possibly ibutilide are in this category, although sotalol's effects are also mediated by beta-blockade and early reports suggested that ibutilide may also enhance late sodium current,[4] an issue that is discussed further later. Other potassium channel blocking antiarrhythmics have additional cardiac electrophysiologic effects, such as blocking of sodium or calcium channels: amiodarone, dronedarone, and quinidine are in this category. Accordingly, predicting the whole-heart effects of these drugs is especially complex, reflecting the fact that some effects prolong QT and others shorten it. In addition, flecainide and propafenone, generally classified as fairly pure sodium channel blockers, also have potassium channel blocking effects and can prolong QT intervals in humans.

A wealth of data supports the idea that the major mechanism whereby potassium channel blocking drugs, whether pure or mixed, prolong the QT interval is by inhibiting a major repolarizing potassium current in heart, I_{Kr}.[5-7] Thus, a discussion of variability in the clinical actions of I_{Kr} blockers focuses on variability, whether genetic or other, in factors that modulate the interactions of drugs with the Kv11.1 channel (encoded by KCNH2, formerly termed Human Ether-a-go-go-Related Gene [HERG]) responsible for I_{Kr} and its resultant effect on QT interval prolongation. These factors include delivery of the drug to the channel, the number of channels present, and the number of other repolarizing and depolarizing channels present. Further, as discussed later in this article, recent work has identified alternate mechanisms whereby even pure potassium channel blockers may modulate cardiac repolarization. Thus, even a simple interaction of a drug with a singular molecular target, such as the Kv11.1 channel, can introduce important complexities in analysis of variability of drug actions.

Two fundamental processes can lead to variability in drug action. The first is pharmacokinetic variability caused by variability in drug concentrations at the target sites of action. The second source of variability is pharmacodynamic; here, drug concentrations at the site of action are constant but there is variability in drug action at the cellular, tissue, whole-organ, or whole-organism level.[1]

PHARMACOKINETIC MECHANISMS

Pharmacokinetic effects are generally analyzed in terms of 4 fundamental processes that determine such drug concentrations: absorption, distribution, metabolism, and elimination. Nongenetic factors such as coadministration of inhibiting drugs or dysfunction of excretory organs can perturb these processes. For example, sotalol and dofetilide are not metabolized but are excreted largely unchanged by the kidneys. The drug transporter responsible for this excretion has not been definitively identified, but, as a general rule, patients with decreased renal function must have the drug doses reduced or the drug stopped to avoid very high drug concentrations, excessive QT interval prolongation, and torsades de pointes. Genetic factors may also play a role. For example, among noncardiovascular potassium channel blockers, the antipsychotic thioridazine is metabolized by the enzyme CYP2D6, and poor metabolizers (5%–10% of white and African people), who lack active enzyme, develop higher than usual drug concentrations at ordinary drug doses and some data suggest that this is associated with an increased risk of torsades de pointes.[8] Similarly, poor metabolizers for CYP2B6 may be at increased risk for methadone-induced torsades de pointes.[9]

It is thought that drugs blocking the Kv11.1 channel must access the drug binding site from the interior of the cell, so it is possible that variability in intracellular drug concentrations, caused by variable drug uptake or efflux, could account for variability in drug action. In vitro experiments have shown that manipulating the function of drug uptake or efflux transport molecules can produce such variability in Kv11.1 block,[10,11] but DNA variants that generate this effect in human patients have not yet been reported.

PHARMACODYNAMICS

Multiple biological mechanisms may underlie pharmacodynamic variability. These mechanisms include variability in expression or function of the target molecules with which drugs interact to achieve their effects and/or variability in the broad biological context, (including genetic alterations contributing to the disease being studied) in which drugs act. In the case of potassium channel blockers, variability in effects might be caused by variability in the number of Kv11.1 channels in the membrane, or by genetic or other mechanisms (such as phosphorylation or interaction with modulating proteins) that interfere with channel function or with drug access or binding to its target sites of actions. In addition, net drug action in a cell may be modulated by the number or function of other channels that also contribute to repolarization. For example, reduction in I_{Ks}, a second major cardiac repolarizing potassium current, may render the heart more dependent on robust I_{Kr} function to accomplish normal repolarization. In this situation, administration of an I_{Kr} blocker may unmask this dependency by producing exaggerated QT prolongation and torsades.

This is one example of the general phenomenon of repolarization reserve.[12–14] It is postulated that normal cardiac repolarization is accomplished by multiple partially redundant processes such as I_{Ks} and I_{Kr}. A reduction in function in one of these processes may be subclinical at baseline (because other mechanisms are still present to accomplish normal repolarization), but revealed, by exaggerated QT prolongation and torsades de pointes, by I_{Kr} block.

Heart disease may modulate the number or function of channels and thus lead to altered drug actions; it is likely that clinical risk factors for torsades, such as congenital long QT syndromes, heart failure, left ventricular hypertrophy, female gender, or after cardioversion of atrial fibrillation, act in this fashion.[7] There are many other settings in which marked lability in QT duration or morphology have been consistently reported: these include stress cardiomyopathy,[15] postpacing or bundle branch block (memory) changes,[16,17] diabetes,[18–20] and subarachnoid hemorrhage.[21] The fundamental mechanisms leading to these QT changes are not well understood, and whether they increase torsades risk is uncertain, but changes in critical signaling pathways that regulate channel synthesis or function seem likely.

METHODOLOGIC CONSIDERATIONS IN STUDYING THE GENOMICS OF DRUG-INDUCED QT INTERVAL PROLONGATION

Two general approaches have been used in this area. One is to study the extent to which drug exposure prolongs the QT interval across a population and to relate variability in this metric to genetic variants. A second approach is to study patients who develop exaggerated QT prolongation (corrected QT [QTc] >480 or 500 milliseconds or some other cutoff) and/or torsades de pointes and compare them with a large sample drawn from a representative population or a sample of

patients exposed to the same drugs without developing marked QT prolongation.

The specific genetic analysis in these settings is often constrained by sample size. For small samples, it is unrealistic to look for associations across large numbers of genetic variants and so investigators often choose a small number of common variants in logically chosen candidate genes and compare their frequency across a population or in cases and controls. Candidate genes for modulating variability in the effects of I_{Kr} blockers include pharmacokinetic and pharmacodynamic genes: the latter include *KCNH2*, genes encoding other repolarizing potassium channels in heart, genes encoding depolarizing sodium or calcium channels in heart, genes controlling sodium-calcium or sodium-potassium fluxes, and genes identified as modulators of baseline QT by unbiased approaches (discussed later).

The candidate gene approach has the advantage that it makes physiologic sense, but experience has shown that candidate gene associations are often not replicated when larger numbers of study subjects are accrued.[22] Accumulation of very large sets of study subjects can enable unbiased approaches, such as the genome-wide association study (GWAS), to identify new associations between genetic loci and human traits.[23] For example, in a very large GWAS analysis of baseline QT variability, the top association was with single nucleotide polymorphisms (SNPs) near *NOS1AP*, which encodes a subunit for neuronal nitric oxide synthase.[24] The mechanism of the association has not been definitively established but *NOS1AP* has been reported to modulate sodium, potassium, and calcium channel function.[25,26] The advantage of this approach is that new modulators of human traits may be identified, as in the case of NOS1AP and the QT. However, although these associations are highly statistically significant, each SNP contributes a very small amount to the trait under study. For example, the association between NOS1AP variants and QT has a *P* value of 10^{-213}, but the effect size is ~ 3 milliseconds per allele.

For a rare adverse drug effect, such as torsades de pointes, it is often not possible to generate very large numbers of affected subjects (by definition) so unbiased approaches may be limited by small sample sizes. As in any contemporary genetic analysis, correction for potential confounders such as ancestry, gender, extent, or type of underlying heart disease, or even specific drug exposure, is generally required.

WHAT IS THE EVIDENCE THAT DRUG-INDUCED LONG QT SYNDROME IS A GENETIC PROBLEM?

The occasional patients who develop marked QT interval prolongation and torsades de pointes present a problem for clinicians because the reaction is idiosyncric (ie, unanticipated in that patient). Shortly after the initial cloning of major congenital long QT syndrome disease genes came a series of case reports that rare disease-associated variants in these genes were occasionally found in patients with drug-induced arrhythmias (ie, subclinical congenital long QT syndrome seems to be a risk factor for the drug-induced form).[27,28] This observation is in keeping with the reduced repolarization reserve concept outlined earlier and points to genetic predisposition as a contributor to the idiosyncratic nature of diLQTS. Another observation supporting the idea that individuals vary in specific susceptibility was from Kääb and colleagues,[29] who studied 22 subjects with drug-induced torsades de pointes. After clinical stabilization and return of the QT interval to normal, these subjects were rechallenged in a coronary care unit with intravenous sotalol, and marked QT interval prolongation was again observed, and not seen in a group of control subjects.

PHARMACOGENOMIC STUDIES IN THE DRUG-INDUCED LONG QT SYNDROME

Complex in silico models of multiple physiologically based ion channel behaviors can predict the cellular consequences of a range of pathophysiologic interventions (changes in rate, potassium, drug exposure, and so forth). The original Luo-Rudy model was used to show that reduction in I_{Kr} not only produced action potential prolongation (as expected) but also generated early afterdepolarizations that the model could then attribute to reactivation of L-type calcium channels,[30] as also predicted from experimental data.[31] Similarly, slight reduction in I_{Ks} produces minimal action potential prolongation, but markedly exaggerates the effects of an I_{Kr} blocker.[32] This finding is an example of reduced repolarization reserve.

Pharmacogenetic studies of diLQTS have used both candidate gene and genome-wide approaches (**Table 1**). The frequency of subclinical

---

Table 1
Identifying possible risk variants predisposing to drug-induced long QT syndrome

Approach	Outcome	References
Sequencing congenital LQTS disease genes in diLQTS cases	Rare variants (possible subclinical congenital LQTS) in ~5%–30%	33,35–38
Examine associations with large numbers of SNPs in candidate genes	*KCNE1* D85N identified as a risk allele (1.8%–29% in controls; 8.6% in cases; odds ratio 9–12)	39
	NOS1AP variant as modulator of amiodarone-induced diLQTS	40
	NOS1AP and *NUBPL* variants as potential modulators of QT prolongation by antipsychotics	46
GWAS of QT prolongation by drugs	Variant in NRG3 as potential modulator of iloperidone effect	45
	Variant in *SLC22A23* as potential modulator of quetiapine effect	46
	Variant near *NRG3* as potential modulator of sotalol effect	44
GWAS of diLQTS	No variants at genome-wide significance in 216 diLQTS cases and 771 controls	41
Exome sequencing	Variants in *KCNE1* and *ACN9* reach significance. Slightly more rare variants in K$^+$ channel genes in cases (37%) vs controls (21%)	42
Identifying mutant zebrafish lines with exaggerated or blunted responses to dofetilide challenge	Variants in *GINS3* (implicated in control of baseline QT[24]) as potential diLQTS risk	47

Abbreviations: GWAS, genome-wide association study; LQTS, long QT syndrome.
  Data from Refs.[33,35–42,44–47]

congenital long QT syndrome mutations has been examined in patients with the drug-induced form of the arrhythmia. One study sought sequence variants in KCNE2, a potassium channel subunit modulating Kv11.1 function, in 98 subjects with diLQTS and found 3 rare variants and 1 polymorphism (T8A),[33] now recognized to occur in 0.3% of the population.[34] The rare variants were associated with decreased potassium current even before drug use, whereas potassium channels reconstituted by coexpression of Kv11.1 and the T8A variant KCNE2 showed normal potassium current at baseline but exaggerated block by sulfamethoxazole, the drug that produced diLQTS in the affected patient. Surveys of other potassium and sodium channel congenital long QT syndrome disease genes have suggested that 5% to 40% of patients with diLQTS may have subclinical versions of the congenital syndrome.[35–38]

With accumulation of larger sets of cases and controls, surveys of larger numbers of candidate polymorphisms were enabled. One such study examined 1424 SNPs in 18 candidate genes in 176 patients with documented torsades de pointes during treatment with a QT-prolonging drug, 207 patients exposed to QT-prolonging drugs with minimal QT prolongation, and 837 population controls.[39] A single SNP in KCNE1, encoding a potassium channel–modulating subunit, was present in 8.6% of diLQTS cases and 1.8% to 2.9% of controls, giving an odds ratio of 9.0; the direction of the signal was replicated in a second set.[39]

In an analysis of 167 SNPs across the NOS1AP locus in 58 subjects with diLQTS and 87 controls (all white), 1 variant, rs10800397, was associated with diLQTS risk, particularly in subjects with amiodarone-induced torsades de pointes.[40] A GWAS analysis of 216 cases and 771 ancestry-matched controls failed to identify any signal at genome-wide significance.[41] Whether this result reflects low case numbers, a large contribution by nongenetic factors, or other experimental variables is not known. As might be expected from a GWAS involving small numbers of cases, the study was underpowered and could identify only variants occurring with a minor allele frequency greater than 10% and conferring an odds ratio greater than 2.7.

One other possibility is that torsades de pointes risk is modulated by multiple rare variants across multiple ion channel or other genes. Accordingly, in an exome sequencing experiment involving 65 patients with diLQTS and 148 drug-exposed ancestry-matched controls, rare variants were sought across all genes, and across subsets of genes associated with arrhythmias,[42] with

replication in 551 subjects in the exome sequencing project.[43] There were significant associations between non-synonymous variants in KCNE1 and ACN9 in the diLQTS cases. The KCNE1 signal replicates the candidate gene study described earlier; ACN9 is a gene involving gluconeogenesis and its relationship to cardiac arrhythmias remains to be determined. When a specifically predefined set of 7 congenital long QT syndrome genes encoding potassium channels or their modulatory subunits were examined, rare non-synonymous variants were commoner among subjects (37%) compared with controls (21%, $P = .009$). These data further support the idea that subclinical congenital long QT syndrome disease genes do predispose to diLQTS, but are not found in most patients.

Another approach is to examine variants associated with variability in the extent to which drug exposure prolongs QT interval. Although this method does not explicitly consider patients with torsades de pointes, it does allow larger numbers of subjects to be enrolled. One study, a GWAS analysis of 404 European-American subjects, all exposed to sotalol and ascertained via an electronic medical record, identified associations at near genome-wide significance in NRG3, a gene known to be involved in cardiac development.[44] A previous GWAS had identified variants in NRG3 as contributing to diLQTS risk after exposure to the antipsychotic drug iloperidone.[45] A candidate gene analysis of change in QT during antipsychotic therapy implicated NOS1AP, previously associated with baseline QTc, and NUBPL, associated with iloperidone change in QTc.[46] A GWAS of the same data set also implicated variants in the drug transporter SLC22A23 in variable quetiapine effects.[46]

Animal models have also been used to identify genes modulating QT interval prolongation by drugs. Zebrafish in which the orthologue of KCNH2 has been knocked out show marked action potential prolongation, whereas heterozygotes show only minimal action potential prolongation but do show exaggerated action potential prolongation on exposure to dofetilide.[47] This experiment suggests that zebrafish action potentials can be used to search for new genes involved in QT prolongation by drugs. Dofetilide exposure in zebrafish with random mutations across the genome identified lines with exaggerated QT prolongation that was transmissible across generations,[47] and subsequent analyses implicated variants in GINS3 as potential modulators of QT prolongation in this model. GWAS has identified the GINS3 locus as a modulator of baseline QT interval in humans.[24] The function of this gene and its associated biological pathways remains to be determined but the series of studies shows the way in which human population data can be combined with model organism data to discover new pathways in QT regulation and other biological processes.

CURRENT STATE OF THE ART

For some adverse drug reactions, single variants, often in the human leucocyte antigen-B (HLA-B) locus (for immunologically mediated reactions) contribute strongly to,[48,49] or completely define, risk. In contrast, in diLQTS the data sets outlined earlier support the idea that rare variants play a role in multiple pathways, including ion channels and perhaps other electrical signaling pathways whose function has not yet been well defined (eg, GINS3 or NRG3). However, another possibility is that the adverse drug reaction is determined not simply by germline genomic variation interacting with drug exposure but also by environmental influences, specifically signaling pathways modulated by underlying heart disease or other known diLQTS risk factors.

One potential example is variability in gene expression or function conferred by microRNAs. Xiao and colleagues[50] reported that prolonged exposure to dofetilide in canine cardiomyocytes resulted in an unexpected shortening of action potential duration. Subsequent investigation attributed this change to a decrease in 2 microRNAs and a consequent increase in the other repolarizing current, I_{Ks}.

Lu and colleagues[51] noted that the tyrosine kinase inhibitor nilotinib, which is associated with QT prolongation in patients, does not acutely block I_{Kr}. However, with chronic exposure, action potentials in canine cardiomyocytes were prolonged and this change was attributed to downregulation of important repolarizing potassium currents (I_{Kr} and I_{Ks}) as well as increases in the late sodium current. Our group then went on to show that hours of exposure to pure I_{Kr} blockers, such as dofetilide, strikingly increased late sodium current and produced arrhythmogenic afterdepolarizations in mouse myocytes; acute dofetilide exposure produced no change in action potential in mouse cardiomyocytes as expected because I_{Kr} plays no role in repolarization in these cells.[52] Intracellular perfusion with phosphatidyl (3,4,5)-triphosphate (PIP3) the downstream effector of phosphoinositide (PI) 3-kinase (PI3K) signaling, reversed the effect, implicating inhibited PI3K signaling as a major proximate mechanism underlying the increasing late sodium current. Other reports indicate that increased late sodium current (reversible by pipette PIP3) may also underlie

increased action potential duration in diabetes.[19] Further, mice with the alpha isoform of PI3K (which mediates the change in late sodium current[53]) show increased susceptibility to atrial fibrillation.[54] These findings suggest a molecular basis for the link between structural heart disease and diLQTS susceptibility.

Another well-recognized risk factor is hypokalemia. We have shown that decreased extracellular potassium strikingly increases the I_{Kr}-blocking potency of dofetilide or quinidine.[55] The underlying mechanism likely represents a potassium-induced shift in the balance between open and inactivated states of the channel during depolarization[56] or to increased block by extracellular sodium when extracellular potassium is decreased.[57] Another report suggested that hypokalemia generated arrhythmias by inhibiting Na-K-ATPase and activating calmodulin-dependent kinase, thereby enhancing late sodium current, prolonging repolarization, and generating arrhythmias; dofetilide potentiated this effect.[58]

Another interesting model system that is now being introduced into this area is the development of technologies to derive cardiomyocytes from human patients via induced pluripotent stem cells (iPSCs). In cells derived from patients with congenital long QT syndrome, action potentials are longer than those seen in patients without mutations, and the cells show marked action potential prolongation and arrhythmogenic afterdepolarizations on exposure to very low concentrations of I_{Kr}-blocking drugs.[59] Another approach to translating the effects of drugs on individual ion channels to effect in the whole heart is systematic exploration of the ECG effects of drugs known to be pure or mixed potassium channel blockers; initial studies suggest that Kv11.1 block produces consist changes in T-wave morphology regardless of whether other pharmacologic properties are superimposed.[60] Recent proposals from the pharmaceutical industry and the US Food and Drug Administration suggest that these new approaches, including the use of iPSC-derived cardiomyocytes, systematic ECG analyses, and in silico modeling, may complement or supplant current approaches to evaluating the potential of a new drug entity to cause diLQTS.[61]

SUMMARY

The QT interval on the surface ECG serves as an interesting model of a multicomponent integrated readout of many different biological systems, including ion channels, modulatory subunits, the signaling systems that modulate their activity, and the mechanisms that regulate the expression of their responsible genes. A highly integrated system like this behaves in a fairly consistent way in normal humans, and in people harboring congenital long QT syndrome disease mutations; most heart beats do not trigger fatal cardiac arrhythmias. The problem of drug exposure causing exaggerated QT interval prolongation and torsades de pointes has evolved from a historical curiosity as an idiosyncratic drug action to a set of genomic and model system experiments that highlight the multicomponent nature of cardiac repolarization and the way in which simple perturbations can, in some patients, yield exaggerated responses. Future directions will involve cellular approaches coupled to evolving technologies that can interrogate not just cells but multicellular systems up to and including the whole heart, and provide an increasingly sophisticated view of mechanisms in this previously idiosyncratic drug reaction.

REFERENCES

1. Roden DM, Johnson JA, Kimmel SE, et al. Cardiovascular pharmacogenomics. Circ Res 2011;109:807–20.
2. Sattiraju S, Reyes S, Kane GC, et al. K(ATP) channel pharmacogenomics: from bench to bedside. Clin Pharmacol Ther 2008;83:354–7.
3. Lugaresi A. Pharmacology and clinical efficacy of dalfampridine for treating multiple sclerosis. Expert Opin Drug Metab Toxicol 2015;11:295–306.
4. Lee KS. Ibutilide, a new compound with potent class III antiarrhythmic activity, activates a slow inward Na+ current in guinea pig ventricular cells. J Pharmacol Exp Ther 1992;262:99–108.
5. Sanguinetti MC, Jurkiewicz NK. Two components of cardiac delayed rectifier K+ current: differential sensitivity to block by class III antiarrhythmic agents. J Gen Physiol 1990;96:195–215.
6. Sanguinetti MC, Jiang C, Curran ME, et al. A mechanistic link between an inherited and an acquired cardiac arrhythmia: HERG encodes the I Kr potassium channel. Cell 1995;81:299–307.
7. Roden DM. Long QT syndrome: reduced repolarization reserve and the genetic link. J Intern Med 2006;259:59–69.
8. Llerena A, Berecz R, de la Rubia A, et al. QTc interval lengthening is related to CYP2D6 hydroxylation capacity and plasma concentration of thioridazine in patients. J Psychopharmacol 2002;16:361–4.
9. Eap CB, Crettol S, Rougier JS, et al. Stereoselective block of hERG channel by (S)-methadone and QT interval prolongation in CYP2B6 slow metabolizers. Clin Pharmacol Ther 2007;81:719–28.
10. McBride BF, Yang T, Roden DM. Influence of the G2677T/C3435T haplotype of MDR1 on P-glycoprotein trafficking and ibutilide-induced block of HERG. Pharmacogenomics J 2009;9:194–201.
11. McBride BF, Yang T, Liu K, et al. The organic cation transporter, OCTN1, expressed in the human heart, potentiates antagonism of the HERG potassium channel. J Cardiovasc Pharmacol 2009;54:63–71.
12. Roden DM. Taking the idio out of idiosyncratic - predicting torsades de pointes. Pacing Clin Electrophysiol 1998;21:1029–34.
13. Roden DM. Repolarization reserve: a moving target. Circulation 2008;118:981–2.
14. Wu L, Rajamani S, Li H, et al. Reduction of repolarization reserve unmasks the proarrhythmic role of endogenous late Na(+) current in the heart. Am J Physiol Heart Circ Physiol 2009;297:H1048–57.
15. Samuelov-Kinori L, Kinori M, Kogan Y, et al. Takotsubo cardiomyopathy and QT interval prolongation: who are the patients at risk for torsades de pointes? J Electrocardiol 2009;42(4):353–7.e1.
16. Coronel R, Opthof T, Plotnikov AN, et al. Long-term cardiac memory in canine heart is associated with the evolution of a transmural repolarization gradient. Cardiovasc Res 2007;74:416–25.
17. Rosso R, Adler A, Strasberg B, et al. Long QT syndrome complicating atrioventricular block: arrhythmogenic effects of cardiac memory. Circ Arrhythm Electrophysiol 2014;7:1129–35.
18. Christensen PK, Gall MA, Major-Pedersen A, et al. QTc interval length and QT dispersion as predictors of mortality in patients with non-insulin-dependent diabetes. Scand J Clin Lab Invest 2000;60:323–32.
19. Lu Z, Jiang YP, Wu CY, et al. Increased persistent sodium current due to decreased PI3K signaling contributes to QT prolongation in the diabetic heart. Diabetes 2013;62:4257–65.
20. Heller S, Darpö B, Mitchell MI, et al. Considerations for assessing the potential effects of antidiabetes drugs on cardiac ventricular repolarization: a report from the Cardiac Safety Research Consortium. Am Heart J 2015;170:23–35.
21. Rudehill A, Sundqvist K, Sylven C. QT and QT-peak interval measurements: a methodological study in patients with subarachnoid haemorrhage compared to a reference group. Clin Physiol 1986;6:23–37.
22. McCarthy MI, Abecasis GR, Cardon LR, et al. Genome-wide association studies for complex traits: consensus, uncertainty and challenges. Nat Rev Genet 2008;9:356–69.
23. Manolio TA. Genomewide association studies and assessment of the risk of disease. N Engl J Med 2010;363:166–76.
24. Arking DE, Pulit SL, Crotti L, et al. Genetic association study of QT interval highlights role for calcium signaling pathways in myocardial repolarization. Nat Genet 2014;46:826–36.

25. Chang KC, Barth AS, Sasano T, et al. CAPON modulates cardiac repolarization via neuronal nitric oxide synthase signaling in the heart. Proc Natl Acad Sci U S A 2008;105:4477–82.

26. Kapoor A, Sekar RB, Hansen NF, et al. An enhancer polymorphism at the cardiomyocyte intercalated disc protein NOS1AP locus is a major regulator of the QT interval. Am J Hum Genet 2014;94:854–69.

27. Donger C, Denjoy I, Berthet M, et al. KVLQT1 C-terminal missense mutation causes a forme fruste long-QT syndrome. Circulation 1997;96:2778–81.

28. Napolitano C, Schwartz PJ, Brown AM, et al. Evidence for a cardiac ion channel mutation underlying drug-induced QT prolongation and life-threatening arrhythmias. J Cardiovasc Electrophysiol 2000;11:691–6.

29. Kääb S, Hinterseer M, Nabauer M, et al. Sotalol testing unmasks altered repolarization in patients with suspected acquired long-QT-syndrome–a case-control pilot study using I.V. sotalol. Eur Heart J 2003;24:649–57.

30. Viswanathan P, Rudy Y. Pause induced early afterdepolarizations in the long QT syndrome: a simulation study. Cardiovasc Res 1999;42:530–42.

31. January CT, Riddle JM. Early afterdepolarizations: mechanism of induction and block: a role for L-type Ca 2+ current. Circ Res 1989;64:977–90.

32. Roden DM, Viswanathan PC. Genetics of acquired long QT syndrome. J Clin Invest 2005;115:2025–32.

33. Sesti F, Abbott GW, Wei J, et al. A common polymorphism associated with antibiotic-induced cardiac arrhythmia. Proc Natl Acad Sci U S A 2000;97:10613–8.

34. Exome Aggregation Consortium (ExAC). Available at: http://exac.broadinstitute.org. Accessed November 4, 2015.

35. Yang P, Kanki H, Drolet B, et al. Allelic variants in Long QT disease genes in patients with drug-associated torsades de pointes. Circulation 2002;105:1943–8.

36. Paulussen AD, Gilissen RA, Armstrong M, et al. Genetic variations of KCNQ1, KCNH2, SCN5A, KCNE1, and KCNE2 in drug-induced long QT syndrome patients. J Mol Med 2004;82:182–8.

37. Itoh H, Sakaguchi T, Ding WG, et al. Latent genetic backgrounds and molecular pathogenesis in drug-induced long QT syndrome. Circ Arrhythm Electrophysiol 2009;2:511–23.

38. Itoh H, Crotti L, Aiba T, et al. The genetics underlying acquired long QT syndrome: impact for genetic screening. Eur Heart J 2015. [Epub ahead of print].

39. Kääb S, Crawford DC, Sinner MF, et al. A large candidate gene survey identifies the KCNE1 D85N polymorphism as a possible modulator of drug-induced torsades de pointes. Circ Cardiovasc Genet 2012;5:91–9.

40. Jamshidi Y, Nolte IM, Dalageorgou C, et al. Common variation in the NOS1AP gene is associated with drug-induced QT prolongation and ventricular arrhythmia. J Am Coll Cardiol 2012;60(9):841–50.

41. Behr ER, Ritchie MD, Tanaka T, et al. Genome wide analysis of drug-induced torsades de pointes: lack of common variants with large effect sizes. PLoS One 2013;8:e78511.

42. Weeke P, Mosley JD, Hanna D, et al. Exome sequencing implicates an increased burden of rare potassium channel variants in the risk of drug-induced long QT interval syndrome. J Am Coll Cardiol 2014;63:1430–7.

43. Tennessen JA, Bigham AW, O'Connor TD, et al. Evolution and functional impact of rare coding variation from deep sequencing of human exomes. Science 2012;337:64–9.

44. Weeke P, Delaney J, Mosley JD, et al. Genetic variants associated with QT prolongation in patients exposed to sotalol: a genome wide association study. AHA 2012 Scientific Sessions. Circulation 2012;126:A18723.

45. Volpi S, Heaton C, Mack K, et al. Whole genome association study identifies polymorphisms associated with QT prolongation during iloperidone treatment of schizophrenia. Mol Psychiatry 2009;14(11):1024–31.

46. Aberg K, Adkins DE, Liu Y, et al. Genome-wide association study of antipsychotic-induced QTc interval prolongation. Pharmacogenomics J 2012;12:165–72.

47. Milan DJ, Kim AM, Winterfield JR, et al. Drug-sensitized zebrafish screen identifies multiple genes, including GINS3, as regulators of myocardial repolarization. Circulation 2009;120:553–9.

48. Daly AK, Donaldson PT, Bhatnagar P, et al. HLA-B*5701 genotype is a major determinant of drug-induced liver injury due to flucloxacillin. Nat Genet 2009;41:816–9.

49. Mallal S, Phillips E, Carosi G, et al. HLA-B*5701 screening for hypersensitivity to abacavir. N Engl J Med 2008;358:568–79.

50. Xiao L, Xiao J, Luo X, et al. Feedback remodeling of cardiac potassium current expression: a novel potential mechanism for control of repolarization reserve. Circulation 2008;118:983–92.

51. Lu Z, Wu CY, Jiang YP, et al. Suppression of phosphoinositide 3-kinase signaling and alteration of multiple ion currents in drug-induced long QT syndrome. Sci Transl Med 2012;4:131ra50.

52. Yang T, Chun YW, Stroud DM, et al. Screening for acute IKr block is insufficient to detect torsades de pointes liability: role of late sodium current. Circulation 2014;130:224–34.

53. Yang T, Hong CC, Roden DM. Inhibition of the α-subunit of PI3 kinase increases late sodium

current (INa-L) and generates arrhythmias. Heart Rhythm 2015;12:S150.

54. Pretorius L, Du X-J, Woodcock EA, et al. Reduced phosphoinositide 3-kinase (p110α) activation increases the susceptibility to atrial fibrillation. Am J Pathol 2009;175:998–1009.

55. Yang T, Roden DM. Extracellular potassium modulation of drug block of I Kr: implications for torsades de pointes and reverse use-dependence. Circulation 1996;93:407–11.

56. Yang T, Snyders DJ, Roden DM. Rapid inactivation determines the rectification and [K+]o dependence of the rapid component of the delayed rectifier K+ current in cardiac cells. Circ Res 1997;80: 782–9.

57. Mullins FM, Stepanovic SZ, Gillani NB, et al. Functional interaction between extracellular sodium,

potassium and inactivation gating in HERG channels. J Physiol 2004;558:729–44.

58. Pezhouman A, Singh N, Song Z, et al. Molecular basis of hypokalemia-induced ventricular fibrillation. Circulation 2015;132:1528–37.

59. Liang P, Lan F, Lee AS, et al. Drug screening using a library of human induced pluripotent stem cell–derived cardiomyocytes reveals disease-specific patterns of cardiotoxicity. Circulation 2013;127:1677–91.

60. Vicente J, Johannesen L, Mason JW, et al. Comprehensive T wave morphology assessment in a randomized clinical study of dofetilide, quinidine, ranolazine, and verapamil. J Am Heart Assoc 2015;4.

61. Darpo B, Garnett C, Keirns J, et al. Implications of the IQ-CSRC prospective study: time to revise ICH E14. Drug Saf 2015;38:773–80.

Mechanism of Proarrhythmic Effects of Potassium Channel Blockers

Lasse Skibsbye, PhD[a], Ursula Ravens, MD[b],*

KEYWORDS

- Cardiac action potentials • K[+] channels blockers • Antiarrhythmic drugs • Proarrhythmic effects
- Mechanism of arrhythmia

KEY POINTS

- Prolongation of the cardiac action potential by K[+] channel blockers is well recognized as an antiarrhythmic mechanism, but can exacerbate to life-threatening arrhythmia.
- The risk for drug-induced torsades de pointes arrhythmia and subsequent ventricular fibrillation is best documented for Kv11.1 (hERG) and Kv7.1 (KvLQT1) channel blockers.
- Potassium channels with predominant expression in the atrial myocardium may be beneficial in supraventricular arrhythmias without proarrhythmic risk in the ventricles.
- Many compounds target K[+] channels that were only recently discovered to also be expressed in the heart (eg, K2P and SK channels). The antiarrhythmic and proarrhythmic potential of such compounds is discussed.

INTRODUCTION
Excitability of the Heart: Basic Cardiac Electrophysiology

To accomplish its life-supporting function of pumping oxygenated blood around the body, the heart contracts and relaxes in a regulated fashion. This contraction process is preceded by electrical excitation that is initiated in the sinoatrial node and spreads throughout the heart in an orderly manner via the specialized cardiac conduction system. The action potential (AP) of the working myocardium lasts for several hundreds of milliseconds, with the delayed repolarization securing a refractory state for new excitations throughout the entire contraction phase. The sequence of ventricular excitation ensures that the cardiac contraction wave travels from the apex to the base and from endocardial to epicardial layers, whereas repolarization and relaxation take the reverse direction. Thus, the AP duration is shorter in epicardial than endocardial muscle and also shorter in the basal than the apical region. This heterogeneity of AP duration safeguards against bulging of the ventricles during a pumping cycle.

Action potentials and repolarization reserve
The shape of the cardiac AP is governed by voltage-dependent and time-dependent changes in ion movements across the cell membrane via selective ion channels, transporters, exchangers, and pumps.[1] Ion channels are hydrophobic protein complexes that span across the cell membrane and contain a hydrophilic pore that can open and close as the channel passes through an activated, inactivated, or deactivated stage in a voltage-dependent and time-dependent fashion.

Conflicts of Interest: U. Ravens is consultant to Xention Limited. BT.
[a] Danish Arrhythmia Research Centre, Faculty of Health and Medical Sciences, University of Copenhagen, 3 Blegdamsvej, 3 Copenhagen N DK-2200, Denmark; [b] Department of Pharmacology and Toxicology, Medical Faculty Carl Gustav Carus, Institut für Pharmakologie und Toxikologie, TU Dresden, Fetscherstrasse 74, Dresden D-01307, Germany
* Corresponding author.
E-mail address: ravens@mail.zih.tu-dresden.de

The driving force for current flow through an open channel is determined by the transmembrane concentration gradients for a particular ion species as well as by the membrane potential. Inward and outward flow of cations causes depolarization and repolarization, respectively. AP initiation of the cardiomyocyte happens as a response to the activation of voltage-gated Na^+ channels causing a fast depolarizing upstroke. The initial repolarization is caused by inactivating Na^+ current and the rapidly activating transient outward current. During the long plateau phase of the cardiac AP inward current mainly via L-type Ca^{2+} channels and outward current via a large variety of K^+ channels will temporarily be in balance until eventually K^+ currents prevail causing final repolarization. Delayed repolarization in human myocardium relies mainly on the large diversity of cardiac K^+ channels (**Fig. 1**), but also on a particular redundancy in the heart known as the "repolarization reserve," in which one current is taking over if another one should fail.[2]

Potassium channels

Potassium channels form a large family of ion channel proteins (see Nerbonne JM: Molecular Basis of Functional Myocardial Potassium Channel Diversity, in this issue) that are involved in controlling both resting membrane potential and AP shape and duration. The K^+ currents that play a role in the heart are listed in **Fig. 1**, which also contains the nomenclature of the gene encoding the pore-forming α-subunit of a particular K^+ channel.

Classification of K^+ channels is based on their rectifier properties describing how the channel is passing current better in one direction than the other, and on their kinetic function, although auxiliary subunits (β-subunits) also modify channel behavior. The outward rectifier K^+ channels (Kv channels) are formed by 4 α-subunits, each consisting of 6 transmembrane segments.[1] The inwardly rectifying K^+ channels (Kir family) are composed of 4 α-subunits that contain only 2 transmembrane segments.[3] In addition, weak inward rectifier channels have been detected and

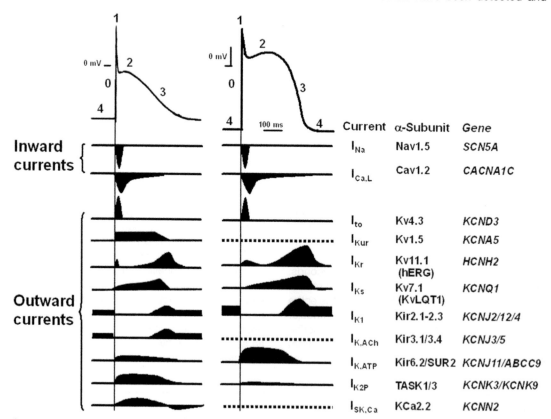

Current	α-Subunit	Gene
I_{Na}	Nav1.5	SCN5A
$I_{Ca,L}$	Cav1.2	CACNA1C
I_{to}	Kv4.3	KCND3
I_{Kur}	Kv1.5	KCNA5
I_{Kr}	Kv11.1 (hERG)	HCNH2
I_{Ks}	Kv7.1 (KvLQT1)	KCNQ1
I_{K1}	Kir2.1-2.3	KCNJ2/12/4
$I_{K,ACh}$	Kir3.1/3.4	KCNJ3/5
$I_{K,ATP}$	Kir6.2/SUR2	KCNJ11/ABCC9
I_{K2P}	TASK1/3	KCNK3/KCNK9
$I_{SK,Ca}$	KCa2.2	KCNN2

Fig. 1. Inward, depolarizing and outward, repolarizing currents that underlie the atrial and ventricular AP. Inward currents: I_{Na}, sodium current; $I_{Ca,L}$, L-type calcium current; I_{to}, transient outward current; I_{Kur}, ultra rapidly activating delayed rectifier current; I_{Kr} and I_{Ks}, rapidly and slowly activating delayed rectifier current; I_{K1}, inward rectifier current; $I_{K,ACh}$, acetylcholine-activated potassium current. Note, that I_{Kur} is present in atria only. Phase 0, rapid depolarization; phase 1, rapid early repolarization phase; phase 2, slow repolarization phase ("plateau" phase); phase 3, rapid late repolarization phase; phase 4, resting membrane potential. (*Adapted from* Ravens U, Cerbai E. Role of potassium currents in cardiac arrhythmias. Europace 2008;10(10):1134; with permission.)

were named according to their unusual structure; that is, TWIK-1 for "*T*andem of P domains in a *W*eak *I*nward rectifying *K*$^+$ channel."[4] The channels consist of only 2 α-subunits, each with 4 transmembrane-spanning regions but 2 pore domains (K2P channels). Of the family of Ca^{2+}-activated K$^+$ channels, the only channels with small single-channel K$^+$ conductance (SK) are expressed in the heart.[5] SK channels also consist of 4 α-subunits with 6 transmembrane-spanning segments, but are unique in that they are voltage-independent and solely gated by an increase in intracellular Ca^{2+}.[6]

Causes of Arrhythmia

Dysfunctional impulse formation (abnormal Ca^{2+} handling) and impulse conduction

Cardiac arrhythmia is a "multiscale" problem, involving both functional and structural aberrations at the molecular, cellular, tissue, and organism levels.[7] Basically, regular excitation of the heart can be perturbed by dysfunctional excitability and abnormal impulse conduction. Enhanced

rate of spontaneous diastolic depolarization as observed with increased sympathetic stimulation (**Fig. 2**A) may cause tachyarrhythmia. Abnormal excitations (extrasystoles, focal activity) are usually associated with unstable membrane potential either at the resting potential or at the AP plateau and early part of final repolarization, referred to as delayed and early afterdepolarizations, respectively (DAD, EAD), and can serve as triggers for ectopic activity (**Fig. 2**B, C). During critical prolongation of the AP plateau phase, inactivated Na$^+$ and/or Ca^{2+} channels may reopen, providing the extra depolarizing current for EAD.[8] On the organ scale, EAD may induce torsades de pointes arrhythmia (TdP), a type of polymorphic ventricular tachycardia,[9] which may evolve into ventricular fibrillation (**Fig. 2**D). DADs are linked to abnormalities in cellular Ca^{2+} handling.[10] Enhanced cellular Ca^{2+} load, for instance, is compensated by increased intracellular Ca^{2+} removal via the Na$^+$/Ca^{2+}-exchanger operating in its forward mode giving rise to a transient inward current due to the exchanging stoichiometry of 3/1 Na$^+$/Ca^{2+} with a depolarizing force of 1 net current. The

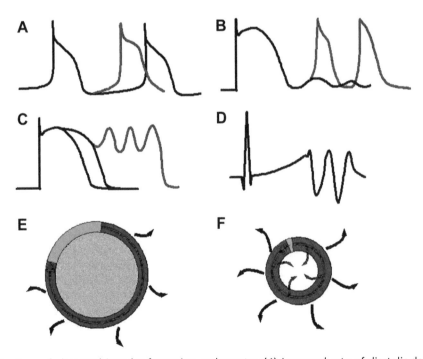

Fig. 2. Mechanisms of abnormal impulse formation and reentry. (*A*) Increased rate of diastolic depolarization accelerates automatic rhythm. Red color represents abnormal action potential conduction. (*B*) Delayed afterdepolarizations caused by transient inward currents via NCX (Na$^+$/Ca^{2+} exchanger) may reach threshold for a propagated extrasystole. Red color represents abnormal action potential conduction. (*C*) Early afterdepolarizations on excessive AP prolongation is due to reactivation of Na$^+$ channels or L-type Ca^{2+} channels. Red color represents abnormal action potential conduction. (*D*) Electrocardiogram with very long QT-interval exacerbating into TdP. (*E*) Reentry circuit around a scar. Red color represents tissue refractoriness. (*F*) Reentry around a functional obstacle; green, excitatory gap. The small arrows symbolize impulse conduction into the surrounding tissue. Red color represents tissue refractoriness.

resulting DAD initiates an extrasystole when the membrane potential reaches the threshold of sodium channel activation and the propagation of an AP (see **Fig. 2**C).

Impulse propagation can be impaired on an electrophysiological scale by reduced sodium current (I_{Na}) during the upstroke of the AP, at the (inter) cellular level by decoupled gap junctions between adjacent myocytes, and at the anatomic level by structural obstacles such as fibrosis or scar formation. Such impairments of electrical conduction may by arrhythmogenic by providing a functional substrate for arrhythmias to perpetuate.

Reentry phenomena

For an arrhythmia to establish, a triggering event must encounter a susceptible substrate to initiate self-sustained AP propagation. Propagation of an abnormal excitatory impulse around an anatomic (**Fig. 2**E) or functional obstacle (**Fig. 2**F) can perpetuate as reentry.[11] Fibrillation-developed propagation becomes chaotic, producing wavelets and high-frequency rotating waves ("rotors").[12]

Normally an impulse spreads in every direction and the tissue immediately behind each excitation front is refractory owing to the long-lasting AP (excitatory gap; see **Fig. 2**E, F). The pathway that an excitation front must travel before it can re-excite its origin is determined by the product of conduction velocity and effective refractory period ("wavelength").[13] The shorter the wavelength, the more prone a heart is to reentry arrhythmias. Any slowing of conduction velocity irrespective of its mechanism is associated with abbreviated reentry wavelengths and enhanced susceptibility to tachyarrhythmia. Shortening of the AP by increased K^+ currents reduces the functional refractory period, which also facilitates reentry. To this end, tissue heterogeneity in refractoriness is seen as a strong enhancer of arrhythmia vulnerability.[14]

Causes of arrhythmia should not be confused with the actual mechanism of rhythm disturbance.[7] These investigators emphasize that *causes* for arrhythmia include molecular factors like within channels and transporters, genetic precursors, and acquired diseases or side effects of a plethora of drugs for cardiac as well as for noncardiac indications. They also stress that "arrhythmias are no molecules but *behaviors* of an integrated dynamical system, namely the excitable medium of cardiac tissue." In addition, structural (fibrosis and other nonconducting tissue) and electrophysiological (heterogeneity of channel expression) peculiarities are incorporated as "fixed" factors that add another level of complexity.[7]

In summary, the major trigger mechanisms for arrhythmia are abnormal Ca^{2+} handling, and, may be somewhat counterintuitive, both excessive shortening *and* prolongation of the AP. Although excessive AP shortening is pro-arrhythmic by abbreviating wavelength, excessive AP prolongation may cause EADs, thereby providing a trigger for ectopic impulse formation.

Antiarrhythmic Drug Targets

Based on the causes outlined previously, strategies that target excessive Ca^{2+} entry, abnormal cell excitability, reduced refractoriness, and impaired coupling between cells are expected to suppress arrhythmias. Indeed, antiarrhythmic drugs of class I according to Vaughan Williams[15] are Na^+ channel blockers that suppress excitability and prolong postexcitation refractoriness thereby suppressing ectopic foci; class II drugs (β-adrenoceptor blockers) reduce spontaneous diastolic depolarization and suppress increased Ca^{2+} entry due to excessive β-adrenergic stimulation; class III drugs are defined as AP duration-lengthening agents. They prolong effective refractory period and hence terminate reentry arrhythmia; class IV agents block Ca^{2+} channels and prevent spontaneous activity due to Ca^{2+} overload. Each of these mechanisms provides protection against arrhythmias only within a limited range of change, but may become proarrhythmic when excessive. Treatment with established antiarrhythmic drugs is also associated with a disappointingly low efficacy and high incidence of cardiac and extracardiac side effects, again illustrating that our present understanding of the complexities of arrhythmias is far from complete.

Proarrhythmic Effects of Ion Channel Blockers

All approved antiarrhythmic drugs are potentially proarrhythmic. Na^+ channel blockers decrease Na^+ channel availability and therefore reduce conduction velocity, which is a function of Na^+ current and cellular coupling. Sodium channel blockers are clinically applied for their antiarrhythmic properties due to decreased rotor activity and spiral core excitability,[16] but impaired conduction also reduces wavelength, thereby facilitating reentry arrhythmias.[13] Most K^+ channel blockers prolong action potential duration (APD) and effective refractory period (ERP) and suppress reentry arrhythmias by increased wavelength. However, very long AP plateau phases also render the myocardium susceptible to EAD with a high risk of deterioration to TdP arrhythmias.[17] Finally, excessive slowing of spontaneous diastolic depolarization by β-adrenoceptor blockers or L-type Ca^{2+} channel blockers may cause severe bradycardia and atrioventricular nodal conduction delays, especially when combined with β-adrenoceptor blockers.[18]

The propensity of antiarrhythmic drugs to life-threatening arrhythmias was clinically detected in the CAST (Cardiac Arrhythmia Suppression Trial) study that tested whether suppression of extrasystoles by Na$^+$ channel blockers could improve survival after myocardial infarction.[19] The unexpected negative result sparked off the development of selective K$^+$ channel blockers as safe antiarrhythmic drugs. One of the first marketed antiarrhythmic drugs targeting hERG channels was clinically tested in the SWORD (Survival With Oral D-sotalol) trial, assessing the efficacy of the class III antiarrhythmic agent D-sotalol. The trial was terminated prematurely because of an increased mortality in the drug-treated relative to the placebo-treated group.[17] Today it is recognized that most conventional class III antiarrhythmic agents increase the risk for polymorphic ventricular tachycardia (TdP, Fig. 3). This vulnerability occurs largely due to heterogeneity in repolarization at a time when some of the myocardium is depolarized, some is incompletely repolarized, and some is completely repolarized, which are excellent conditions for arrhythmias to establish.

The QT interval of the electrocardiogram serves as a surrogate of the integrated durations of all cellular APs of the ventricles. Therefore, long QT intervals, like AP prolongations, present a risk for TdP arrhythmias. In addition, the proarrhythmic effects of delayed final repolarization are exacerbated by numerous clinical factors (**Box 1**), including age; sex; cardiac disease, such as myocardial ischemia,[20] hypertrophy, and heart failure; bradycardia; acquired or inherited QT interval[21]; reduced repolarization reserve; silent gene mutations; hypomagnesemia; and hypokalemia/hyperkalemia.[22]

Because lengthening of APD without instability or triangulation is not proarrhythmic in itself but rather antiarrhythmic,[23] and because not all patients with a long QT interval develop arrhythmias, Hondeghem[24] introduced the acronym "TRIaD" as a proarrhythmic risk estimate for AP-prolonging drugs, which stands for *Triangulation*, *Reverse use-dependency*, *Instability* and *Dispersion* of the AP, as a more integrated estimate of proarrhythmic effects of drugs. *Triangulation* of the AP is associated with proarrhythmic effects, because the delta time, at which the cells are most prone to reactivation during repolarization, is increased. This means that the time duration for reactivation of inactivated depolarizing channels (Ca^{2+} and Na$^+$) is increased and thus the likelihood for the induction of EADs will be enhanced. Prolonged APs with a rectangular configuration due to plateau prolongation and rapid final repolarization provide a rather safe antiarrhythmic mechanism, increasing the functional

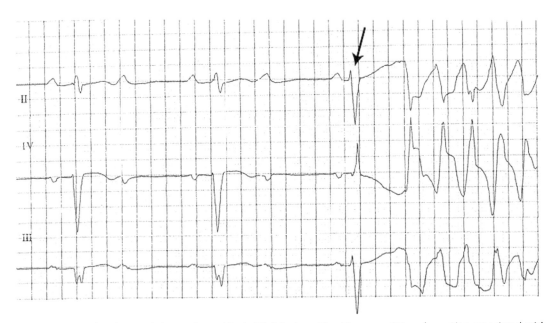

Fig. 3. An example of second-degree heart block (Mobitz type 2) with severe QT prolongation associated with sotalol therapy. A ventricular ectopic beat occurs (*arrow*) with associated severe QT prolongation and an augmented and elevated T-wave followed by a late-coupled initiation of TdP. (*From* Behr ER, Roden D. Drug-induced arrhythmia: pharmacogenomic prescribing? Eur Heart J 2013;34(2):92; with permission.)

Box 1
Clinical risk factors of drug-induced Torsades de Pointes

- Age
- Female sex
- Heart disease
  - Left ventricular hypertrophy
  - Heart failure
- Bradycardia
- Long QT Syndrome (LQTS)
  - Congenital LQTS
  - Acquired LQTS
- Electrolytes
- Hypokalemia
- Liver disease
- Renal dysfunction

refractory period without increasing the proarrhythmic time frame of repolarization.[25] *Reverse frequency-dependence* of K^+ channel blockers (often incorrectly referred to as *reverse "use" dependence*) implies that AP and ERP prolongation due to channel block are most pronounced at slow heart rate, and decrease with increasing heart rate. Because class III agents in general and hERG channel blockers in particular display strong reverse frequency–dependent effects,[26] patients with bradycardia are highly susceptible to drug-induced proarrhythmia. *Instability and dispersion* of repolarization and refractoriness across ventricular walls and between the ventricles presents a proarrhythmic substrate and favors the likelihood for electrical reentry in tissue regions with heterogeneous excitability and heterogeneously distributed repolarization.[27] All of these factors are believed to be important and to work in synergy in the genesis of acquired TdP arrhythmias.

SPECIFIC POTASSIUM CHANNELS AND EFFECTS OF BLOCKERS

In the following sections, the known or putative proarrhythmic effects of selective blockers are discussed for each cardiac K^+ channel (see also **Fig. 1** for nomenclature).

Delayed Rectifier K^+ Channels

Kv11.1 (hERG1): rapid delayed outward rectifier K^+ current I_{Kr}

The delayed rectifier Kv11.1 (*hERG1*) channel, encoded by the *KCNH2* gene, conducts the I_{Kr} current and is characterized by specific gating properties and binding affinity of diverse cardiac and noncardiac drugs. The conformational transition from a closed to an open state on depolarization is a fast process, but the subsequent inactivation is even faster. Consequently, the channel will almost immediately reach an inactivated, nonconducting state, not contributing substantially to the initial repolarization or plateau phase. However, in later repolarization stages, the channels are released from inactivation at a fast rate to an open state, whereas deactivation from an open to a closed state by a conformational change is a slow process.[28,29] This gives rise to the delayed "tail current," which is responsible for the relatively large contribution of I_{Kr} to the final part *phase 3* of repolarization and to the early part of the diastolic *phase 4*.

Mutations of the *hERG* gene may cause dysfunction of this rapidly activating delayed rectifier and thus lead to cardiac arrhythmia, such as congenital type 2 long QT syndrome (LQTS).[30] The major cause of acquired LQTS is due to pharmacologic block of *hERG* channels.[31,32]

Drug-induced TdP arrhythmias have mostly been associated with antiarrhythmic drug therapy, including D-sotalol[17] and dofetilide.[33] However, numerous noncardiac drugs also block hERG channels and cause acquired LQTS.[34] They belong to many different drug classes including antibiotics (macrolides [eg, erythromycin], and fluoroquinolones [eg, moxifloxacin]), antifungal imidazolines (ketoconazole), neuroleptics (chlorpromazine, haloperidol), antihistamines (terfenadine, astemizole), and gastrointestinal drugs (cisapride and domperidone).[35] The estimated incidence of drug-induced TdP and deaths associated with noncardiac drugs is 1 to 10 per 100,000 and much lower compared with the antiarrhythmic drug risk. Nevertheless, the accumulated risk could be as high as 3% of all prescribed medications that are potentially associated with proarrhythmic effects.[36]

Loss of hERG channel function in congenital and drug-induced LQTS can involve different mechanisms including interference with synthesis of channels and protein trafficking and other posttranslational modifications, with channel gating or K^+ permeation. Direct block of hERG channels is caused by drug-binding at the inner mouth of the ion-conducting pore. Unlike other Kv channels, hERG channels feature easy access to 2 aromatic amino acids in this pore region, which provides a high-affinity binding site for a large diversity of chemical structures[31,37] (especially 2 aromatic residues are important for channel binding and blockage).[38] This explains the surprisingly large variety of drugs that are hERG channel blockers. Impaired trafficking of otherwise normal channel protein was described as a cause of acquired LQTS for the antineoplastic agent arsenic trioxide or for the antiviral drug pentamidine.[39,40] Recently, yet another mechanism of drug-induced LQT was described for the cholesterol-lowering drug probucol, in which probucol downregulates a protein involved in the protein degradation signal cascade causing excess ubiquitination of hERG with subsequent enhanced endocytosis and channel degradation.[41]

Kv7.1 (KCNQ1): slow delayed outward rectifier K$^+$ current I$_{Ks}$

The slow outward rectifier Kv7.1 *(KCNQ1)* channel, together with its regulatory β-subunits of the *KCNE* family, of which KCNE1 and KCNE4 are the most abundant in the heart, give rise to native cardiac I$_{Ks}$.[42,43] I$_{Ks}$ is slowly activated on depolarization, with channel gating occurring at more depolarized potentials (right-shifted activation curve) showing only limited inactivation.[44,45] These properties allow I$_{Ks}$ to build up slowly over time contributing primarily to repolarization at *phase 3*. Accumulation of I$_{Ks}$ is considered crucial for AP shortening at fast heart rates.[44] I$_{Ks}$ also participates in the AP shortening on sympathetic stimulation, because the current is strongly regulated by β-adrenoceptor signaling[46] and probably also by α$_1$-adrenoceptor–mediated regulation of I$_{Ks}$ via Ca^{2+}-dependent protein kinase C.[47] Loss of function mutations in the KCNQ1 or KCNE genes constitutes major causes of lethal phenotypes of congenital LQTS.[48]

Although I$_{Ks}$ (KCNQ1) blockers have antiarrhythmic potential,[49] and several selective blockers have been developed as potential therapeutic agents,[50–52] these compounds possess an inherent proarrhythmic risk especially in situations of reduced I$_{Kr}$ or any other situation of reduced repolarization reserve.[53] This was observed experimentally in a study of LQT2 rabbits during isoflurane or propofol anesthesia (I$_{Ks}$ blockers), which resulted in polymorphic ventricular tachycardia.[54] I$_{Ks}$ blockage alone is rarely associated with proarrhythmic risk, which could be because I$_{Ks}$ is highly active during fast heart rates, keeping the AP short, while not producing much repolarizing current at slow heart rates, which is where the heart would be prone to a reduced repolarizing force.

Kv1.5 (KCNA5): ultrarapid delayed outward rectifier K$^+$ current I$_{Kur}$

The ultrarapidly activating delayed rectifier Kv1.5 channel conducts I$_{Kur}$. The Kv1.5 channel is predominantly expressed in atrial tissue and gives rise to an ultrarapidly activating "delayed" outward rectifier current.[55] Although Kv1.5 transcripts[56] and Kv1.5 protein[57] have also been detected in the human ventricle, no current corresponding to functional channels has been reported.[58] Therefore, blockers of I$_{Kur}$ are expected to prolong APD and ERP only in the atria and leave the ventricles unaffected, thus providing "atrial selectivity" when treating atrial fibrillation.[59]

This concept has inspired drug companies to develop new compounds for selective block of Kv1.5 channels.[60] In human atrial tissue from patients in sinus rhythm, block of I$_{Kur}$ causes marked elevation of the plateau phase, but APD and ERP are in fact *shortened* at physiologic pacing rates of 1 second^{-1}.[61,62] However, with the highly selective I$_{Kur}$ blocker XEN-D0103, we could demonstrate that the APD/EFP *shortening* effect at low stimulation rates actually converts into a *prolonging* effect at rates higher than 3 to 4 seconds^{-1}, which are more likely to be encountered in atrial fibrillation (Ford and colleagues[63] accepted Heart Rhythm 2015). This hitherto unknown positive frequency-dependent action of pure I$_{Kur}$ blockers may also be the reason why the first-in-humans study with the selective I$_{Kur}$ blocker MK-0448 revealed lack of effect on atrial ERP in healthy volunteers; that is, the cycle lengths (ie, >400 ms) used were probably too long.[64] On the other hand, so far no evidence for proarrhythmic activity of selective I$_{Kur}$ blockers has been reported.[64,65]

The only approved antiarrhythmic drug targeting I$_{Kur}$ is vernakalant,[66] although I$_{Kur}$ block was absent in human atrial cardiomyocytes. Vernakalant did not elevate the human atrial AP plateau phase that is characteristic of selective I$_{Kur}$ blockers.[67] The efficacy of vernakalant in acute cardioversion of AF is likely due to multiple-channel block, including inhibition of I$_{Na}$ and I$_{K,ACh}$ at clinically relevant concentrations.[68] Although marketed as an atrial selective drug, it is not completely free of ventricular side effects, including QTc prolongation and some cases of TdP and ventricular tachycardia described in Tsuji and Dobrev.[69] Kv1.5 protein may contribute to electrical activity in the ventricle through the formation of heteromultimeric K$^+$ channels with other Shaker-like subunits.[57]

Kv4.2 (KCND2), Kv4.3 (KCND3): transient outward current I$_{to}$

In the human myocardium, Kv4.2 and Kv4.3 channels encoded by *KCND2* and *KCND3*, respectively, conduct the rapidly activating and inactivating transient outward K$^+$ current I$_{to}$ that recovers rapidly from inactivation. The biophysical properties of the channels are modulated by diverse accessory subunits including KChIP and proteins of the KCNE family. In addition, cardiac I$_{to}$ channels are components of macromolecular protein complexes with regulatory proteins that influence channel expression and interaction with the actin cytoskeleton.[70] I_{to} governs the early rapid repolarization phase of the AP and, much like I_{Kur}, is also important for the plateau phase by setting the membrane potential for activation of L-type Ca^{2+} current.[71]

Currently, no selective blockers of I_{to} are known, although many compounds block this current along with others. High concentrations of 4-aminopyridine inhibit I_{to} in human atrial cardiomyocytes.[62] The antimalarial drug mefloquine inhibits I_{to} in rat ventricular myocytes and in Chinese hamster ovary (CHO) cells cotransfected with human Kv4.3 and its accessory subunit hKChIP2C.[72]

Sufficiently large I_{to} can suppress EADs, and a wide range of intermediate I_{to} properties can promote EADs by influencing the temporal evolution of other currents affecting late repolarization reserve. These findings raise caution in targeting I_{to} as an antiarrhythmic strategy.[73]

Nicotine blocks I_{to} in Kv4.2 and Kv4.3 channels expressed in Xenopus oocytes by direct channel interactions.[74] Tedisamil is a drug with potent bradycardic and therefore anti-ischemic properties that blocks I_{to} and I_{Ks} leading to AP prolongation and termination of atrial fibrillation.[75,76]

Inward Rectifier K+ Channels

Several pathophysiological conditions, such as gain-of-function mutations in the respective ion channels, ischemia, or chronic atrial fibrillation are accompanied by an upregulation of inward rectifier currents and enhance the cardiac propensity to develop and maintain reentrant tachyarrhythmias. Experimental and computational evidence suggests that enhanced inward rectifier current will hyperpolarize the membrane and enhance the frequency and stability of reentrant arrhythmias.[77,78] Blockers of inward rectifier channels should possess an antiarrhythmic, rather than a proarrhythmic potential. Because inward rectifiers are crucial for maintaining the resting membrane potential, inhibition of these currents depolarizes the cell membrane and will therefore reduce excitability and impulse propagation due to reduced Na+ channel availability.

Kir2.1/Kir2.3: I_{K1} inward rectifier K+ current

Kir channels are open regardless of the membrane potential. Rectification of these channels is accomplished through inhibition of outward current by divalent cations, primarily Mg^{2+} or polyamines such as spermine and spermidine.[3] The major background of inward rectifier current I_{K1} is that it passes through heteromeric channels of the Kir2.1 and Kir2.2 subunits. Selective blockers

of I_{K1} channels have only been developed for experimental purposes, although many drugs impair I_{K1} channels as a side effect to their main action. Because of their dominant role in setting the resting membrane potential, Kir2.1/2.3 channels cannot be blocked without destabilizing almost all excitable cells in the body. Electrophysiological remodeling in heart failure comprises decreased I_{K1}, which together with altered Ca^{2+} handling predisposes ventricular cardiomyocytes to DAD and triggered activity.[79] The pentamidine analogue PA-6 has been reported to selectively block I_{K1} and to prolong APD in isolated canine ventricular myocytes.[80] In an unpublished study, PA-6 prolonged the ventricular APD and ERP in the Langendorff rat heart and increased both short-term and long-term variability, which are correlated with ventricular proarrhythmicity.

Kir3.1/Kir3.4 (KCNJ3/KCNJ5): acetylcholine-activated inward rectifier K+ current $I_{K,ACh}$

The acetylcholine-activated inward rectifier conducting $I_{K,ACh}$ is composed of heteromers of Kir3.1 and Kir3.4 (GIRK1 and GIRK4) with a 2:2 stoichiometry.[81,82] Stimulation of the parasympathetic nervous system leads to release of acetylcholine that activates $I_{K,ACh}$ channels via G_i-protein coupled muscarinic type 2 (M_2) receptors. On stimulation of M_2 receptors, the heterotrimeric inhibitory G_i proteins dissociate into $G\alpha_i$ and $G\beta\gamma$ subunits of which the latter directly bind to Kir3.1/3.4 channels to enhance their open probability.[83,84] The resulting shortening of the cardiac APD increases the atrial susceptibility to tachyarrhythmia. By reversing this shortening, blockers of $I_{K,ACh}$ have an antiarrhythmic potential, which theoretically could be exploited to normalize the shortened APD in chronic atrial fibrillation, as expression and function of Kir3.2/3.4 channels is less abundant in ventricular (although functional currents have been reported)[85,86] than atrial cardiomyocytes.[81] Interestingly, several antiarrhythmic agents, including dofetilide, ibutilide, sotalol, terikalant, and amiodarone, are known blockers of $I_{K,ACh}$.[87,88] $I_{K,ACh}$ blockers are not expected to cause proarrhythmic effects, although side effects from the central nervous system are likely unless drugs are designed to not pass the blood-brain barrier.

Compelling evidence indicates that constitutively active $I_{K,ACh}$ channels develop during atrial fibrillation as part of the electrical remodeling processes and are considered to contribute to the maintenance of the rhythm.[89,90] $I_{K,ACh}$ is regarded as an atrial-selective drug target (see Voigt N, Dobrev D: Atrial-Selective Potassium Channel Blockers, in this issue), and there is considerable interest in developing selective compounds preferably targeting constitutively active $I_{K,ACh}$ channels only.[65] One selective inhibitor of I_{KACh}, NTC-801, showed good efficacy in preventing and suppressing atrial fibrillation in several animal models[91]; however, clinical development of the compound was stopped for unknown reasons.[92]

Kir6.1/Kir6.2 plus SUR1/SUR2: ATP-activated K$^+$ current $I_{K,ATP}$

Kir6.1 and Kir6.2 channels in association with the sulfonylurea receptors SUR1 and SUR2 conduct weakly inward-rectifying current, $I_{K,ATP}$.[93] The ATP-sensitive K$^+$ (K_{ATP}) channels activate when the intracellular ATP concentration decreases.[94]

K_{ATP} channels have been extensively reviewed (see Nichols CG: ATP-sensitive Potassium Currents in Heart Disease and Cardioprotection, in this issue). Here they are mentioned briefly in the context of arrhythmias. Activation of cardiac K_{ATP} channels under conditions of metabolic blockade[95] or during ischemia and hypoxia is associated with strong abbreviation of the cardiac AP and depolarization of the membrane due to extracellular K$^+$ accumulation. The short APD may limit excess Ca^{2+} entry and thus could be protective against ischemic damage.[96] On the other hand, AP shortening facilitates reentry and increases the cardiac vulnerability to life-threatening ventricular tachyarrhythmias.[97] If fully activated by complete metabolic blockade, K_{ATP} channels can lead to cessation of cardiac electrical activity and contractile failure.[98] Therefore, blocking the ischemia-induced opening of K_{ATP} channels seems to be a promising antiarrhythmic approach.

Block of the sulfonylurea receptor isoforms as the regulatory subunits of K_{ATP} channels reduces $I_{K,ATP}$ and arrhythmogenic risk of $I_{K,ATP}$ activation under many experimental conditions. For instance, the antidiabetic drug glibenclamide (pancreatic $I_{K,ATP}$ inhibition) reduced the risk of asystole in a canine model,[99] the compound HM1883 (myocardial $I_{K,ATP}$ inhibition) reduced the APD shortening during AMI in pigs,[100] and SUR1 blocker gliclazide (also myocardial $I_{K,ATP}$ inhibition) resulted in cardioprotective effects in experimentally induced ischemic injury of the rat heart.[101] These experimental results are encouraging; nevertheless, they do not preclude proarrhythmic effects of K_{ATP} channel blockers.

Weak Inward Rectifiers K2P Channels

TWIK-1 (KCNK1); TREK-1 (KCNK2 or K$_{2P}$2.1), TASK-1 (KCNK3 or K$_{2P}$3.1); TASK-3 (KCNK9 or K$_{2P}$9.1) – I_{K2P}

Of the 15 known different K2P α-subunits, TWIK-1 and TASK channels (*TWIK*-related *A*cid-*S*ensitive

K$^+$ [TASK-1; TASK-3] channels) were found in human atria and are recognized to play a role in cardiac electrophysiology and some inherited forms of arrhythmias.[102] Heterologous expression of these channels gives rise to instantaneous, non-inactivating K$^+$ current that displays little or no voltage dependence, suggesting that they might contribute to background or leak currents. These background leak channels, which are highly regulated and control excitability, stabilize membrane potential below firing threshold and shorten ERP.[103] They are robustly expressed in the cardiovascular system and are involved in multiple physiologic functions, including cardioprotection, regulation of cardiac rhythm, and mechanical stress.[104] Blockage of these K$^+$ background channels prolongs APD[105] and could contribute to arrhythmogenesis via initiation of EAD leading to TdP and fibrillation, although so far there is little experimental proof for these theoretic considerations. Currently, it is not known whether K2P channels could be promising antiarrhythmic drug targets. Human cardiac K$_{2P}$3.1 (TASK-1) potassium leak channels heterologously expressed in *Xenopus* oocytes were blocked by amiodarone in therapeutically relevant concentrations.[106] In addition to their primary mechanism of action, many other antiarrhythmic drugs, including many Kv1.5 blockers[107] and mexiletine, propafenone, carvedilol, AVE0118, and dronedarone, also block TASK-1 at high therapeutic plasma concentration indicating a possible contribution to their therapeutic effect.[65]

Calcium-Activated K$^+$ Channels of Small Conductance

SK1, SK2, SK3 (KCNN1, KCNN2, KCNN3) channels - Ca^{2+}-activated K$^+$ current $I_{SK,Ca}$

The family of Ca^{2+}-activated K$^+$ channels includes 3 classes according to their single-channel K$^+$ conductance (big, intermediate, and small; BK, IK, and SK, respectively). The 3 subtypes of Ca^{2+}-activating K$^+$ channels with small conductance (SK1, SK2, and SK3 or KCa2.1, KCa2.2, KCa2.3 channels) are expressed in the heart, but are mainly physiologically functional in the atria.[5,108] SK2 is abundantly and selectively distributed in the atria.[109]

Like in vascular smooth muscle, the physiologic function of SK channels in the heart is probably to limit excessive Ca^{2+} entry.[110] Theoretically, activation of SK channels can have both antiarrhythmic and proarrhythmic effects because they protect against DADs and extrasystoles by preventing intracellular Ca^{2+} leakage or overload, but facilitate reentry by shortening the AP duration. Indeed, the role of SK channels in the genesis of cardiac arrhythmias is increasingly recognized.[111–113]

Owing to their predominant expression in the atria,[109] SK channels are attributed with atrial electrophysiology and have been proposed to contribute in AF remodeling.[114–116] In genetically engineered mice, increase in SK2 abbreviated APs, whereas loss of SK2 function prolonged AP duration and induced EAD. Clinically, the role of atrial SK channels is also conflicting, because both I_{KCa} upregulation[117] and downregulation[5,118] have been reported in patients with persistent and permanent AF. In the ventricles, SK channels have limited function except under pathophysiological conditions, such as human heart failure[119,120] and heart failure–associated ventricular arrhythmias.[121] In patients with heart failure, SK channels and I_{KCa} are consistently upregulated,[14] which supposedly serves as a protective mechanism securing sufficient ventricular repolarization reserve and eliminating DADs by reducing triggered activity or through stabilization of ventricular repolarization.[14,119,122] Heterogeneous distribution of upregulated SK channels may be proarrhythmic.[120]

Although the physiologic role of SK channels in the heart remains debated, larger animal model reports consistently show SK channel inhibition to protect against AF.[108,113] In the same way as the physiologic role of cardiac SK channels in atria is controversial and debated, the same holds true for the pathophysiological role. There is no general consensus whether block of SK channels provides protection against or facilitates ventricular arrhythmias. In the isolated rabbit heart, the SK channel blocker apamin prolongs the ventricular AP, rendering the ventricles prone to arrhythmia. However, in other studies, apamin and other SK inhibitors eliminated recurrent ventricular fibrillation.[108,123] In line with these observations, SK channel inhibition in a rat study of acute myocardial infarction showed prolonged ventricular refractoriness and protective effects on ventricular arrhythmias.[124] In various ex vivo and in vivo studies, small animal models of experimental AF SK channel blockers (NS8593, UCL1684, ICA) exhibited antiarrhythmic effects.[125–128] However, atrial proarrhythmic effects of SK channel block also have been proposed, supposedly as a result of increased APD heterogeneity.[129]

SYNERGISTIC DRUG EFFECTS IN PROLONGING THE QT INTERVAL
Synergistic Pharmacodynamics Effects

Lethal arrhythmias are provoked when repolarization reserve is used up by concomitant administration of several QTc prolonging drugs that inhibit different K^+ channels.[130] Therefore, robust information about the QT-prolonging potential of all drugs is required and indeed requested by official agencies for drug approval. Comprehensive lists of drugs with reported or suspected risk for TdP are available on the Internet (for instance, http://www.qtdrugs.org/).

Patients with manifest congenital LQTS and also silent gene mutations are at a particularly high risk for drug-induced TdP. Even in asymptomatic patients, a genetic predisposition related to congenital LQTS may exacerbate drug action that turns the otherwise borderline QT interval into overt prolongation. Some polymorphisms, for instance in the gene encoding for a common ancillary subunit (ie, the KCNE2 gene), have normal function at baseline but are susceptible to block by sulfamethoxazole that imposes no prolongation in healthy individuals.[131]

Vagal nerve stimulation may provoke atrial fibrillation via acetylcholine release that activates $I_{K,ACh}$ and shortens AP duration and ERP, facilitating reentry. In comparison, drugs that shorten APD by activating K^+ currents are expected to predispose to atrial fibrillation. Much less is known about the actual incidence of drug-induced atrial fibrillation than of TdP in the case of LQTS. As outlined previously, prolongation in atrial APD by block of K^+ channels may also trigger atrial fibrillation; however, unlike ventricular fibrillation, these are not immediately life threatening.

Synergistic Pharmacokinetic Effects

Arrhythmogenic exacerbation frequently occurs due to pharmacokinetic interactions by coadministered drugs that interfere with biotransformation and excretion of a previously tolerated drug resulting in excessive plasma concentrations. If the parent compound is more effective than the metabolite in producing a proarrhythmic event, inhibition of drug-metabolizing enzymes will enhance arrhythmogenicity. Conversely, if the metabolite is more effective, induction of enzymes is proarrhythmogenic.

Drugs with high affinity to the hERG channels are often bound to CYP3A4, the isoform of the cytochrome P450 enzyme that is responsible for metabolic degradation of approximately 50% of all therapeutically relevant drugs. Drugs that are substrates for CYP3A4 compete for binding and therefore interfere with biodegradation of each other and raise the plasma concentrations for both drugs.[132] How pharmacokinetic interaction between 2 comedicated drugs can cause acquired LQTS is illustrated with the following example: The hERG channel blocker terfenadine is transformed by CYP3A4 into the nonblocking metabolite norterfenadine, which retains the anti-histaminic action. If a patient on terfenadine therapy is concomitantly treated with erythromycin, which blocks hERG channels and is a CYP3A4-blocking drug, the plasma concentration of the parent compound terfenadine increases and together with erythromycin's own hERG channel blocking capacity grossly and increasing the risk of developing TdP.[133] Similar interactions between terfenadine and CYP3A4 inhibitors were described for antifungal drugs (ketoconazole), protease inhibitors (ritonavir), and even grapefruit juice.[134,135]

SUMMARY

The regular heartbeat depends on generation and ordered propagation of electrical activity that triggers and coordinates the contractile function of the heart. Any disturbance of impulse formation and conduction or repolarization can lead to rhythm disorders. The cardiac AP is characterized by a long plateau phase that protects the myocardium from new excitations as long as the contraction cycle is lasting (ERP). Of the diverse ion channels, transporters, exchangers, and pumps that maintain the shape of the AP, K$^+$ channels play a prominent role in securing the delayed repolarization. Both loss and gain of K$^+$ channel function, either by genetic deviation or pharmacologic intervention, can cause detrimental arrhythmias. Although pharmacologic manipulation of ion channels may exert antiarrhythmic effects within certain limits, numerous cardiac and noncardiac drugs are known to have proarrhythmic effects, mainly through excessive inhibition of cardiac K$^+$ channels causing loss of repolarization reserve. In this review, we described the causes and mechanisms of proarrhythmic effects that arise as a response to blockers of cardiac K$^+$ channels. The largest and chemically most diverse group of compounds targets hERG and Kv7.1 (KvLQT1) channels. Finally, the propensity of atrial-selective K$^+$ blockers inhibiting Kv1.5, Kir3.1/3.4, SK, and K2P channels was discussed.

REFERENCES

1. Nerbonne JM, Kass RS. Molecular physiology of cardiac repolarization. Physiol Rev 2005;85(4): 1205–53.
2. Roden DM. Taking the "idio" out of "idiosyncratic": predicting torsades de pointes. Pacing Clin Electrophysiol 1998;21(5):1029–34.
3. Lopatin AN, Nichols CG. Inward rectifiers in the heart: an update on I(K1). J Mol Cell Cardiol 2001;33(4):625–38.
4. Lesage F, Guillemare E, Fink M, et al. TWIK-1, a ubiquitous human weakly inward rectifying K+ channel with a novel structure. EMBO J 1996; 15(5):1004–11.
5. Skibsbye L, Poulet C, Diness JG, et al. Small-conductance calcium-activated potassium (SK) channels contribute to action potential repolarization in human atria. Cardiovasc Res 2014;103(1): 156–67.
6. Schumacher MA, Rivard AF, Bachinger HP, et al. Structure of the gating domain of a Ca2+-activated K+ channel complexed with Ca2+/calmodulin. Nature 2001;410(6832):1120–4.
7. Weiss JN, Garfinkel A, Karagueuzian HS, et al. Perspective: a dynamics-based classification of ventricular arrhythmias. J Mol Cell Cardiol 2015; 82:136–52.
8. Zeng J, Rudy Y. Early afterdepolarizations in cardiac myocytes: mechanism and rate dependence. Biophys J 1995;68(3):949–64.
9. Dessertenne F. Ventricular tachycardia with 2 variable opposing foci. Arch Mal Coeur Vaiss 1966; 59(2):263–72 [in French].
10. Dobrev D. Atrial Ca2+ signaling in atrial fibrillation as an antiarrhythmic drug target. Naunyn Schmiedebergs Arch Pharmacol 2010;381(3):195–206.
11. Jalife J. Ventricular fibrillation: mechanisms of initiation and maintenance. Annu Rev Physiol 2000;62: 25–50.
12. Vaquero M, Calvo D, Jalife J. Cardiac fibrillation: from ion channels to rotors in the human heart. Heart Rhythm 2008;5(6):872–9.
13. Allessie MA, Bonke FI, Schopman FJ. Circus movement in rabbit atrial muscle as a mechanism of tachycardia. III. The "leading circle" concept: a new model of circus movement in cardiac tissue without the involvement of an anatomical obstacle. Circ Res 1977;41(1):9–18.
14. Yu CC, Corr C, Shen C, et al. Small conductance calcium-activated potassium current is important in transmural repolarization of failing human ventricles. Circ Arrhythm Electrophysiol 2015;8(3):667–76.
15. Vaughan Williams EM. Classification of antidysrhythmic drugs. Pharmacol Ther B 1975;1(1): 115–38.
16. Comtois P, Kneller J, Nattel S. Of circles and spirals: bridging the gap between the leading circle and spiral wave concepts of cardiac reentry. Europace 2005;7(Suppl 2):10–20.
17. Waldo AL, Camm AJ, deRuyter H, et al. Effect of d-sotalol on mortality in patients with left ventricular dysfunction after recent and remote myocardial infarction. The SWORD Investigators. Survival with oral d-sotalol. Lancet 1996;348(9019):7–12.

18. Winniford MD, Fulton KL, Hillis LD. Symptomatic sinus bradycardia during concomitant propranolol-
verapamil administration. Am Heart J 1985;
110(2):498.

19. Echt DS, Liebson PR, Mitchell LB, et al. Mortality
and morbidity in patients receiving encainide,
flecainide, or placebo. The cardiac arrhythmia suppression trial. N Engl J Med 1991;324(12):781–8.

20. Spann JF Jr, Moellering RC Jr, Haber E, et al.
Arrhythmias in acute myocardial infarction; a study
utilizing an electrocardiographic monitor for automatic detection and recording of arrhythmias.
N Engl J Med 1964;271:427–31.

21. Sanguinetti MC, Jiang C, Curran ME, et al.
A mechanistic link between an inherited and an
acquired cardiac arrhythmia: HERG encodes the
IKr potassium channel. Cell 1995;81(2):299–307.

22. El-Sherif N, Turitto G. Electrolyte disorders and
arrhythmogenesis. Cardiol J 2011;18(3):233–45.

23. Hondeghem LM, Carlsson L, Duker G. Instability
and triangulation of the action potential predict
serious proarrhythmia, but action potential duration
prolongation is antiarrhythmic. Circulation 2001;
103(15):2004–13.

24. Hondeghem LM. TRIad: foundation for proarrhythmia (triangulation, reverse use dependence and
instability). Novartis Found Symp 2005;266:235–
44 [discussion: 244–50].

25. Frommeyer G, Eckardt L. Drug-induced proarrhythmia: risk factors and electrophysiological
mechanisms. Nat Rev Cardiol 2016;13(1):36–47.

26. Hondeghem LM, Snyders DJ. Class III antiarrhythmic agents have a lot of potential but a long
way to go. Reduced effectiveness and dangers of
reverse use dependence. Circulation 1990;81(2):
686–90.

27. Verduyn SC, Vos MA, van der Zande J, et al. Role
of interventricular dispersion of repolarization in acquired torsade-de-pointes arrhythmias: reversal by
magnesium. Cardiovasc Res 1997;34(3):453–63.

28. Piper DR, Hinz WA, Tallurri CK, et al. Regional
specificity of human ether-a'-go-go-related gene
channel activation and inactivation gating. J Biol
Chem 2005;280(8):7206–17.

29. Sanguinetti MC, Tristani-Firouzi M. hERG potassium channels and cardiac arrhythmia. Nature
2006;440(7083):463–9.

30. Curran ME, Splawski I, Timothy KW, et al.
A molecular basis for cardiac arrhythmia: HERG
mutations cause long QT syndrome. Cell 1995;
80(5):795–803.

31. Mitcheson JS, Chen J, Sanguinetti MC. Trapping of
a methanesulfonanilide by closure of the HERG potassium channel activation gate. J Gen Physiol
2000;115(3):229–40.

32. Perrin MJ, Kuchel PW, Campbell TJ, et al. Drug
binding to the inactivated state is necessary but

not sufficient for high-affinity binding to human
ether-a-go-go-related gene channels. Mol Pharmacol 2008;74(5):1443–52.

33. Jaiswal A, Goldbarg S. Dofetilide induced torsade
de pointes: mechanism, risk factors and management strategies. Indian Heart J 2014;66(6):640–8.

34. Haverkamp W, Breithardt G, Camm AJ, et al. The
potential for QT prolongation and pro-arrhythmia
by non-anti-arrhythmic drugs: clinical and regulatory implications. Report on a Policy Conference of
the European Society of Cardiology. Cardiovasc
Res 2000;47(2):219–33.

35. Kannankeril P, Roden DM, Darbar D. Drug-induced
long QT syndrome. Pharmacol Rev 2010;62(4):
760–81.

36. Behr ER, Roden D. Drug-induced arrhythmia: pharmacogenomic prescribing? Eur Heart J 2013;
34(2):89–95.

37. Choe H, Nah KH, Lee SN, et al. A novel hypothesis
for the binding mode of HERG channel blockers.
Biochem Biophys Res Commun 2006;344(1):72–8.

38. Perry M, de Groot MJ, Helliwell R, et al. Structural
determinants of HERG channel block by clofilium
and ibutilide. Mol Pharmacol 2004;66(2):240–9.

39. Ficker E, Kuryshev YA, Dennis AT, et al. Mechanisms of arsenic-induced prolongation of cardiac
repolarization. Mol Pharmacol 2004;66(1):33–44.

40. Cordes JS, Sun Z, Lloyd DB, et al. Pentamidine reduces hERG expression to prolong the QT interval.
Br J Pharmacol 2005;145(1):15–23.

41. Shi YQ, Yan CC, Zhang X, et al. Mechanisms underlying probucol-induced hERG-channel deficiency. Drug Des Devel Ther 2015;9:3695–704.

42. McCrossan ZA, Abbott GW. The MinK-related peptides. Neuropharmacology 2004;47(6):787–821.

43. Jespersen T, Grunnet M, Olesen SP. The KCNQ1
potassium channel: from gene to physiological
function. Physiology (Bethesda) 2005;20:408–16.

44. Werry D, Eldstrom J, Wang Z, et al. Single-channel
basis for the slow activation of the repolarizing cardiac potassium current, I(Ks). Proc Natl Acad Sci U
S A 2013;110(11):E996–1005.

45. Splawski I, Tristani-Firouzi M, Lehmann MH, et al.
Mutations in the hminK gene cause long QT syndrome and suppress IKs function. Nat Genet
1997;17(3):338–40.

46. Sanguinetti MC, Jurkiewicz NK, Scott A, et al.
Isoproterenol antagonizes prolongation of refractory period by the class III antiarrhythmic agent
E-4031 in guinea pig myocytes. Mechanism of
action. Circ Res 1991;68(1):77–84.

47. Uchi J, Rice JJ, Ruwald MH, et al. Impaired IKs
channel activation by Ca(2+)-dependent PKC
shows correlation with emotion/arousal-triggered
events in LQT1. J Mol Cell Cardiol 2015;79:203–11.

48. Fodstad H, Swan H, Laitinen P, et al. Four potassium
channel mutations account for 73% of the genetic

spectrum underlying long-QT syndrome (LQTS) and provide evidence for a strong founder effect in Finland. Ann Med 2004;36(Suppl 1):53–63.

49. Kato S, Honjo H, Takemoto Y, et al. Pharmacological blockade of IKs destabilizes spiral-wave reentry under beta-adrenergic stimulation in favor of its early termination. J Pharmacol Sci 2012; 119(1):52–63.

50. Bauer A, Becker R, Freigang KD, et al. Electrophysiologic effects of the new I(Ks)-blocking agent chromanol 293b in the postinfarction canine heart. Preserved positive use-dependence and preferential prolongation of refractoriness in the infarct zone. Basic Res Cardiol 2000;95(4):324–32.

51. Gogelein H, Bruggemann A, Gerlach U, et al. Inhibition of IKs channels by HMR 1556. Naunyn Schmiedebergs Arch Pharmacol 2000;362(6): 480–8.

52. Thomas GP, Gerlach U, Antzelevitch C. HMR 1556, a potent and selective blocker of slowly activating delayed rectifier potassium current. J Cardiovasc Pharmacol 2003;41(1):140–7.

53. Varro A, Baczko I. Cardiac ventricular repolarization reserve: a principle for understanding drug-related proarrhythmic risk. Br J Pharmacol 2011; 164(1):14–36.

54. Odening KE, Hyder O, Chaves L, et al. Pharmacogenomics of anesthetic drugs in transgenic LQT1 and LQT2 rabbits reveal genotype-specific differential effects on cardiac repolarization. Am J Physiol Heart Circ Physiol 2008;295(6):H2264–72.

55. Ravens U, Wettwer E. Ultra-rapid delayed rectifier channels: molecular basis and therapeutic implications. Cardiovasc Res 2011;89(4):776–85.

56. Fedida D, Wible B, Wang Z, et al. Identity of a novel delayed rectifier current from human heart with a cloned K+ channel current. Circ Res 1993;73(1): 210–6.

57. Mays DJ, Foose JM, Philipson LH, et al. Localization of the Kv1.5 K+ channel protein in explanted cardiac tissue. J Clin Invest 1995;96(1):282–92.

58. Li GR, Feng J, Yue L, et al. Evidence for two components of delayed rectifier K+ current in human ventricular myocytes. Circ Res 1996;78(4):689–96.

59. Ravens U, Poulet C, Wettwer E, et al. Atrial selectivity of antiarrhythmic drugs. J Physiol 2013;591: 4087–97.

60. Ford JW, Milnes JT. New drugs targeting the cardiac ultra-rapid delayed-rectifier current (I Kur): rationale, pharmacology and evidence for potential therapeutic value. J Cardiovasc Pharmacol 2008; 52(2):105–20.

61. Courtemanche M, Ramirez RJ, Nattel S. Ionic targets for drug therapy and atrial fibrillation-induced electrical remodeling: insights from a mathematical model. Cardiovasc Res 1999;42(2): 477–89.

62. Wettwer E, Hala O, Christ T, et al. Role of IKur in controlling action potential shape and contractility in the human atrium: influence of chronic atrial fibrillation. Circulation 2004;110(16):2299–306.

63. Ford J, Milnes J, El Haou S, et al. The positive frequency-dependent electrophysiological effects of the IKur inhibitor XEN-D0103 are desirable for the treatment of atrial fibrillation. Heart Rhythm 2016; 13(2):555–64.

64. Pavri BB, Greenberg HE, Kraft WK, et al. MK-0448, a specific Kv1.5 inhibitor: safety, pharmacokinetics, and pharmacodynamic electrophysiology in experimental animal models and humans. Circ Arrhythm Electrophysiol 2012;5(6):1193–201.

65. El-Haou S, Ford JW, Milnes JT. Novel K+ channel targets in atrial fibrillation drug development— where are we? J Cardiovasc Pharmacol 2015; 66(5):412–31.

66. Fedida D, Orth PM, Chen JY, et al. The mechanism of atrial antiarrhythmic action of RSD1235. J Cardiovasc Electrophysiol 2005;16(11):1227–38.

67. Wettwer E, Christ T, Endig S, et al. The new antiarrhythmic drug vernakalant: ex vivo study of human atrial tissue from sinus rhythm and chronic atrial fibrillation. Cardiovasc Res 2013;98(1):145–54.

68. Roy D, Pratt CM, Torp-Pedersen C, et al. Vernakalant hydrochloride for rapid conversion of atrial fibrillation: a phase 3, randomized, placebo-controlled trial. Circulation 2008;117(12):1518–25.

69. Tsuji Y, Dobrev D. Safety and efficacy of vernakalant for acute cardioversion of atrial fibrillation: an update. Vasc Health Risk Manag 2013;9: 165–75.

70. Niwa N, Nerbonne JM. Molecular determinants of cardiac transient outward potassium current (I(to)) expression and regulation. J Mol Cell Cardiol 2010;48(1):12–25.

71. Wettwer E, Terlau H. Pharmacology of voltage-gated potassium channel Kv1.5–impact on cardiac excitability. Curr Opin Pharmacol 2014;15:115–21.

72. Perez-Cortes EJ, Islas AA, Arevalo JP, et al. Modulation of the transient outward current (Ito) in rat cardiac myocytes and human Kv4.3 channels by mefloquine. Toxicol Appl Pharmacol 2015;288(2): 203–12.

73. Nguyen TP, Singh N, Xie Y, et al. Repolarization reserve evolves dynamically during the cardiac action potential: effects of transient outward currents on early afterdepolarizations. Circ Arrhythm Electrophysiol 2015;8(3):694–702.

74. Wang H, Shi H, Zhang L, et al. Nicotine is a potent blocker of the cardiac A-type K(+) channels. Effects on cloned Kv4.3 channels and native transient outward current. Circulation 2000;102(10): 1165–71.

75. Dukes ID, Cleemann L, Morad M. Tedisamil blocks the transient and delayed rectifier K+ currents in

mammalian cardiac and glial cells. J Pharmacol Exp Ther 1990;254(2):560–9.

76. Wettwer E, Himmel HM, Amos GJ, et al. Mechanism of block by tedisamil of transient outward current in human ventricular subepicardial myocytes. Br J Pharmacol 1998;125(4):659–66.

77. Dhamoon AS, Jalife J. The inward rectifier current (IK1) controls cardiac excitability and is involved in arrhythmogenesis. Heart Rhythm 2005;2(3): 316–24.

78. Pandit SV, Berenfeld O, Anumonwo JM, et al. Ionic determinants of functional reentry in a 2-D model of human atrial cells during simulated chronic atrial fibrillation. Biophys J 2005;88(6):3806–21.

79. Myles RC, Wang L, Bers DM, et al. Decreased inward rectifying K+ current and increased ryanodine receptor sensitivity synergistically contribute to sustained focal arrhythmia in the intact rabbit heart. J Physiol 2015;593(6):1479–93.

80. Takanari H, Nalos L, Stary-Weinzinger A, et al. Efficient and specific cardiac IK(1) inhibition by a new pentamidine analogue. Cardiovasc Res 2013;99(1):203–14.

81. Krapivinsky G, Gordon EA, Wickman K, et al. The G-protein-gated atrial K+ channel IKACh is a heteromultimer of two inwardly rectifying K(+)-channel proteins. Nature 1995;374(6518): 135–41.

82. Silverman SK, Lester HA, Dougherty DA. Subunit stoichiometry of a heteromultimeric G protein-coupled inward-rectifier K+ channel. J Biol Chem 1996;271(48):30524–8.

83. Whorton MR, MacKinnon R. Crystal structure of the mammalian GIRK2 K+ channel and gating regulation by G proteins, PIP2, and sodium. Cell 2011; 147(1):199–208.

84. Yamada M, Inanobe A, Kurachi Y. G protein regulation of potassium ion channels. Pharmacol Rev 1998;50(4):723–60.

85. Koumi S, Wasserstrom JA. Acetylcholine-sensitive muscarinic K+ channels in mammalian ventricular myocytes. Am J Physiol 1994;266(5 Pt 2):H1812–21.

86. Liang B, Nissen JD, Laursen M, et al. G-protein-coupled inward rectifier potassium current contributes to ventricular repolarization. Cardiovasc Res 2014;101(1):175–84.

87. Mori K, Hara Y, Saito T, et al. Anticholinergic effects of class III antiarrhythmic drugs in guinea pig atrial cells. Different molecular mechanisms. Circulation 1995;91(11):2834–43.

88. Watanabe Y, Hara Y, Tamagawa M, et al. Inhibitory effect of amiodarone on the muscarinic acetylcholine receptor-operated potassium current in guinea pig atrial cells. J Pharmacol Exp Ther 1996;279(2): 617–24.

89. Dobrev D, Friedrich A, Voigt N, et al. The G protein-gated potassium current I(K,ACh) is constitutively active in patients with chronic atrial fibrillation. Circulation 2005;112(24):3697–706.

90. Voigt N, Makary S, Nattel S, et al. Voltage-clamp-based methods for the detection of constitutively active acetylcholine-gated I(K,ACh) channels in the diseased heart. Methods Enzymol 2010;484: 653–75.

91. Machida T, Hashimoto N, Kuwahara I, et al. Effects of a highly selective acetylcholine-activated K+ channel blocker on experimental atrial fibrillation. Circ Arrhythm Electrophysiol 2011;4(1):94–102.

92. Zhao HP, Xiang BR. Discontinued cardiovascular drugs in 2013 and 2014. Expert Opin Investig Drugs 2015;24(8):1083–92.

93. Seino S. ATP-sensitive potassium channels: a model of heteromultimeric potassium channel/receptor assemblies. Annu Rev Physiol 1999;61: 337–62.

94. Zhang H, Flagg TP, Nichols CG. Cardiac sarcolemmal K(ATP) channels: latest twists in a questing tale! J Mol Cell Cardiol 2010;48(1):71–5.

95. Noma A. ATP-regulated K+ channels in cardiac muscle. Nature 1983;305(5930):147–8.

96. Flagg TP, Enkvetchakul D, Koster JC, et al. Muscle KATP channels: recent insights to energy sensing and myoprotection. Physiol Rev 2010; 90(3):799–829.

97. Fujita A, Kurachi Y. Molecular aspects of ATP-sensitive K+ channels in the cardiovascular system and K+ channel openers. Pharmacol Ther 2000;85(1):39–53.

98. Nichols CG, Lederer WJ. The regulation of ATP-sensitive K+ channel activity in intact and permeabilized rat ventricular myocytes. J Physiol 1990; 423:91–110.

99. Taylor TG, Venable PW, Shibayama J, et al. Role of KATP channel in electrical depression and asystole during long-duration ventricular fibrillation in ex vivo canine heart. Am J Physiol Heart Circ Physiol 2012;302(11):H2396–409.

100. Wirth KJ, Uhde J, Rosenstein B, et al. K(ATP) channel blocker HMR 1883 reduces monophasic action potential shortening during coronary ischemia in anesthetised pigs. Naunyn Schmiedebergs Arch Pharmacol 2000;361(2):155–60.

101. Bao Y, Sun X, Yerong Y, et al. Blockers of sulfonylureas receptor 1 subunits may lead to cardiac protection against isoprenaline-induced injury in obese rats. Eur J Pharmacol 2012;690(1–3):142–8.

102. Decher N, Kiper AK, Rolfes C, et al. The role of acid-sensitive two-pore domain potassium channels in cardiac electrophysiology: focus on arrhythmias. Pflugers Arch 2015;467(5):1055–67.

103. Goldstein SA, Bockenhauer D, O'Kelly I, et al. Potassium leak channels and the KCNK family of two-P-domain subunits. Nat Rev Neurosci 2001; 2(3):175–84.

104. Gierten J, Ficker E, Bloehs R, et al. Regulation of two-pore-domain (K2P) potassium leak channels by the tyrosine kinase inhibitor genistein. Br J Pharmacol 2008;154(8):1680–90.

105. Putzke C, Wemhoner K, Sachse FB, et al. The acid-sensitive potassium channel TASK-1 in rat cardiac muscle. Cardiovasc Res 2007;75(1):59–68.

106. Gierten J, Ficker E, Bloehs R, et al. The human cardiac K2P3.1 (TASK-1) potassium leak channel is a molecular target for the class III antiarrhythmic drug amiodarone. Naunyn Schmiedebergs Arch Pharmacol 2010;381(3):261–70.

107. Kiper AK, Rinne S, Rolfes C, et al. Kv1.5 blockers preferentially inhibit TASK-1 channels: TASK-1 as a target against atrial fibrillation and obstructive sleep apnea? Pflugers Arch 2015;467(5):1081–90.

108. Diness JG, Bentzen BH, Sorensen US, et al. Role of calcium activated potassium channels in AF pathophysiology and therapy. J Cardiovasc Pharmacol 2015;66(5):441–8.

109. Xu Y, Tuteja D, Zhang Z, et al. Molecular identification and functional roles of a Ca(2+)-activated K+ channel in human and mouse hearts. J Biol Chem 2003;278(49):49085–94.

110. Ledoux J, Werner ME, Brayden JE, et al. Calcium-activated potassium channels and the regulation of vascular tone. Physiology (Bethesda) 2006;21:69–78.

111. Zhang XD, Lieu DK, Chiamvimonvat N. Small-conductance Ca(2+)-activated K(+) channels and cardiac arrhythmias. Heart Rhythm 2015;12(8):1845–51.

112. Skibsbye L. Antiarrhythmic principle of SK channel inhibition in atrial fibrillation. Dan Med J 2015;62(6).

113. Diness JG, Bentzen BH, Sørensen US, et al. Role of calcium-activated potassium channels in atrial fibrillation pathophysiology and therapy. J Cardiovasc Pharmacol 2015;66(5):441–8.

114. Nattel S. Calcium-activated potassium current: a novel ion channel candidate in atrial fibrillation. J Physiol 2009;587(Pt 7):1385–6.

115. Ozgen N, Dun W, Sosunov EA, et al. Early electrical remodeling in rabbit pulmonary vein results from trafficking of intracellular SK2 channels to membrane sites. Cardiovasc Res 2007;75(4):758–69.

116. Li N, Timofeyev V, Tuteja D, et al. Ablation of a Ca2+-activated K+ channel (SK2 channel) results in action potential prolongation in atrial myocytes and atrial fibrillation. J Physiol 2009;587(Pt 5):1087–100.

117. Li ML, Li T, Lei M, et al. Increased small conductance calcium-activated potassium channel (SK2 channel) current in atrial myocytes of patients with persistent atrial fibrillation. Zhonghua Xin Xue Guan Bing Za Zhi 2011;39(2):147–51 [in Chinese].

118. Ling TY, Wang XL, Chai Q, et al. Regulation of the SK3 channel by microRNA-499—Potential role in atrial fibrillation. Heart Rhythm 2013;10(7):1001–9.

119. Bonilla IM, Long VP III, Vargas-Pinto P, et al. Calcium-activated potassium current modulates ventricular repolarization in chronic heart failure. PLoS One 2014;9(10):e108824.

120. Chang PC, Turker I, Lopshire JC, et al. Heterogeneous upregulation of apamin-sensitive potassium currents in failing human ventricles. J Am Heart Assoc 2013;2(1):e004713.

121. Mizukami K, Yokoshiki H, Mitsuyama H, et al. Small conductance Ca2+-activated K+ current is upregulated via the phosphorylation of CaMKII in cardiac hypertrophy from spontaneously hypertensive rats. Am J Physiol Heart Circ Physiol 2015;309(6):H1066–74.

122. Terentyev D, Rochira JA, Terentyeva R, et al. Sarcoplasmic reticulum Ca2+ release is both necessary and sufficient for SK channel activation in ventricular myocytes. Am J Physiol Heart Circ Physiol 2014;306(5):H738–46.

123. Chua SK, Chang PC, Maruyama M, et al. Small-conductance calcium-activated potassium channel and recurrent ventricular fibrillation in failing rabbit ventricles. Circ Res 2011;108(8):971–9.

124. Gui L, Bao Z, Jia Y, et al. Ventricular tachyarrhythmias in rats with acute myocardial infarction involves activation of small-conductance Ca2+-activated K+ channels. Am J Physiol Heart Circ Physiol 2013;304(1):H118–30.

125. Skibsbye L, Wang X, Axelsen LN, et al. Antiarrhythmic Mechanisms of SK Channel Inhibition in the Rat Atrium. J Cardiovasc Pharmacol 2015;66(2):165–76.

126. Diness JG, Sorensen US, Nissen JD, et al. Inhibition of small-conductance Ca2+-activated K+ channels terminates and protects against atrial fibrillation. Circ Arrhythm Electrophysiol 2010;3(4):380–90.

127. Diness JG, Skibsbye L, Jespersen T, et al. Effects on atrial fibrillation in aged hypertensive rats by Ca(2+)-activated K(+) channel inhibition. Hypertension 2011;57(6):1129–35.

128. Skibsbye L, Diness JG, Sorensen US, et al. The duration of pacing-induced atrial fibrillation is reduced in vivo by inhibition of small conductance Ca(2+)-activated K(+) channels. J Cardiovasc Pharmacol 2011;57(6):672–81.

129. Hsueh CH, Chang PC, Hsieh YC, et al. Proarrhythmic effect of blocking the small conductance calcium activated potassium channel in isolated canine left atrium. Heart Rhythm 2013;10(6):891–8.

130. Sarkar AX, Sobie EA. Quantification of repolarization reserve to understand interpatient variability in the response to proarrhythmic drugs: a computational analysis. Heart Rhythm 2011; 8(11):1749–55.

131. Sesti F, Abbott GW, Wei J, et al. A common polymorphism associated with antibiotic-induced cardiac arrhythmia. Proc Natl Acad Sci U S A 2000; 97(19):10613–8.

132. Boxenbaum H. Cytochrome P450 3A4 in vivo ketoconazole competitive inhibition: determination of Ki and dangers associated with high clearance drugs in general. J Pharm Pharm Sci 1999;2(2): 47–52.

133. Biglin KE, Faraon MS, Constance TD, et al. Drug-induced torsades de pointes: a possible interaction of terfenadine and erythromycin. Ann Pharmacother 1994;28(2):282.

134. Dresser GK, Spence JD, Bailey DG. Pharmacokinetic-pharmacodynamic consequences and clinical relevance of cytochrome P450 3A4 inhibition. Clin Pharmacokinet 2000;38(1): 41–57.

135. Wang YJ, Yu CF, Chen LC, et al. Ketoconazole potentiates terfenadine-induced apoptosis in human Hep G2 cells through inhibition of cytochrome p450 3A4 activity. J Cell Biochem 2002;87(2): 147–59.

Atrial-Selective Potassium Channel Blockers

Niels Voigt, MD, Dobromir Dobrev, MD*

KEYWORDS

- $I_{K,ACh}$ • I_{Kur} • K2P channels • SK channels • Kv1.1 channels • Atrial fibrillation

KEY POINTS

- Atrial selective K^+ channels largely contribute to differences in the shape of the atrial versus ventricular action potential.
- Acetylcholine-activated inward-rectifier K^+ current ($I_{K,ACh}$) and ultrarapid delayed-rectifier K^+ current (I_{Kur}) represent classical atrial-selective K^+ currents, which are absent in ventricular myocytes.
- None of the "pure" blockers of I_{Kur} or $I_{K,ACh}$ passed phase II clinical trials yet.
- K2P channels, SK channels, and Kv1.1 channels have been shown recently to contribute to atrial repolarization and may represent novel atrial-selective drug targets.
- Because multichannel blockers are established compounds for treatment of atrial fibrillation, specific combinations of ion channel blockade may be an additional promising approach.

INTRODUCTION

Atrial fibrillation (AF), the most frequent cardiac arrhythmia, is associated with increased morbidity and mortality.[1] Currently available pharmacologic interventions for AF have major limitations, including limited efficacy and risk of life-threatening ventricular proarrhythmic side effects.[2–4] Amiodarone, a classical K^+ channel blocker that affects also a wide range of other ion channels and receptors, is currently the most frequently prescribed antiarrhythmic compound for AF therapy, suggesting that blocking of K^+ channels may be a promising therapeutic principle for AF.

The shape of a cardiac action potential (AP) is determined by the fine-tuned balance between depolarizing inward currents ($I_{Ca,L}$ and I_{Na}) and repolarizing outward currents (K^+ currents; **Fig. 1**). In patients with long-standing persistent and permanent (chronic) AF (cAF), the predominance of K^+ currents is supposed to lead to AP shortening, a major hallmark of electrical remodeling.[5,6] Because AP shortening promotes the maintenance of reentry excitations, it is assumed that inhibition of repolarizing K^+ currents may prevent the maintenance of AF.[2–4] Conversely, inhibition of ventricular K^+ channels may lead to extensive AP prolongation in the ventricle, which may promote the occurrence of "torsades de pointes" ventricular arrhythmias.[7] Therefore, atrial-selective inhibition of cardiac K^+ channels is a major goal in development of novel anti-AF K^+ channel blockers.

Disclosure Statement: D. Dobrev is an advisor and educational lecturer for Daiichi Sankyo, Servier, OMEICOS and Boston Scientific. N. Voigt has received financial support for experimental studies from NISSAN Chemical Industries.
The author's research is supported by the German Federal Ministry of Education and Research through DZHK (German Center for Cardiovascular Research) and the European Union (European Network for Translational Research in Atrial Fibrillation, EUTRAF, grant 261057).
Institute of Pharmacology, West German Heart and Vascular Center, University Duisburg-Essen, Hufelandstr. 55, Essen 45122, Germany
* Corresponding author.
E-mail address: dobromir.dobrev@uk-essen.de

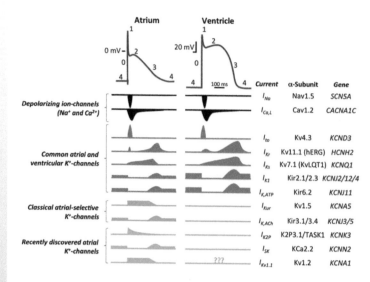

Fig. 1. Contribution of depolarizing inward and repolarizing outward currents to the atrial and ventricular action potential (AP). Activity of inward currents ($I_{Ca,L}$, L-type Ca^{2+}-current; I_{Na}, sodium current) and outward currents during the cardiac AP is displayed together with underlying channel α-subunit and corresponding gene. Outward currents are mediated by potassium (K^+) channels, which are expressed in both atrium and ventricle ($I_{K,ATP}$, adenosine triphosphate-sensitive inward-rectifier K^+ current; I_{K1}, inward-rectifier K^+ current; I_{Kr} and I_{Ks}, rapidly and slowly activating delayed-rectifier current; I_{to}, transient outward), and by K^+ currents, which are predominantly expressed in the atria ($I_{K,ACh}$, acetylcholine-activated inward-rectifier K^+ current; I_{K2P} 2-pore domain channel mediated K^+ current; I_{Kur}, ultrarapidly delayed-rectifier K^+ current; $I_{Kv1.1}$, Kv1.1 channel mediated K^+ current; I_{SK}, SK2-channel mediated K^+ current). The contribution of I_{K2P}, I_{SK}, and $I_{Kv1.1}$ has been estimated based on recent publications.[10,13,89] (*Adapted from* The Sicilian gambit. A new approach to the classification of antiarrhythmic drugs based on their actions on arrhythmogenic mechanisms. Task Force of the Working Group on Arrhythmias of the European Society of Cardiology. Circulation 1991;84(4):1831–51 and Ravens U and Cerbai E. Role of potassium currents in cardiac arrhythmias. Europace 2008;10(10):1133–7; with permission.)

The differences in AP shape between atria and ventricles are mainly owing to the atrial-selective occurrence of K^+ channels, which provide a potential target for atrial-selective antiarrhythmic therapy.[8] The best validated atrial-specific ion currents are the acetylcholine-activated inward-rectifier K^+ current ($I_{K,ACh}$) and ultrarapid delayed-rectifier K^+ current (I_{Kur}), which are absent in ventricular myocytes. Recent publications show that 2-pore domain K^+ channels (K2P channels),[9,10] small-conductance Ca^{2+}-activated K^+ channels (SK channels),[11,12] and Kv1.1 channels[13] may also contribute to the atrial repolarization, potentially representing atrial-specific drug targets (**Fig. 2**).

Herein we review the molecular and electrophysiologic characteristics of atrial-selective K^+ channels and their potential pathophysiologic role in AF. We summarize the currently available K^+ channel blockers focusing on the most important compounds that highlight general principles or that have been evaluated in clinical studies (**Fig. 3**). For a detailed overview we refer the interested readers to a recent excellent review by El-Haou and colleagues.[14]

CLASSICAL ATRIAL-SELECTIVE K^+ CHANNELS
Acetylcholine-Activated Inward-Rectifier K^+ Current

The hallmark of inward-rectifier K^+ channels is the high conductance of K^+ ions into the cell, whereas the physiologically more relevant outward conductance is relatively low (see **Fig. 2B**).[15] Despite this relatively small outward conductance at physiologic potentials, inward-rectifier K^+ channels are major contributors to the late AP repolarization and play a major role in stabilizing the resting membrane potential.[8,16] Increased inward-rectifier K^+ currents have been shown to contribute to APD shortening in cAF patients and to stabilization of reentrant excitations.[3,5] In addition to basal inward-rectifier K^+ current I_{K1}, atrial, but not ventricular myocytes express $I_{K,ACh}$ channels, which are physiologically activated by the vagal neurotransmitter acetylcholine in a muscarinic (M)-receptor-dependent manner.[15,17–19] The $I_{K,ACh}$ channel is a heterotetramer composed of 2 Kir3.1- and 2 Kir3.4 subunits[20] and binding of G-protein βγ-subunits to the N- and C-terminus leads to a stronger interaction of phosphatidylinositol 4,5-bisphosphate with the channel, resulting in channel activation.[21,22] In cAF, $I_{K,ACh}$ develops agonist-independent (constitutive) activity, which has been suggested to contribute to the increased total inward-rectifier K^+ current.[23,24] Because $I_{K,ACh}$ is atrial selective, constitutively active $I_{K,ACh}$ currents represent a potential atrial- and pathology-specific drug target of AF.[2,25]

Blockers
Several antiarrhythmic drugs like amiodarone, flecainide, quinidine, chloroquine, and verapamil possess $I_{K,ACh}$-blocking effects that may

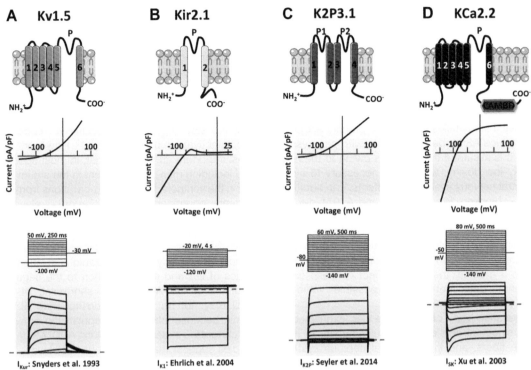

Fig. 2. Membrane topology and current-voltage relationships of voltage-activated (*A*), inward-rectifier (*B*), 2-pore domain (*C*), and small-conductance Ca^{2+}-dependent K^+ currents (*D*). Membrane topology (*upper panels*) shows typical single K^+ channel subunits with numbered transmembrane domains and pore regions (P). External side facing upward. IV-curves (*middle panels*) represent idealized examplaric visualization. Bottom panel shows representative current responses to voltage-steps for I_{Kur} (*A*),[90] I_{K1} (*B*),[91] I_{K2P} (*C*),[92] and I_{SK} (*D*) currents.[89] CAMBD, calmodulin-binding domain. (*Adapted from* Goldstein SA, Bockenhauer D, O'Kelly I, et al. Potassium leak channels and the KCNK family of two-P-domain subunits. Nat Rev Neurosci 2001;2(3):178; with permission.)

contribute to their clinical efficacy.[15,26–29] Based on the putative role of $I_{K,ACh}$ in cAF, a large number of selective $I_{K,ACh}$ inhibitors have been developed during the last years.[14] Tertiapin, a peptidic component of the venom of the European honey bee (*Apis melifera*), is the most widely known representative,[30] but several newer compounds

are currently being evaluated in preclinical and clinical studies.[14]

NIP-142 was the first moderately selective $I_{K,ACh}$ blocker and has been shown to terminate carbachol- and aconitine-induced AF in dogs.[31] The follow-up compound NIP-151, which features higher potency and selectivity over hERG, also

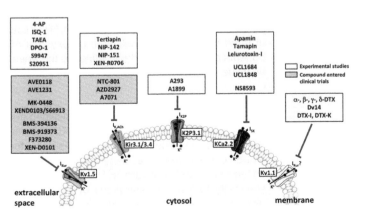

Fig. 3. Atrial-selective K^+ channels and specific blockers. See text for further details. 4-AP, 4-aminopyridine; DPO-1, diphenylphosphine oxide; DTX, dendrotoxin; $I_{K,ACh}$, acetylcholine-activated inward-rectifier K^+ current; I_{K2P}, 2-pore domain channel mediated K^+ current; I_{Kur}, ultrarapid delayed-rectifier K^+ current; $I_{Kv1.1}$, Kv1.1 channel–mediated K^+ current; I_{SK}, SK channel–mediated K^+ current; ISQ-3, isoquinoline-3-nitrile; TAEA, triarylethanolamine.

effectively terminates AF in animal models and intravenous infusion of even 10 times of the maximal effective dose did not prolong QTc interval in vivo.[32,33]

NTC-801 is a selective $I_{K,ACh}$ blocker that effectively prevents atrial tachypacing or vagally induced (mediated) AF. NTC-801 was the first $I_{K,ACh}$ blocker investigated in clinical studies.[34] A phase II study failed to meet the primary endpoint to reduce AF burden in patients with paroxysmal AF. It is assumed that this was owing to the relatively low dosing, which was necessary to avoid central nervous system side effects.[14] In addition, $I_{K,ACh}$ blockers like AZD2927 and A7071 did not affect atrial repolarization in atrial flutter patients.[35] However, because electrical remodeling reverses within 48 hours of AF termination and these patients had been in sinus rhythm (SR) for longer than 3 months, the lack of effect of these compounds does not exclude possible value of $I_{K,ACh}$-blockade in AF.

Because $I_{K,ACh}$ channels are also expressed in the sinoatrial and atrioventricular nodes, in Purkinje fibers, and in the central nervous system, general inhibition of $I_{K,ACh}$ may cause unwanted side effects in these systems. In addition, an improved understanding the molecular basis of the development of agonist-independent constitutive $I_{K,ACh}$ activity may provide effective $I_{K,ACh}$ blockers with limited side effects.[17,36] A number of mechanisms have been suggested to be involved in constitutive $I_{K,ACh}$ activity, including a disbalance between protein kinase C isoforms, increased activity of the nucleoside diphosphate kinase B, or changes in channel stoichiometry.[22,37,38] The last mechanism is supported by experiments with XEN-R0706, the first compound that inhibits Kir3.4 homotetramers with similar potency as Kir3.1/Kir3.4 heterotetramers.[14] In contrast with other $I_{K,ACh}$ blockers, which preferentially inhibit Kir3.1/Kir3.4 heterotetramers, XEN-R0706 prolonged APD in human atrial trabeculae preparations from patients with cAF but not from patients with SR. Although further work is warranted to confirm these observations, these data suggest that Kir3.4 homotetramers may be involved in the development of constitutive $I_{K,ACh}$ activity and compounds preferentially targeting Kir3.4 homotetramers may provide specific anti-AF effects.

Ultrarapid Delayed-Rectifier K+ Current

In contrast with inward-rectifier K+ channels, voltage-gated outward-rectifying K+ channels are closed at resting membrane potential and require membrane depolarization for activation

(see **Fig. 2A**).[8] Outwardly rectifying currents with rapid activation kinetics and little or no inactivation were identified in atrial myocytes from several species, including man.[39] These channels differ from the other voltage-activated outward K+ currents present in the human atrium, that is, the transient outward K+ current (I_{to}), which exhibits strong time-dependent inactivation and from the rapid (I_{Kr}) and slow (I_{Ks}) delayed-rectifier K+ currents, which activate much slower.[40,41] However, the most important difference is that, in most species and including man, I_{Kur} is present in the atrium but not in the ventricle.[42] In atrial preparations from SR patients, pharmacologic inhibition of I_{Kur} elevates the AP plateau but abbreviates the APD,[43] which may facilitate maintenance of reentry excitations.[44,45] Whereas the first observation can be concluded directly from the rapid activation kinetics of I_{Kur} and its contribution to the negative potential of the AP plateau, shortening of the APD may not be a direct consequence of I_{Kur} block, because inhibition of repolarizing outward K+ currents is expected to prolong APD. Modeling studies suggest that the pronounced elevation of the AP plateau results in a stronger activation of other repolarizing K+ currents, such as I_{Kr} and I_{Ks}, thereby shortening the AP.[26,43,46] In contrast, I_{Kur} inhibition in atrial cardiomyocytes from patients with cAF results in a prolongation of the typical triangular AP. The AF-typical triangular shape is the result of extensive electrical remodeling of major ion currents, including reductions of I_{to} and L-type Ca^{2+} currents ($I_{Ca,L}$) and an increase in I_{K1}.[5,6] As a result of the imbalance between ion currents, the putative secondary effects of I_{Kur} block may be reduced resulting in reentry-preventing AP prolongation.[26,43] Although I_{Kur} block is expected to prolong APD in remodeled tissue particularly at rapid rates,[47] I_{Kur} downregulation in cAF patients may limit the effect of I_{Kur} inhibition in these patient populations. In addition, computational modeling has shown that I_{Kur} inhibition may cause EADs during enhanced autonomic tone.[48] Clearly, more studies performed for AF prevention or termination and looking at AP effects at rapid atrial rates particularly in paroxysmal AF patients are needed to further define the therapeutic value of selective I_{Kur} block for AF.

Blockers

I_{Kur} is carried by a channel complex consisting of 4 Kv1.5α subunits that are encoded by KCNA5 and various ancillary β-subunits.[39] Experimentally, the Kv1.5 current may be separated from other voltage-activated outward K+ currents by its sensitivity to low concentrations of 4-aminopyridine (see **Fig. 3**).[26,43] In vivo, 4-aminopyridine neither terminates sustained AF nor prevents the initiation of acetylcholine-induced AF at concentrations that specifically block I_{Kur}, suggesting that pure I_{Kur} block may not suffice to suppress AF effectively.[44] Despite the uncertainty of I_{Kur} as an effective anti-AF target, more than 50 Kv1.5-blocking compounds have been identified during the last decades.[49] It is assumed that most of the tested compounds bind to the inner cavity of the Kv1.5 channel pore and compete with binding of the β-subunits.

The biphenyl derivate AVE0118 effectively prevents inducibility and maintenance of AF in a goat model.[50,51] However, although AVE0118 effectively blocks I_{Kur} in atrial cardiomyocytes from SR patients, it also inhibits I_{to} and $I_{K,ACh}$. In contrast, likely owing to remodeling, AVE0118 has no effect on I_{Kur}, I_{to}, or $I_{K,ACh}$ in atrial cardiomyocytes from cAF patients.[26] Other agents (AVE1231, ISQ-1, TAEA, diphenylphosphine oxide) suppress AF, but these agents also block other ion channels at concentrations that effectively control AF.[42] In atrial multicellular preparations from SR patients, inhibition of I_{Kur} with MK-0448 elevates the AP plateau but abbreviates the APD[52] and, consistent with these in vitro findings, MK-0448 did not prolong atrial repolarization in healthy volunteers.[53] However, in multicellular preparations from cAF patients, MK-0448 prolonged APD in preparations, likely because of reduced repolarization reserve owing to AF-induced remodeling. To the best of our knowledge, XEN-D0103 is currently the most selective Kv1.5 inhibitor with a more than 250-fold higher potency against Kv1.5 than other cardiac ion channels (Kir3.1/3.4, hERG, Kv4.3, Kir2.1, Cav1.2, Nav1.5, and Kv7.1). XEN-D0103 prevents tachypacing-induced AF in dogs and has just completed a phase I clinical trial, but the results are not disclosed yet.[33] Two phase II clinical trials assessing the efficacy of the compound are ongoing.[14]

Atrial selectivity of I_{Kur} block can be increased during the rapid atrial rate in AF and compounds like XEN-D0103, S9947, S20951, and diphenylphosphine oxide inhibit I_{Kur} with increasing effectivity at higher stimulation frequencies.[54] This "use-dependence" approach may be an additional approach to increase the safety profile and limit proarrhythmic side effects.[2]

Overall, although a large number of I_{Kur}-blocking compounds have been developed and 6 selective I_{Kur} drugs (BMS-394136, BMS-919373, MK-0448, F373280, XEN-D0101, and XEND0103/S66913) have entered clinical development, none of them has been launched for therapeutics.[14] Therefore, it still needs to be determined whether "pure" I_{Kur}

blockers are useful for antiarrhythmic therapy in AF.

RECENTLY DISCOVERED ATRIAL K⁺ CHANNELS

Human atrial myocytes from both SR and cAF patients exhibit a substantial noninactivating late outward K⁺ current component, which is commonly defined as part of I_{Kur} but that is insensitive to Kv1.5 blockers like AVE0118.[26,39] The molecular basis of this current is currently unknown but recent publications suggest that K2P, SK, and Kv1.1 channels, which were previously unrecognized to contribute to atrial electrophysiology, may at least partially mediate the AVE0118-insensitive component of I_{Kur}.

Two-Pore Domain K⁺ Channels

Commonly described cardiac K⁺ channels feature a tetrameric structure assembled from 4 identical (homologous) or structural related nonidentical (heterologous) subunits.[55] In voltage-gated ion channels such as I_{Kr}, I_{Ks}, I_{to}, and I_{Kur}, each subunit consists of 6 transmembrane domains (TMD) and a distinctive pore-forming loop structure, which is located between the fifth and sixth TMD and is responsible for the K⁺ selectivity (see **Fig. 2A**). Similarly, subunits of inward-rectifier K⁺ channels I_{K1} and $I_{K,ACh}$ exhibit 1 pore-forming loop but only 2 TMD (see **Fig. 2B**). In contrast, K2P channels are assumed to be dimers consisting of 2 subunits each consisting of 4 TMD and 2 pore-forming loops (see **Fig. 2C**).[56] A recent study showed that, of all identified human K2P-isoforms (K2P1.1-K2P7.1, K2P9.1, K2P10.1, K2P12.1, K2P13.1, and K2P15.1-K2P18.1), K2P1.1 and K2P3.1 are expressed predominantly in the atrium.[9,10] Therefore, it has been assumed that atrial K2P channels may contribute to the rapidly activating, noninactivating K⁺ current defined as I_{Kur}.[9] Furthermore, cAF was associated with an increased expression of K2P3.1 but not K2P1.1. Accordingly, selective inhibition of K2P3.1-mediated current using the pharmacologic compound A293 prolonged APD in cardiomyocytes from cAF patients but not in SR patients bringing K2P3.1 into spotlight as an atrial- and pathology-specific drug target in patients with cAF.[57]

Blockers

Amiodarone has been shown to inhibit K2P channels in therapeutically relevant concentrations, suggesting that inhibition of K2P channels may at least partially contribute to its affectivity in AF.[58] More specifically, the aromatic carbonamide A293 (Sanofi-Aventis) has been developed for pharmacologic K2P channel inhibition (see **Fig. 3**).[9,10,59] At a concentration of 1 μmol/L, A293 inhibited 90% and 50% of K2P3.1 and K2P9.1 channel–mediated currents, respectively, in expression systems. In contrast, inhibition of other K2P channels and major cardiac ion channels was less than 10%, revealing A293 as a selective blocker of K2P3.1 and K2P9.1 channels. Another compound, A1899, has been used as a highly selective blocker of K2P3.1 channels and specific binding sites within the channel pore have been identified.[60] Further insights into the specific 3-dimensional structure of K2P channels, such as the recently discovered crystal structure of K2P1 channels, will fuel extensive ongoing efforts to develop K2P channel inhibitors as novel compounds for treatment of arrhythmias and neuronal disorders.[56,61]

Small-Conductance Ca^{2+}-Activated K$^+$ Channels

SK channels are voltage insensitive but possess a high sensitivity to intracellular Ca^{2+} (<1 μmol/L).[62] Their single-channel conductance between 4 and 14 pS is well below the calculated conductance of intermediate (IK)- or big (BK)-conductance Ca^{2+}-activated K$^+$ channels.[63] The 3 isoforms of the channel subunits SK1-SK3 consist of 6 TMD and 1 pore-forming loop between the fifth and sixth TMD responsible for K$^+$ selectivity (see **Fig. 2**C). Four subunits are necessary to form a functional SK channel.[62] The Ca^{2+} sensitivity is mediated by highly conserved calmodulin-binding sites at the proximal C-terminus of each α-subunit.[64] Ca^{2+} binding to calmodulin induces conformational rearrangements of calmodulin, which are transferred to the α-subunits and result in SK channel activation.[62] SK channel–mediated currents show inward rectification thereby limiting the physiologic relevant outward current branch. Similar to the classical inward-rectifier K$^+$ currents divalent cations such as Ca^{2+} or Mg^{2+} may account for this inward rectification.[12,63]

The activation of SK channels limits excitability in neuronal cells by hyperpolarization that closes voltage-gated Ca^{2+} channels. In contrast, hyperpolarization in response to SK channel activation increases driving force for Ca^{2+} entry through non–voltage-gated Ca^{2+} channels, leading to an increased intracellular Ca^{2+} concentration.[62] Recent evidence suggests that SK channels are expressed in mouse and human hearts, with the SK2 subunit being most predominant in the atria. SK2 knockout in mice resulted in atrial APD prolongation with no significant changes in the ventricles of the same animals.[65] In experimental studies in guinea pigs, aged hypertensive rats and dogs with atrial tachycardia remodeling pharmacologic inhibition of SK channels prolongs APD and prevents burst pacing-induced AF.[12,66,67] However, the role of SK channels in cAF patients is controversial. Both upregulation and downregulation of SK currents has been observed in cAF patients.[3,68–70] In addition, loss of SK channel function has been associated with AF-promoting EADs[65] and block of SK channels has been shown to favor alternans, wavebreak, and atrial arrhythmias in isolated dog atrium.[71]

Blockers

Several compounds have been developed to selectively target SK channels. Here we focus on compounds that are used in experimental studies or that may act as lead structures for development of new SK channel-selective agents. For a more extensive review, see Girault and colleagues' report.[63]

SK channels are selectively blocked by apamin, an 18 amino acid peptide from the honey bee (*Apis mellifera*) venom, making it possible to separate them from IK and BK channels (see **Fig. 3**).[72] Several other peptides from scorpion venom, such as tamapin and leiurotoxin-I, block SK channels with very low median inhibition concentration values (24 and 200 pmol/L, respectively).[63,73] It is assumed that positively charged arginine residues interact with negatively charged aspartate located in the outer pore region of the SK channels. Similarly, several nonpeptide blockers such as UCL1684 and UCL1848 also possess a permanent cationic structure and are assumed to directly block the channel pore region.[74,75] Another approach to modifying SK channel activity in patients with AF may be the modulation of Ca^{2+} sensitivity of SK channels, especially because Ca^{2+} handling abnormalities associated with AF may contribute to SK channel dysregulation.[76,77] Along these lines, NS8593 was the first SK channel inhibitor that acts by decreasing Ca^{2+} sensitivity of SK channels.[78] However, these drugs do not possess clear isoform selectivity and may therefore also cause arrhythmogenic ventricular side effects.[63] Finally, it remains to be seen whether targeting cardiac SK channels can be achieved without significant detrimental effects on other organ systems in which SK channels play important roles.[12]

Voltage-Gated Kv1.1 Channels

Kv1.1 channels encoded by the KCNA1 gene are widely expressed throughout the brain and the peripheral nervous system and their dysfunction has been associated with neurologic diseases including epilepsy and episodic ataxia type 1.[79] Although Kv1.1 channels are commonly seen as neural-specific K^+ channels Kv1.1 messenger RNA and protein has been detected in the mouse atria and ventricles.[80] Accordingly, we recently showed messenger RNA and protein expression of Kv1.1 channels in human right atrial tissue homogenates from patients with SR and detected a rapidly activating and only partially inactivating current, which was sensitive to the Kv1.1-selective blocker dendrotoxin (DTX)-K.[13] These data suggest that DTX-K–sensitive currents may represent a previously unrecognized Kv1.1-mediated current contributing to I_{Kur} in human atrial cardiomyocytes. Furthermore, in cAF patients Kv1.1 protein expression as well as DTX-K–sensitive current component were increased in tissue homogenates and atrial cardiomyocytes, respectively, thereby likely contributing to electrical remodeling in cAF. Although the concurrent increase in Kv1.1 protein expression and Kv1.1-mediated outward currents provides one of the first examples of cAF-associated upregulation of a voltage-dependent K^+ channel, it is unclear whether Kv1.1 may represent an atrial-selective drug target; it is unknown whether Kv1.1 channels are also expressed in the human ventricle. In addition, general inhibition of Kv1.1 channels may cause severe side effects in the central nervous system.

Blockers

In 1980, Harvey and Karlson[81] identified DTX as the active component of the Eastern green mamba (*Dendroaspis angusticeps*) venom, which increases the twitch height of isolated nerve muscle preparations (see **Fig. 3**). It has since been shown that DTX is a potent blocker of neuronal voltage-dependent K^+ channels. DTX or α-DTX is a small protein consisting of 59 amino acids with 3 disulphide bridges. Subsequently, several homologues between 57 to 61 amino acids have been identified in the Eastern green mamba venom (β-, γ- and δ-DTX), in the Western green mamba venom (Dv14), and in the venom of the black mamba (DTX-I and DTX-K).[82]

Although a detailed analysis of the selectivity of the 7 DTX is beyond the scope of this article (for a review, see Harvey[82]), Kv1.1- and Kv1.2-mediated ion currents seem to be the major targets of these toxins with median inhibition concentration values between 1 and 50 nmol/L. Other K^+ currents mediated by Kv1.3, Kv1.4, and Kv1.5 channel subunits are inhibited at 10 to 100 times higher concentrations. Kv1.6 is also blocked by α-DTX.[83] δ-DTK and DTX-K may have a higher selectivity for Kv1.1 than Kv1.2,[84] whereas other DTXs show no clear selectivity for Kv1.1 or Kv1.2 (α-DTX, β-DTX).[85] However, caution has to be taken; selectivity data were usually obtained in expression systems, where channel composition does not necessarily resemble the physiologic situation. In addition, data describing the effects of other non–α-DTX homologues are by far not complete and blocking effects on other K^+ channels cannot be excluded.

SUMMARY

K^+ channels are the most diverse ion channel group in the heart. In addition to K^+ channels such as I_{to}, I_{Kr}, I_{Ks}, and I_{K1}, which are expressed in the ventricles, atrial cardiomyocytes possess a specific subset of K^+ channels ($I_{K,ACh}$, I_{Kur}), which are absent in the ventricle and which determine the typical shape of the atrial AP. Because modulation of atrial-specific K^+ channels does not carry the risk of proarrhythmic ventricular side effects,[86] extensive efforts have been made to develop pharmacologic agents for modulation of atrial-specific channels. In addition, recent studies provide evidence for existence of additional potentially atrial-selective K^+ channels such as K2P channels, SK channels, and Kv1.1 channels. Although atrial-selective K^+ channels seem to be promising antiarrhythmic targets, none of the "pure" blockers of I_{Kur} or $I_{K,ACh}$ have passed phase II clinical trials yet. In contrast, multichannel blockers such as amiodarone and vernakalant are established compounds for treatment of AF.[2,87] Thus, future research will show whether inhibition of a single atrial-specific K^+ channel or the identification of specific combinations of ion channel blockade is needed to improve antiarrhythmic drug efficacy and safety.[88] The main challenge to latter approach is the precise identification of the suitable channel-blocking profile.

REFERENCES

1. Andrade J, Khairy P, Dobrev D, et al. The clinical profile and pathophysiology of atrial fibrillation: relationships among clinical features, epidemiology, and mechanisms. Circ Res 2014;114(9): 1453–68.
2. Dobrev D, Carlsson L, Nattel S. Novel molecular targets for atrial fibrillation therapy. Nat Rev Drug Discov 2012;11(4):275–91.
3. Heijman J, Voigt N, Dobrev D. New directions in antiarrhythmic drug therapy for atrial fibrillation. Future Cardiol 2013;9(1):71–88.
4. Woods CE, Olgin J. Atrial fibrillation therapy now and in the future: drugs, biologicals, and ablation. Circ Res 2014;114(9):1532–46.

5. Wakili R, Voigt N, Kaab S, et al. Recent advances in the molecular pathophysiology of atrial fibrillation. J Clin Invest 2011;121(8):2955–68.

6. Heijman J, Voigt N, Nattel S, et al. Cellular and molecular electrophysiology of atrial fibrillation initiation, maintenance, and progression. Circ Res 2014; 114(9):1483–99.

7. Qu Z, Xie LH, Olcese R, et al. Early afterdepolarizations in cardiac myocytes: beyond reduced repolarization reserve. Cardiovasc Res 2013; 99(1):6–15.

8. Ravens U, Cerbai E. Role of potassium currents in cardiac arrhythmias. Europace 2008;10(10): 1133–7.

9. Limberg SH, Netter MF, Rolfes C, et al. TASK-1 channels may modulate action potential duration of human atrial cardiomyocytes. Cell Physiol Biochem 2011;28(4):613–24.

10. Schmidt C, Wiedmann F, Voigt N, et al. Upregulation of $K_{2P}3.1$ K^+ current causes action potential shortening in patients with chronic atrial fibrillation. Circulation 2015;132(2):82–92.

11. Zhou XB, Voigt N, Wieland T, et al. Enhanced frequency-dependent retrograde trafficking of small conductance Ca^{2+}-activated channels may contribute to electrical remodeling in human atrial fibrillation. Heart Rhythm 2012;9(5S):S319.

12. Qi XY, Diness JG, Brundel BJ, et al. Role of small-conductance calcium-activated potassium channels in atrial electrophysiology and fibrillation in the dog. Circulation 2014;129(4):430–40.

13. Glasscock E, Voigt N, McCauley MD, et al. Expression and function of Kv1.1 potassium channels in human atria from patients with atrial fibrillation. Basic Res Cardiol 2015;110(5):505.

14. El-Haou S, Ford JW, Milnes JT. Novel K^+ channel targets in atrial fibrillation drug development - where are we? J Cardiovasc Pharmacol 2015; 66(5):412–31.

15. Hibino H, Inanobe A, Furutani K, et al. Inwardly rectifying potassium channels: their structure, function, and physiological roles. Physiol Rev 2010;90(1): 291–366.

16. Pandit SV, Berenfeld O, Anumonwo JM, et al. Ionic determinants of functional reentry in a 2-D model of human atrial cells during simulated chronic atrial fibrillation. Biophys J 2005;88(6):3806–21.

17. Voigt N, Abu-Taha I, Heijman J, et al. Constitutive activity of the acetylcholine-activated potassium current $I_{K,ACh}$ in cardiomyocytes. Adv Pharmacol 2014;70:393–409.

18. Gaborit N, Le Bouter S, Szuts V, et al. Regional and tissue specific transcript signatures of ion channel genes in the non-diseased human heart. J Physiol 2007;582(Pt 2):675–93.

19. Voigt N, Trausch A, Knaut M, et al. Left-to-right atrial inward rectifier potassium current gradients in patients with paroxysmal versus chronic atrial fibrillation. Circ Arrhythm Electrophysiol 2010;3(5): 472–80.

20. Krapivinsky G, Gordon EA, Wickman K, et al. The G-protein-gated atrial K^+ channel I_{KACh} is a heteromultimer of two inwardly rectifying K^+-channel proteins. Nature 1995;374(6518):135–41.

21. Rosenhouse-Dantsker A, Sui JL, Zhao Q, et al. A sodium-mediated structural switch that controls the sensitivity of Kir channels to PIP_2. Nat Chem Biol 2008;4(10):624–31.

22. Voigt N, Heijman J, Trausch A, et al. Impaired Na^+-dependent regulation of acetylcholine-activated inward-rectifier K^+ current modulates action potential rate dependence in patients with chronic atrial fibrillation. J Mol Cell Cardiol 2013;61:142–52.

23. Dobrev D, Friedrich A, Voigt N, et al. The G protein-gated potassium current $I_{K,ACh}$ is constitutively active in patients with chronic atrial fibrillation. Circulation 2005;112(24):3697–706.

24. Voigt N, Maguy A, Yeh YH, et al. Changes in $I_{K,ACh}$ single-channel activity with atrial tachycardia remodelling in canine atrial cardiomyocytes. Cardiovasc Res 2008;77(1):35–43.

25. Dobrev D, Nattel S. New antiarrhythmic drugs for treatment of atrial fibrillation. Lancet 2010; 375(9721):1212–23.

26. Christ T, Wettwer E, Voigt N, et al. Pathology-specific effects of the $I_{Kur}/I_{to}/I_{K,ACh}$ blocker AVE0118 on ion channels in human chronic atrial fibrillation. Br J Pharmacol 2008;154(8):1619–30.

27. Voigt N, Rozmaritsa N, Trausch A, et al. Inhibition of $I_{K,ACh}$ current may contribute to clinical efficacy of class I and class III antiarrhythmic drugs in patients with atrial fibrillation. Naunyn Schmiedebergs Arch Pharmacol 2010;381(3):251–9.

28. Kurachi Y, Nakajima T, Ito H, et al. AN-132, a new class I anti-arrhythmic agent, depresses the acetylcholine-induced K^+ current in atrial myocytes. Eur J Pharmacol 1989;165(2–3):319–22.

29. Kurachi Y, Nakajima T, Sugimoto T. Quinidine inhibition of the muscarine receptor-activated K^+ channel current in atrial cells of guinea pig. Naunyn Schmiedebergs Arch Pharmacol 1987;335(2): 216–8.

30. Jin W, Klem AM, Lewis JH, et al. Mechanisms of inward-rectifier K^+ channel inhibition by tertiapin-Q. Biochemistry 1999;38(43):14294–301.

31. Tanaka H, Hashimoto N. A multiple ion channel blocker, NIP-142, for the treatment of atrial fibrillation. Cardiovasc Drug Rev 2007;25(4):342–56.

32. Hashimoto N, Yamashita T, Tsuruzoe N. Characterization of in vivo and in vitro electrophysiological and antiarrhythmic effects of a novel I_{KACh} blocker, NIP-151: a comparison with an I_{Kr}-blocker dofetilide. J Cardiovasc Pharmacol 2008;51(2): 162–9.

33. Milnes JT, Madge DJ, Ford JW. New pharmacological approaches to atrial fibrillation. Drug Discov Today 2012;17(13–14):654–9.

34. Machida T, Hashimoto N, Kuwahara I, et al. Effects of a highly selective acetylcholine-activated K^+ channel blocker on experimental atrial fibrillation. Circ Arrhythm Electrophysiol 2011;4(1):94–102.

35. Walfridsson H, Anfinsen OG, Berggren A, et al. Is the acetylcholine-regulated inwardly rectifying potassium current a viable antiarrhythmic target? translational discrepancies of AZD2927 and A7071 in dogs and humans. Europace 2015;17(3):473–82.

36. Voigt N, Makary S, Nattel S, et al. Voltage-clamp-based methods for the detection of constitutively active acetylcholine-gated $I_{K,ACh}$ channels in the diseased heart. Methods Enzymol 2010;484: 653–75.

37. Voigt N, Friedrich A, Bock M, et al. Differential phosphorylation-dependent regulation of constitutively active and muscarinic receptor-activated $I_{K,ACh}$ channels in patients with chronic atrial fibrillation. Cardiovasc Res 2007;74(3):426–37.

38. Makary S, Voigt N, Maguy A, et al. Differential protein kinase C isoform regulation and increased constitutive activity of acetylcholine-regulated potassium channels in atrial remodeling. Circ Res 2011;109(9):1031–43.

39. Ravens U, Wettwer E. Ultra-rapid delayed rectifier channels: molecular basis and therapeutic implications. Cardiovasc Res 2011;89(4):776–85.

40. Feng J, Xu D, Wang Z, et al. Ultrarapid delayed rectifier current inactivation in human atrial myocytes: properties and consequences. Am J Physiol 1998;275(5 Pt 2):H1717–25.

41. Wang Z, Fermini B, Nattel S. Sustained depolarization-induced outward current in human atrial myocytes. Evidence for a novel delayed rectifier K^+ current similar to Kv1.5 cloned channel currents. Circ Res 1993;73(6):1061–76.

42. Aliot E, Capucci A, Crijns HJ, et al. Twenty-five years in the making: flecainide is safe and effective for the management of atrial fibrillation. Europace 2011; 13(2):161–73.

43. Wettwer E, Hala O, Christ T, et al. Role of I_{Kur} in controlling action potential shape and contractility in the human atrium: influence of chronic atrial fibrillation. Circulation 2004;110(16):2299–306.

44. Burashnikov A, Antzelevitch C. Can inhibition of I_{Kur} promote atrial fibrillation? Heart Rhythm 2008;5(9): 1304–9.

45. Johnson NC, Morgan MW. An unusual case of 4-aminopyridine toxicity. J Emerg Med 2006;30(2): 175–7.

46. Shibata EF, Drury T, Refsum H, et al. Contributions of a transient outward current to repolarization in human atrium. Am J Physiol 1989;257(6 Pt 2): H1773–81.

47. Courtemanche M, Ramirez RJ, Nattel S. Ionic targets for drug therapy and atrial fibrillation-induced electrical remodeling: insights from a mathematical model. Cardiovasc Res 1999;42(2):477–89.

48. Grandi E, Pandit SV, Voigt N, et al. Human atrial action potential and $Ca2^+$ model: sinus rhythm and chronic atrial fibrillation. Circ Res 2011;109(9): 1055–66.

49. Ford JW, Milnes JT. New drugs targeting the cardiac ultra-rapid delayed-rectifier current (I_{Kur}): rationale, pharmacology and evidence for potential therapeutic value. J Cardiovasc Pharmacol 2008; 52(2):105–20.

50. Blaauw Y, Gogelein H, Tieleman RG, et al. "Early" class III drugs for the treatment of atrial fibrillation: efficacy and atrial selectivity of AVE0118 in remodeled atria of the goat. Circulation 2004;110(13): 1717–24.

51. de Haan S, Greiser M, Harks E, et al. AVE0118, blocker of the transient outward current (I_{to}) and ultrarapid delayed rectifier current (I_{Kur}), fully restores atrial contractility after cardioversion of atrial fibrillation in the goat. Circulation 2006; 114(12):1234–42.

52. Loose S, Mueller J, Wettwer E, et al. Effects of I_{Kur} blocker MK-0448 on human right atrial action potentials from patients in sinus rhythm and in permanent atrial fibrillation. Front Pharmacol 2014;5:26.

53. Pavri BB, Greenberg HE, Kraft WK, et al. MK-0448, a specific Kv1.5 inhibitor: safety, pharmacokinetics, and pharmacodynamic electrophysiology in experimental animal models and humans. Circ Arrhythm Electrophysiol 2012;5(6):1193–201.

54. Ford J, Milnes J, El Haou S, et al. The positive frequency-dependent electrophysiological effects of the I_{Kur} inhibitor Xen-D0103 are desirable for the treatment of atrial fibrillation. Heart Rhythm 2016; 13(2):555–64.

55. Goldstein SA, Bockenhauer D, O'Kelly I, et al. Potassium leak channels and the KCNK family of two-P-domain subunits. Nat Rev Neurosci 2001; 2(3):175–84.

56. Miller AN, Long SB. Crystal structure of the human two-pore domain potassium channel K2P1. Science 2012;335(6067):432–6.

57. Schmidt C, Wiedmann F, Schweizer PA, et al. Inhibition of cardiac two-pore-domain K^+ (K_{2P}) channels–an emerging antiarrhythmic concept. Eur J Pharmacol 2014;738:250–5.

58. Gierten J, Ficker E, Bloehs R, et al. The human cardiac $K_{2P}3.1$ (TASK-1) potassium leak channel is a molecular target for the class III antiarrhythmic drug amiodarone. Naunyn Schmiedebergs Arch Pharmacol 2010;381(3):261–70.

59. Putzke C, Wemhoner K, Sachse FB, et al. The acid-sensitive potassium channel TASK-1 in rat cardiac muscle. Cardiovasc Res 2007;75(1):59–68.

60. Streit AK, Netter MF, Kempf F, et al. A specific two-pore domain potassium channel blocker defines the structure of the TASK-1 open pore. J Biol Chem 2011;286(16):13977–84.

61. Coburn CA, Luo Y, Cui M, et al. Discovery of a pharmacologically active antagonist of the two-pore-domain potassium channel K2P9.1 (TASK-3). ChemMedChem 2012;7(1):123–33.

62. Gueguinou M, Chantome A, Fromont G, et al. KCa and Ca^{2+} channels: the complex thought. Biochim Biophys Acta 2014;1843(10):2322–33.

63. Girault A, Haelters JP, Potier-Cartereau M, et al. Targeting SKCa channels in cancer: potential new therapeutic approaches. Curr Med Chem 2012; 19(5):697–713.

64. Schumacher MA, Rivard AF, Bachinger HP, et al. Structure of the gating domain of a Ca^{2+}-activated K$^+$ channel complexed with Ca^{2+}/calmodulin. Nature 2001;410(6832):1120–4.

65. Li N, Timofeyev V, Tuteja D, et al. Ablation of a Ca^{2+}-activated K$^+$ channel (SK2 channel) results in action potential prolongation in atrial myocytes and atrial fibrillation. J Physiol 2009;587(Pt 5):1087–100.

66. Diness JG, Sorensen US, Nissen JD, et al. Inhibition of small-conductance Ca^{2+}-activated K$^+$ channels terminates and protects against atrial fibrillation. Circ Arrhythm Electrophysiol 2010;3(4):380–90.

67. Skibsbye L, Diness JG, Sorensen US, et al. The duration of pacing-induced atrial fibrillation is reduced in vivo by inhibition of small conductance Ca^{2+}-activated K$^+$ channels. J Cardiovasc Pharmacol 2011;57(6):672–81.

68. Ellinor PT, Lunetta KL, Glazer NL, et al. Common variants in KCNN3 are associated with lone atrial fibrillation. Nat Genet 2010;42(3):240–4.

69. Yu T, Deng C, Wu R, et al. Decreased expression of small-conductance Ca^{2+}-activated K$^+$ channels SK1 and SK2 in human chronic atrial fibrillation. Life Sci 2012;90(5–6):219–27.

70. Skibsbye L, Poulet C, Diness JG, et al. Small-conductance calcium-activated potassium (SK) channels contribute to action potential repolarization in human atria. Cardiovasc Res 2014;103(1): 156–67.

71. Hsueh CH, Chang PC, Hsieh YC, et al. Proarrhythmic effect of blocking the small conductance calcium activated potassium channel in isolated canine left atrium. Heart Rhythm 2013;10(6):891–8.

72. Hugues M, Romey G, Duval D, et al. Apamin as a selective blocker of the calcium-dependent potassium channel in neuroblastoma cells: voltage-clamp and biochemical characterization of the toxin receptor. Proc Natl Acad Sci U S A 1982;79(4): 1308–12.

73. Tan PT, Ranganathan S, Brusic V. Deduction of functional peptide motifs in scorpion toxins. J Pept Sci 2006;12(6):420–7.

74. Chen JQ, Galanakis D, Ganellin CR, et al. bis-Quinolinium cyclophanes: 8,14-diaza-1,7(1,4)-diquinolinacyclotetradecaphane (UCL 1848), a highly potent and selective, nonpeptidic blocker of the apamin-sensitive Ca^{2+}-activated K$^+$ channel. J Med Chem 2000;43(19):3478–81.

75. Rosa JC, Galanakis D, Ganellin CR, et al. Bis-quinolinium cyclophanes: 6,10-diaza-3(1,3),8(1,4)-dibenzena-1,5(1,4)- diquinolinacyclodecaphane (UCL 1684), the first nanomolar, non-peptidic blocker of the apamin-sensitive Ca^{2+}-activated K$^+$ channel. J Med Chem 1998;41(1):2–5.

76. Voigt N, Li N, Wang Q, et al. Enhanced sarcoplasmic reticulum Ca^{2+} leak and increased Na$^+$-Ca^{2+} exchanger function underlie delayed afterdepolarizations in patients with chronic atrial fibrillation. Circulation 2012;125(17):2059–70.

77. Voigt N, Heijman J, Wang Q, et al. Cellular and molecular mechanisms of atrial arrhythmogenesis in patients with paroxysmal atrial fibrillation. Circulation 2014;129(2):145–56.

78. Strobaek D, Hougaard C, Johansen TH, et al. Inhibitory gating modulation of small conductance Ca^{2+}-activated K$^+$ channels by the synthetic compound (R)-N-(benzimidazol-2-yl)-1,2,3,4-tetrahydro-1-naphtylamine (NS8593) reduces after hyperpolarizing current in hippocampal CA1 neurons. Mol Pharmacol 2006;70(5):1771–82.

79. Robbins CA, Tempel BL. Kv1.1 and Kv1.2: similar channels, different seizure models. Epilepsia 2012; 53(Suppl 1):134–41.

80. Glasscock E, Qian J, Kole MJ, et al. Transcompartmental reversal of single fibre hyperexcitability in juxtaparanodal Kv1.1-deficient vagus nerve axons by activation of nodal KCNQ channels. J Physiol 2012;590(Pt 16):3913–26.

81. Harvey AL, Karlsson E. Dendrotoxin from the venom of the green mamba, dendroaspis angusticeps. A neurotoxin that enhances acetylcholine release at neuromuscular junction. Naunyn Schmiedebergs Arch Pharmacol 1980;312(1):1–6.

82. Harvey AL. Twenty years of dendrotoxins. Toxicon 2001;39(1):15–26.

83. Grupe A, Schroter KH, Ruppersberg JP, et al. Cloning and expression of a human voltage-gated potassium channel. A novel member of the RCK potassium channel family. EMBO J 1990;9(6): 1749–56.

84. Robertson B, Owen D, Stow J, et al. Novel effects of dendrotoxin homologues on subtypes of mammalian Kv1 potassium channels expressed in Xenopus oocytes. FEBS Lett 1996;383(1–2):26–30.

85. Hopkins W, Miller J, Miljanich G. Voltage-gated potassium channel inhibitors. Curr Pharm Des 1996; 2:389–96.

86. Heijman J, Voigt N, Carlsson LG, et al. Cardiac safety assays. Curr Opin Pharmacol 2014;15:16–21.

87. Dobrev D, Hamad B, Kirkpatrick P. Vernakalant. Nat Rev Drug Discov 2010;9(12):915–6.
88. Reiffel JA, Camm AJ, Belardinelli L, et al. The HARMONY trial: combined ranolazine and dronedarone in the management of paroxysmal atrial fibrillation: mechanistic and therapeutic synergism. Circ Arrhythm Electrophysiol 2015;8(5):1048–56.
89. Xu Y, Tuteja D, Zhang Z, et al. Molecular identification and functional roles of a Ca^{2+}-activated K^+ channel in human and mouse hearts. J Biol Chem 2003;278(49):49085–94.
90. Snyders DJ, Tamkun MM, Bennett PB. A rapidly activating and slowly inactivating potassium channel cloned from human heart. Functional analysis after stable mammalian cell culture expression. J Gen Physiol 1993;101(4):513–43.
91. Ehrlich JR, Cha TJ, Zhang L, et al. Characterization of a hyperpolarization-activated time-dependent potassium current in canine cardiomyocytes from pulmonary vein myocardial sleeves and left atrium. J Physiol 2004;557(Pt 2):583–97.
92. Seyler C, Li J, Schweizer PA, et al. Inhibition of cardiac two-pore-domain K^+ (K2P) channels by the antiarrhythmic drug vernakalant–comparison with flecainide. Eur J Pharmacol 2014;724:51–7.

Dofetilide: Electrophysiologic Effect, Efficacy, and Safety in Patients with Cardiac Arrhythmias

Fatemah Shenasa, BS, Mohammad Shenasa, MD*

KEYWORDS

- Atrial fibrillation • Atrial flutter • Cardiac arrhythmias • Dofetilide • Heart failure • Proarrhythmias
- Torsades de pointes

KEY POINTS

- Dofetilide is a class III antiarrhythmic agent with a selective blockade of rapid component of delayed rectifier potassium current (IK_r).
- Dofetilide was found to be safe in patients after myocardial infarction and those with congestive heart failure and left ventricular systolic dysfunction (ejection fraction of less than 35%).
- An important adverse effect of dofetilide is its potential proarrhythmic risk of ventricular tachyarrhythmias, mostly torsades de pointes.
- Because dofetilide has about an 80% renal excretion, dose adjustment is required in patients with impaired renal function.
- Dofetilide should not be given or discontinued if the QTc is greater than 500 ms.

INTRODUCTION

Despite many challenges in the medical management of atrial fibrillation (AF) and disappointments in the use of antiarrhythmic drug (AAD) therapy in the maintenance of sinus rhythm, AAD therapy remains the mainstay in the management of AF.[1-3] Because of significant adverse effects of many old and newly developed AAD for rhythm control of AF, development of new AADs has been slow. The last AAD that received US Food Drug Administration (FDA) approval was dronedarone.[4,5] Despite early enthusiasm that dronedarone was effective in preventing hospitalization as a surrogate endpoint, the subsequent analysis of dronedarone showed increased mortality in patients with heart failure and permanent AF.[6,7] Dofetilide, on the other hand, appears reasonably safe and effective when used in appropriately selected patients, that is, the right drug for the right patient. Dofetilide was initially tested in patients with post-myocardial infarction (MI) and in those with congestive heart failure (CHF) and low ejection fraction that constitutes a high-risk patient group.[8-11] Among the different classes of AAD that were developed in the last 2 decades, dofetilide was the first specific K^+ channel blocker. Specific ion channel blockers and atrial selective agents are concepts that are appealing and are becoming more popular for the manufacturers to develop and medical community to test and use.[3,12-19] In this review, the AA properties and safety of dofetilide as a prototype of selective K^+ channel blocker are discussed.

Conflict of Interest and Disclosures: None.
Heart and Rhythm Medical Group, Department of Cardiovascular Services, O'Connor Hospital, 105 North Bascom Avenue, San Jose, CA 95128, USA
* Corresponding author.
E-mail address: Mohammad.shenasa@gmail.com

Card Electrophysiol Clin 8 (2016) 423–436
http://dx.doi.org/10.1016/j.ccep.2016.02.006
1877-9182/16/$ – see front matter © 2016 Elsevier Inc. All rights reserved.

Approval of dofetilide by the FDA was based on the data from the DIAMOND study on the efficacy of dofetilide in the treatment of post-MI and CHF that also had AF and atrial flutter (AFL).[8–11]

ELECTROPHYSIOLOGIC EFFECTS OF DOFETILIDE

Dofetilide, like sotalol, is a methane sulfonanilide derivative[20] and belongs to the class III AAD with a prominent effect of blockade of the rapid component of delayed rectifier potassium channel (I_{Kr}). It also increases the late sodium current activity at lower concentration; therefore, it prolongs action potential duration (APD) in atrial, ventricular, and Purkinje cells. It also increases the atrial effective refractory period (ERP) more than the ventricular ERP.[21,22]

Thus, it is more effective in atrial arrhythmias that are due to re-entry than other mechanisms. In principle, K^+ currents are responsible for most parts of the repolarization and are divided into at least 2 major components: the rapidly activated components I_{Kr} and a slower activating component I_{Ks}.[23] Each component is mediated by separate genes (ie, I_{Kr} by hERG and I_{Ks} by Kv LQT$_1$), respectively.[24,25] There are also other K^+ channels in the atria, such as $I_{K,ATP}$, I_{Kur}, $I_{K,Ach}$, I_{SK}, $I_{SK,Ca}$, and I_{K2P}.[15,26,27] In this regard, dofetilide is a specific blocker of I_{Kr}, and because I_{Kr} is responsible for most of the repolarization blockade of I_{Kr}, produces action potential prolongation, which translates to QT prolongation.[21,22] This effect carries the risk of QT prolongation and can potentially be arrhythmogenic.[28,29]

Ion channel transport during depolarization and repolarization is well described in the articles by Voigt and Dobrev and Skibsbye and Ravens (see Voigt N, Dobrev D: Atrial-selective potassium channel blockers; and Skibsybye L, Ravens U: Mechanism of proarrhythmic effects of potassium channel blockers in this issue) and does not need to be repeated here.

Class III AADs demonstrate a dose-dependent property but have a reverse use dependent effect, that is, the effect is more pronounced at slower than faster rates.[21,30] This effect is counterproductive during clinical arrhythmias such as AF/AFL wherein the drug is less effective at faster heart rates.[31–35] Similarly, lower intracellular K^+ concentrations potentiate effects of K^+ channel blockers, whereas high intracellular K^+ concentrations blunt its effect.[21,35] This effect has clinical relevance in that hypokalemia increases the risk of QT prolongation and proarrhythmias (mainly torsades de pointes [TdP]) more than normal K^+ hemostasis. On the other hand, hyperkalemia reduces the efficacy of class III agents such as dofetilide. Experimental studies by Baskin and Lynch[35] and Sedgwick and colleagues[36] have shown the effect of K^+ channel blockers is higher in atrial than ventricular myocardial cells.[21,37] Some K^+ currents are also present in the sinus node; thus, K^+ channel blockers reduce the spontaneous activity of the sinus node cells causing a sinus bradycardia.[24]

Class III AAD effects on APD are reversible by β-adrenergic stimulation such as isoproterenol.[38]

K^+ channel blockers at higher doses exert antifibrillatory effects.[39]

Dofetilide does not exert negative inotropic effect nor induce hypotension. In other words, dofetilide does not produce significant hemodynamic effect.[40]

EFFECT OF DOFETILIDE ON EXPERIMENTAL MODELS OF ATRIAL ARRHYTHMIAS

In general, class III agents such as dofetilide prolong APD and ERP; therefore, they are more effective against arrhythmias that are due to re-entrant mechanisms than those with triggered activity.[21]

Studies by Li and colleagues[41] investigated the electrophysiologic effect and efficacy of dofetilide in 2 different models of AF, that is, rapid atrial pacing-induced atrial remodeling and tachypaced heart failure model. Interestingly, dofetilide was more effective in the tachypace-induced heart failure AF model where the mechanism of AF was due to macro-re-entry. Where prolongation of the ERP decreases the excitable gap, hence the re-entry does not maintain and thus terminate the tachycardia. In contrast, dofetilide was less effective in the atrial pacing-induced AF model, whereby in this model, the mechanisms of AF was due to multiple wavelet re-entry, whereby dofetilide decreased the number and slowed re-entry circuits but did not terminate AF. This difference was assumed by the investigators because of its different electrophysiologic mechanism of AF in each model.[41]

ANTIARRHYTHMIC EFFECTS OF DOFETILIDE
The Clinical Trials of Dofetilide

The initial studies evaluated dofetilide in a large Danish Trial (Danish Investigation of Arrhythmia and Mortality on Dofetilide [DIAMOND]) in patients with post- MI, CHF with reduced left ventricular (LV) systolic function, and AF (**Table 1**); these are discussed later.

DIAMOND Trials

Antiarrhythmic effects of dofetilide and its clinical efficacy in atrial and ventricular arrhythmias were initially evaluated in the DIAMOND Trial (see **Table 1**).[8–11] The DIAMOND trial included high-risk patient subgroups, that is, patients with heart failure[8] and reduced systolic LV function and those in post-MI.[8] The FDA approved the use of dofetilide based on the data from the DIAMOND trial.[8–11]

DIAMOND-CHF

A total of 1518 patients with symptomatic CHF and severe LV systolic dysfunction were randomized to either dofetilide or placebo.[8] Seven hundred sixty-two patients received dofetilide and 756 received placebo. The median follow-up was 18 months. Follow-up duration was 383 days in the dofetilide group and 371 days in the placebo group. Of the initial 288 patients, those who had AF received 250 μg of dofetilide twice a day, and those who did not have AF received 500 μg twice a day. However, based on observation from other studies on the effect of impaired renal function, dose adjustment was made based on the creatinine clearance. Patients with a clearance of 40 to 60 mL a minute were given 250 μg of dofetilide twice a day, and those with a clearance of 20 to 40 mL a minute were given 250 μg of dofetilide once a day. The result of the DIAMOND-CHF showed that compared with placebo, patients on dofetilide had lower rate of hospitalization for worsening of heart failure and did not increase the risk of death among patients with CHF and reduced LV systolic function. Furthermore, dofetilide was effective in converting and maintaining sinus rhythm in this group of patients. In patients who had AF, the overall conversion of AF to sinus rhythm on dofetilide was 44% and on placebo was 14% (P<.001). Twenty-five patients developed TdP, and most of the episodes (76%) occurred in the first 3 days of dofetilide therapy.

DIAMOND-MI

The DIAMOND-MI trial investigated the effect of dofetilide in a randomized double-blind, placebo-controlled fashion in 1510 patients with severe LV systolic dysfunction and recent MI[9]: 749 patients were receiving dofetilide and 761 received placebo. The primary and secondary endpoints of the trials were all-cause mortality and cardiac or arrhythmic mortality, respectively. The results of this trial showed that there were no significant differences between the 2 groups with respect to all-cause mortality and cardiac or arrhythmic mortality. Eight percent of patients in this group had AF or AFL. Those who were on dofetilide did better than the placebo group. The conclusion of the DIAMOND-MI study was that dofetilide did not increase all-cause mortality nor cardiac or arrhythmic death in this high-risk patient group. In the first 839 patients, the initial dose was 500 μg twice a day for those in sinus rhythm and 250 μg twice a day for those in AF/AFL. Dose adjustment was done according to the creatinine clearance.

DIAMOND-AF

In this substudy of the DIAMOND trial, 506 patients with AF/AFL were randomized on dofetilide (249 patients) or placebo (257 patients).[10] Initially, the patients with AF received 250 μg of either drug twice a day. The dose adjustment was done according to the creatinine clearance. The end point of this study was maintenance of sinus rhythm at 1 year, with 79% of patients on dofetilide and 42% of patients on placebo in sinus rhythm (P<.001). Like the other DIAMOND trials, dofetilide in the DIAMOND-AF trial did not increase all-cause mortality or death. Hospitalization was significantly lower in patients who were on dofetilide.

DIAMOND Summary

The DIAMOND-CHF study,[8] DIAMOND-MI study,[9] and DIAMOND-AF study[10] demonstrated that dofetilide did not increase all-cause mortality, hospitalization, or worsening of heart failure. Similarly, dofetilide was effective in converting AF/AFL to sinus rhythm and preventing its recurrence.[8] Dofetilide did not increase the mortality in all 3 subgroups of the DIAMOND trial. **Fig. 1** compares dofetilide with placebo in the 3 substudies of the DIAMOND trials, respectively, (A) effect of dofetilide on survival compared with placebo; (B) dofetilide with placebo in CHF; (C) dofetilide with placebo in MI; (D) AF recurrences.

The EMERALD Trial

The European and Australian Multicenter Evaluative Research on AF of Dofetilide (EMERALD) trial investigated the safety and efficacy of dofetilide in patients with AF/AFL (see **Table 1**).[42–45] The EMERALD study was a double-blind, randomized, placebo-controlled study of 546 patients with persistent AF. It compared dofetilide at doses of 125 μg, 250 μg, or 500 μg twice a day with sotalol at a dose of 80 μg twice a day or placebo. Three hundred ninety-seven patients received dofetilide of all 3 doses, and 137 patients were randomized to placebo. At 1 year, 30%, 45%, and 51% of the patients on dofetilide at the respective doses were in sinus rhythm and free of AF episodes. Similarly, 38% of the patients on sotalol and 16% of placebo patients were in sinus rhythm and free of AF episodes.

Table 1
Trials on dofetilide

Trial Name	Type	N	Dosage	TdP (%)	Results
DIAMOND	Randomized	3028	—	—	—

DIAMOND-CHF,[8,11] 1999	Double-blind, randomized, placebo-controlled	1518	Dofetilide: 762 patients
			Placebo: 756 patients
			Had AF: 250 µg BID
			No AF: 500 µg BID
			Dose adjustment
			(after 288 patients)
			40–60 mL/min:
			  250 µg BID
			20–40 mL/min:
			  250 µg QD
				3.3	Patients on dofetilide had lower rate of hospitalization for worsening of HF and did not increase the risk of death among patients with CHF and reduced LV systolic function; dofetilide was effective in converting and maintaining sinus rhythm in this group of patients

DIAMOND-MI,[9,11] 2000	Randomized, placebo-controlled	1510	Dofetilide: 749 patients Placebo: 761 patients Had AF: 250 µg BID No AF: 500 µg BID *Dose adjustment* *(after 839 patients)*	0.9	No significant differences between the 2 groups with respect to all-cause mortality and cardiac or arrhythmic mortality; dofetilide did not increase all-cause mortality nor cardiac or arrhythmic death in this high-risk patient group

DIAMOND-AF,[16] 2001	Randomized, placebo-controlled	506	Dofetilide: 249 patients
			Placebo: 257 patients
			Had AF: 250 µg BID
			Dose adjustment
			<40 mL/min:
			  250 µg QD
			<20 mL/min:
			  discontinued
				1.6	Dofetilide did not increase all-cause mortality or death; hospitalization was significantly lower in patients who were on dofetilide

Study	Design	No. of Patients	Dose		Comments
EMERALD,[42,43] 1998	Double-blind, randomized, placebo-controlled	546	Dofetilide: 125 μg, 250 μg, 500 μg BID Sotolol: 80 μg BID	1.0	At 1 y, 30% of 125 μg, 45% of 250 μg, and 51% of 500 μg remained in sinus rhythm and were free of AF, whereas 38% of sotalol and 16% of placebo remained in sinus rhythm and were free of AF
SAFIRE-D,[46] 2000	Double-blind, multicenter, placebo-controlled	325	Dofetilide: 125 μg, 250 μg, or 500 μg BID	1.2	Dofetilide was moderately effective in converting and maintaining AF/AFL to sinus rhythm. In this trial, dofetilide did not have an adverse effect on survival
Post-CABG,[48] 1997	Double-blind, randomized, placebo-controlled	98	Dofetilide: 4 μg/kg IV (33 patients); 8 μg/kg IV (32 patients) Placebo: 33 patients	None	No negative inotropic effect; dofetilide did not exhibit a significant conversion rate over placebo, probably due to high spontaneous conversion rate post-CABG that is well recognized
Cleveland Clinic,[44] 2008–2012	Retrospective observational study	1404	Dofetilide: 500 μg BID	1.2	Dofetilide was effective in converting and maintaining sinus rhythm in patients with AF/AFL; patients who developed TdP had a greater 1-y all-cause mortality than those who did not
Heart & Rhythm Medical Group,[47] 2011	Retrospective observational study	27	Dofetilide: 250–500 μg BID	0.04	Dofetilide was effective in the conversion and maintenance of AF/AFL to sinus rhythm in 67% of patients; one patient with an ICD that showed TdP-type VT with short-long sequence

Abbreviations: BID, twice a day; HF, heart failure.
Data from Refs.[8–11,16,42–44,46–48]

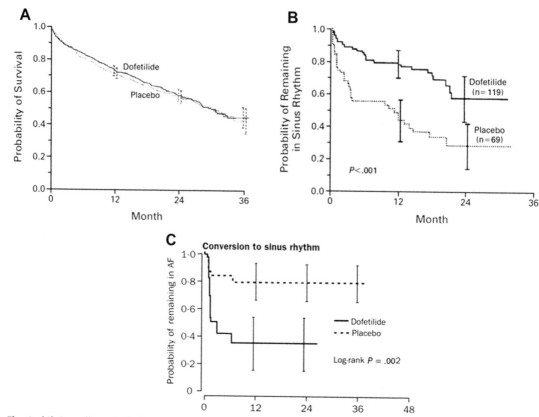

Fig. 1. (*A*) Overall survival of patients who received dofetilide compared with placebo in patients with heart failure and LV systolic dysfunction. (*B*) Dofetilide compared with placebo in maintaining sinus rhythm in patients with CHF and LV systolic dysfunction. (*C*) AF in MI and LV dysfunction. (*Adapted from* Refs.[8,9])

SAFIRE-D Trial

The Symptomatic AF and Randomized Evaluation of Dofetilide (SAFIRE-D) was a double-blind, multicenter, placebo-controlled trial that included 325 patients and was designed to evaluate the efficacy and safety of dofetilide in converting AF and AFL to sinus rhythm (see **Table 1**).[46] The patients were randomized to dofetilide (125, 250, or 500 μg twice a day) or placebo twice a day. The end point of the study was maintaining sinus rhythm at 1 year. Dofetilide dose-adjustment was done according to the QTc prolongation and creatinine clearance. The AF and AFL conversions to sinus rhythm were 6.1%, 9.8%, and 29.8% for dofetilide, respectively, and 1.2% for placebo (*P*<.001). Seventy percent and 91% of the patients converted to sinus rhythm occurred in the first 24 and 36 hours, respectively. There were 2 cases of TdP on day 2 and 3. There was one case of sudden cardiac death that was assumed to be proarrhythmic in the dofetilide group. The conclusion of this trial was that dofetilide was moderately effective in converting and maintaining AF/AFL to sinus rhythm. In this trial, dofetilide did not have an adverse effect on survival.[46]

Cleveland Clinic Report

A recent report by Abraham and colleagues[44] from Cleveland Clinic, a single-center retrospective analysis on a large number of patients (1404) with AF and AFL, demonstrated that dofetilide was effective in converting and maintaining sinus rhythm in patients with AF and AFL (see **Table 1**). Seventy-five percent of patients reported in this study developed QT interval prolongation or TdP. Risk profile in these patients were female sex, 500-μg twice a day dose, patients with reduced LV ejection fraction, and those who had a greater QT interval prolongation at baseline. Patients who developed TdP had a greater 1-year all-cause mortality than those who did not (17.6% vs 3%; *P*>.001). Seventeen patients (1.2%) developed TdP during loading dose while on dofetilide. Of these 17 patients, 10 developed cardiac arrest due to ventricular tachyarrhythmias and one died.[44]

Heart and Rhythm Medical Group Results

Preliminary data from the authors' laboratory reported on the efficacy and safety of dofetilide in 27 patients (15 men; age range 65–92 years) with implantable pacemakers or cardioverter-defibrillators (ICDs) who had documented AF/AFL (see **Table 1**).[47] AF burden, the number and duration of episodes, preterminated episodes, percentage of time in atrial pacing, percentage of time in atrial interventions, and number of episodes of atrial arrhythmias (>6 beats/d) were examined before and after dofetilide derived from device interrogation (**Table 2**). In patients with AFL, the spontaneous and successful atrial pacing overdrive attempts and termination were also examined. Dofetilide was administered orally 250 to 500 μg twice a day. Dose adjustment was done according to the creatinine clearance.

Results

Twenty patients (74%) had AF and 7 (26%) had AFL. Dofetilide converted AF and AFL to sinus rhythm in 10 patients (32%). Furthermore, in 8 patients (30%) dofetilide enhanced the conversion of AF and AFL to sinus rhythm by implantable devices that delivered atrial therapies. In a total of 9 patients (33%), dofetilide had no effect either by device-mediated therapies or with spontaneous termination. Two hundred forty episodes of AF and AFL were subsequently analyzed from device interrogation. The conclusion of this study revealed that dofetilide was effective in the conversion and maintenance of AF/AFL to sinus rhythm in 18 patients (67%, including those with atrial therapies). **Fig. 2** shows an example of termination of AFL in a patient who was treated with 500 μg twice a day. Furthermore, device interrogation with the patients while on dofetilide showed that there were no proarrhythmic effect except in one patient with an ICD that showed TdP-type ventricular tachycardia (VT) with short-long sequence

(**Fig. 3**). The implications of the above study were that the effectiveness and safety of AADs in patients with implantable rhythm devices provide a model for investigation of AADs. In particular, where asymptomatic "silent arrhythmias" pose uncertainty with current monitoring systems, this method may be useful in designing the future AAD trials.[47]

TRIALS ON INTRAVENOUS DOFETILIDE
Post-Coronary Artery Bypass Grafting Trial

In this study, 98 patients who developed AF/AFL after coronary artery bypass grafting (CABG) 1 to 6 days after surgery were included in a double-blind, randomized, placebo-controlled study of intravenous (IV) dofetilide. Thirty-three patients were assigned to dofetilide for 4 μg/kg IV; 32 patients received dofetilide for 8 μg/kg IV, and 33 were assigned to placebo (see **Table 1**).[48] The conversion rates for AF/AFL to sinus rhythm for the 3 groups were 36%, 44%, and 24%, respectively. There were no episodes of TdP nor negative inotropic effect. In this study, dofetilide did not exhibit a significant conversion rate over placebo, probably because of a high spontaneous conversion rate after CABG that is well recognized.[48]

Intravenous Dofetilide

Falk and colleagues[40] studied the efficacy of IV dofetilide in a double-blind, randomized, multicenter, placebo-controlled study in 91 patients with sustained AF (75 patients) or AFL (16 patients). The infusion was carried out over 15 minutes. Body weights of 4 μg/kg or 8 μg/kg

Table 2
Initial interrogation: atrial fibrillation/atrial flutter summary

AF/AFL Summary	Baseline Prior Session 24 July 2008–29 Sept 2008	Dofetilide Last Session 29 Sept 2008–09 Oct 2008
% of time AF/AFL	19.6%	3.5% ↓
Average AF/AFL time/day	4.7 h/d	0.8 h/d ↓
Monitored AF/AFL episodes	10.3/d	0.9/d ↓
Treated AF/AFL episodes	22.6/d	2.5/d ↓
Pace-terminated episodes	64.7%	66.7% ↑
% of time atrial pacing	53.5%	96.0% ↑
% of time atrial intervention	23.6%	<0.1% ↓
Atrial arrhythmias (>6 beats)	243.7/d	29.2/d ↓

AF burden shows the data obtained from interrogation of an ICD of a patient who was treated with dofetilide for recurrent AF/AFL.

↑, increase; ↓, decrease.

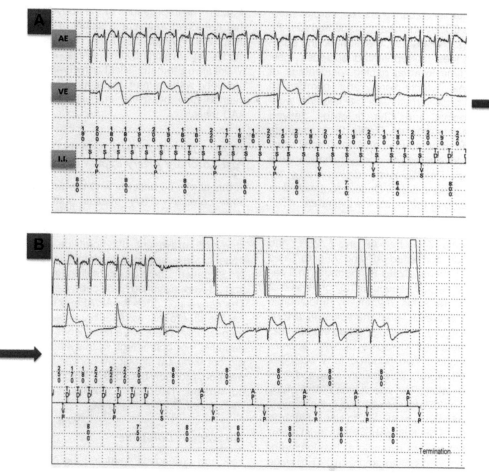

Fig. 2. Termination of AFL in a patient treated with dofetilide 500 μg orally twice a day. (*A*) AFL. (*B*) Conversion of AFL to sinus rhythm. Arrow denotes continuous strip. AE, atrial electrogram; I.I., intracardiac intervals; VE, ventricular electrogram.

were compared with placebo. Compared with patients who received 4 μg/kg (4 of 32 patients; 12.5%), patients who received 8 μg/kg (9 of 29 patients; 31%) had a higher conversion rate of AF/AFL to sinus rhythm (*P*<.001). No patients on placebo converted to sinus rhythm. Patients with AFL had a higher conversion rate to dofetilide compared with those with AF (54% vs 14.5%,

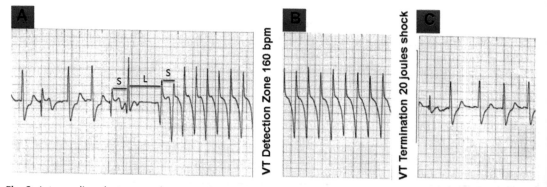

Fig. 3. Intracardiac electrogram from a patient with ICD and AF who was treated with dofetilide 500 μg twice a day. (*A*) A short-long-short RR sequence that triggers a (*B*) fast VT (TdP), (*C*) sinus rhythm established after an ICD-delivered 20-J shock. L, long; S, short.

P<.001). There were 2 cases of TdP during dofetilide infusion (3.2).

Nørgaard and colleagues[49] also investigated the efficacy and safety of IV dofetilide in a multicenter, double-blind, randomized, placebo-controlled trial in 96 patients. Seventy-nine patients had AF and 17 patients had AFL. Sixty-six patients received 8 μg/kg IV dofetilide and 30 were randomized to the placebo arm. The end point of the study was conversion from AF/AFL to sinus rhythm. The conversion rate to sinus rhythm was 30.3% after IV dofetilide and 3.4% after placebo (*P*<.006). Conversion was higher in AFL than in AF: 64% versus 24% (*P* = .012). This finding was similar to the previous trial. VT of TdP form was developed in 2 patients (3%) and IV infusion was discontinued before the end of the study.

A few other trials on IV dofetilide have been carried out and provided similar results.[50,51]

EFFECT OF DOFETILIDE ON THE ELECTROCARDIOGRAM

Dofetilide has no effect on PR interval and QRS duration. In patients with normal baseline value of QT interval and QT dispersion after MI who also had an LV dysfunction, dofetilide was not associated with significant proarrhythmic effect and showed a survival benefit.[52–54]

Dofetilide has no significant effect on AH and H-V interval recorded on intracardiac electrograms.[55] Because dofetilide at the recommended dose predominantly and selectively blocks K^+ currents and prolongs APD and QT interval, dofetilide should not be used (contraindicated) in patients with congenital or acquired long QT syndrome.[56] A more detailed analysis of the electrocardiogram provides further insight into the efficacy and arrhythmogenic effect of dofetilide.[57–59]

PHARMACOKINETICS OF DOFETILIDE

Dofetilide has approximately 100% absorption and more than 90% bioavailability after oral administration.[21,56] Peak plasma concentration is at 2 to 3 hours after oral administration. Dofetilide's half-life is calculated at 8 to 10 hours and has a protein binding of 65%.[60] Dofetilide has a renal excretion of about 80%, and 20% to 30% is metabolized in the liver by CYP3A4 enzymatic pathway.[21] Therefore, dose adjustment is required in patients with impaired renal function.

DRUG INTERACTIONS WITH DOFETILIDE

Dofetilide has significant interactions with the pharmacologic agents, as shown in **Table 3**.

Importantly, dofetilide has no significant drug interactions with digoxin, phenytoin, propranolol, theophylline, and warfarin.[56] Most AADs, including dofetilide, metabolize in the liver via CYP3A4/5 enzymes. Pharmacologic agents that inhibit the CYP3A4/5 agents include erythromycin, ketoconazole, grapefruit juice, amiodarone, and calcium antagonists (specifically verapamil), which will potentiate the effect of dofetilide and increase the risk of TdP.[56] Potassium-wasting diuretics such as the thiazide group also potentiate the effect of dofetilide and increase the risk of TdP. Other pharmacologic agents that potentially interact with dofetilide and increase the risk of TdP include arsenic trioxide, cisapride, domperidone, droperidol, and methadone.

Table 3
Dofetilide selected drug interactions

Interacts with	Results	Mechanism
Cimetidine, ketoconazole	↑ Dofetilide	↓ P-glycoprotein Renal secretion
Grapefruit juice[66]	↑ Dofetilide	↓ Decreases CYP3A4
Ketoconazole, azole antifungals	↑ Dofetilide	Inhibit CYP3A4
Prochlorperazine[67]	↑ Dofetilide	↓ Renal elimination of dofetilide
Thiazides	↑ Dofetilide	↓ P-glycoprotein Renal secretion
Trimethoprim	↑ Dofetilide	↓ P-glycoprotein Renal secretion
Megestrol[67]	↑ Dofetilide	↓ Renal elimination of dofetilide
Verapamil	↑ Dofetilide$_{max}$	Changes absorption

↑, increase; ↓, decrease.
Adapted from Mounsey JP, DiMarco J. Dofetilide. Circulation 2000;102:2665–70.

TORSADOGENIC EFFECT OF DOFETILIDE

All pharmacologic agents that prolong APD and QT interval carry the risk of inducing malignant polymorphic ventricular arrhythmias, that is, TdP. Risk factors for developing TdP are summarized in **Box 1**.[28]

Among the most important risk factor isfemale gender, which demonstrates a higher (14%–22%) concentration of dofetilide than the male gender even after adjusting for body weight and creatinine clearance. Dofetilide demonstrates a dose-dependent fashion in prolongation of QT interval. TdP and other ventricular arrhythmias generally occur in the first 48 to 72 hours after initiation of the drug. Hypokalemia and diuretic therapy also increase the risk of TdP in patients receiving dofetilide.

In general, the occurrence of dofetilide or any other pharmacologic agent that induces TdP is unpredictable. Overall, the risk of TdP in patients receiving dofetilide depends on baseline QT and other factors that are referenced in **Box 1**. However, it ranges from 0.7% to 3.3%. The FDA meta-analysis reports 1.7%.[61]

Box 1
Risk factors for dofetilide-induced torsades de pointes

- Female gender
  - Age
  - Morbid obesity
- Electrocardiogram
  - Prolonged baseline QT interval and QT dispersion
  - Sinus bradycardia, prolonged pauses
    - Short-long sequence
  - T-wave abnormalities
  - T-wave alternans
- Electrolyte imbalance
  - Hypokalemia
  - Hypomagnesemia
  - Impaired renal function
- Congestive heart failure
- Family history
  - History of drug-induced TdP
  - Genetic predisposition
- Other concomitant medications that increase risk of TdP

Mechanisms of Torsadogenic Effect of Dofetilide

The mechanisms of torsadogenic effect of dofetilide are thought to be related to

1. Prolongation of repolarization
2. Producing dispersion of repolarization
3. Triggering factors such as bradycardia (pause-dependent effect) atrial or ventricular extrasystoles (especially those with short-long-short RR intervals; see **Fig. 3**) that predispose for re-entrant arrhythmias.

Patients who are phenotype negative but genotype positive that certain agents may unmask the QT prolongation are also at high risk of developing TdP. Such conditions that upregulate genes related to I_{Kr} and I_{Ks} play an important role in developing TdP. The underlying pathophysiology of these gender differences is not fully understood, but several factors play an important role such as hormonal changes, higher QT interval, and rate adaptation to heart rate changes, as well as a response to exercise.[29,45,62] The mechanisms of TdP effect of class III agents are well described in articles in this issue and do not need to be repeated here (see Skibsybye L, Ravens U: Mechanism of proarrhythmic effects of potassium channel blockers; and McCauley M, Vallabhajosyula S, Darbar D. Proarrhythmic and torsadogenic effects of potassium channel blockers in patients in this issue). Sugrue and colleagues[63] recently reported on the value of the T-wave right slope that correlates strongly with the occurrence of TdP.

Management of Dofetilide-induced Torsades de Pointes

1. Discontinue dofetilide
2. Avoid bradycardia and pauses, especially short-long-short sequences
3. Correct underlying causes (ie, electrolyte imbalances)
4. Adjust for creatinine clearance

DISCUSSION

Dofetilide is an effective AAD in the management of AF and AFL. Importantly, it is safe to use in the so-called high-risk patient group such as those with post-MI, CHF with reduced systolic function, and structural heart disease. Dofetilide exhibits a dose-dependent effect and has a reverse frequency-dependent effect, which is a property of most class III agents. As the prevalence and incidence of asymptomatic AF and its relation to stroke either symptomatic or silent are more recognized, the effectiveness of rhythm control strategies either pharmacologic or with ablative procedure is less defined.

Implantable rhythm management devices, that is, pacemaker and ICDs, provide an excellent and unique opportunity to evaluate rhythm control strategies. Indeed, interrogation of implanted devices provides not only accurate characteristics of AF (ie, incidence, rate, duration) but also information on the proarrhythmic effects of AAD and correlation with patient symptoms.

It is hoped that the future trials on AAD safety and efficacy may be evaluated in patients with implantable devices. An important concern on the use of dofetilide and other class III agents is their torsadogenic effects that account for up to 0.7% to 3.3% (FDA meta-analysis reviewed at 1.7%).[61]

It is important to note that dofetilide did not adversely affect mortality in this high-risk patient group with recent MI, CHF, and reduced ejection fraction. Furthermore, Pritchett and colleagues[64] evaluated the safety of dofetilide in patients with supraventricular arrhythmias and revealed that dofetilide did not pose any adverse effects on survival.

The main concern with dofetilide, like most of the pharmacologic agents that prolong the QT interval, is its torsadogenic effect, which was discussed above (see **Table 3**).

DOFETILIDE IN PREGNANCY

Although there are not enough solid data regarding the adverse effects of dofetilide during pregnancy, the drug insert is labeled as category C.

ADVERSE EFFECTS

Proarrhythmia (TdP), which is dose-related, is discussed above.

Noncardiac side effects include dizziness, headache, chest pain, dyspnea, nausea, severe diarrhea, vomiting, and increased thirst.[56]

GUIDELINES FOR USE OF DOFETILIDE

The current American College of Cardiology (ACC), American Heart Association (AHA), and the Heart Rhythm Society (HRS) guidelines on the use of dofetilide is described (see Gillis A: Guidelines for K+ channel blockers use, in this issue).

Briefly, dofetilide may be considered for rhythm control (conversion and maintenance of sinus rhythm) in patients with AF/AFL with the following conditions[65]:

1. No or minimal structural heart disease
2. Coronary artery disease and post-MI period
3. CHF

4. According to the guidelines, dofetilide should not be used in patients with a baseline QT interval greater than 440 ms (500 ms in patients with ventricular conduction abnormalities) and then should be discontinued at a QT interval of greater than 500 ms
5. Dofetilide should also be avoided in those at risk of TdP or in patients that are taking other medications that can potentially prolong the QT interval

Dofetilide is also contraindicated in

1. Profound bradycardia
2. Creatinine clearance less than 20 mL/min
3. Pre-existing QT prolongation
4. Hypokalemia
5. Hypomagnesemia

Patients who have started dofetilide should have electrocardiogram and QTc interval measurement every 6 months. An evaluation of transient repolarization abnormalities, renal function, and electrolytes, including magnesium every 6 months, should also be measured.[2]

SUMMARY

Dofetilide, a selective K+ channel blocker, is highly effective as a rhythm-control strategy in patients with paroxysmal and persistent AF as well as those with AFL. The average effectiveness at 1 year is about 40% to 65%. Dofetilide is safe and can be used in patients with coronary artery disease, after MI, CHF with diminished LV systolic function, hypertrophic cardiomyopathy, and mild LV hypertrophy.[56] Dofetilide should not be used in severe LV hypertrophy (wall thickness >1.5 cm).[65] A significant adverse effect of dofetilide is its torsadogenic profile that accounts for 0.7% to 3.3% of causes (FDA meta-analysis reviewed at 1.7%).[61]

The risk factors for dofetilide's torsadogenic effect include female gender, age, sinus bradycardia and pauses, previous history of TdP and other ventricular arrhythmias, and others that are listed in **Box 1**.

Thus, dofetilide should be initiated in hospitals under cardiac monitoring. Because 80% of dofetilide is renally cleared, dose-adjustment is required in patients with impaired renal function and according to the corrected QT interval and baseline and during therapy.[21] Dofetilide is approved only in the United States.

ACKNOWLEDGMENT

The authors wish to thank Mariah Smith for her superb assistance in preparation of this article.

REFERENCES

1. Savelieva I, Camm J. Anti-arrhythmic drug therapy for atrial fibrillation: current anti-arrhythmic drugs, investigational agents, and innovative approaches. Europace 2008;10(6):647–65.

2. Savelieva I, Camm AJ. Use of antiarrhythmic drug treatment in atrial fibrillation. In: Shenasa M, Camm AJ, editors. Management of atrial fibrillation. New York: Oxford University Press; 2015. p. 75–98.

3. Ehrlich J, Nattel S. Novel approaches for pharmacological management of atrial fibrillation. Drugs 2009; 69(7):757–74.

4. Hohnloser S, Crijns H, Eickels M, et al. Effect of dronedarone on cardiovascular events in atrial fibrillation. N Engl J Med 2009;360:668–78.

5. Pisters R, Hohnloser SH, Connolly SJ, et al. Effect of dronedarone on clinical end points in patients with atrial fibrillation and coronary heart disease: insights from the ATHENA trial. Europace 2014;16(2):174–81.

6. Hohnloser SH, Crijns HJ, van Eickels M, et al. Dronedarone in patients with congestive heart failure: insights from ATHENA. Eur Heart J 2010;31(14): 1717–21.

7. Connolly S, Camm AJ, Halperin HR, et al. Dronedarone in high-risk permanent atrial fibrillation. N Engl J Med 2011;365:2268–76.

8. Torp-Pedersen C, Moller M, Bloch Thomsen PE, et al. Dofetilide in patients with congestive heart failure and left ventricular dysfunction. N Engl J Med 1999;341:857–65.

9. Køber L, Thomsen PEB, Møller M, et al. Effect of dofetilide in patients with recent myocardial infarction and left-ventricular dysfunction: a randomised trial. Lancet 2000;356:2052–8.

10. Pedersen OD, Bagger H, Keller N, et al. Efficacy of dofetilide in the treatment of atrial fibrillation-flutter in patients with reduced left ventricular function: a Danish Investigations of Arrhythmia and Mortality on Dofetilide (DIAMOND) substudy. Circulation 2001;104:292–6.

11. Camm AJ, Ekht D, Meinertz T, et al. Dofetilide in patients with left ventricular dysfunction and either heart failure or acute myocardial infarction: rationale, design, and patient characteristics of the DIAMOND studies. Clin Cardiol 1997;20(8):704–10.

12. Burashnikov A, Antzelevitch C. New developments in atrial antiarrhythmic drug therapy. Nat Rev Cardiol 2010;7(3):139–48.

13. Ravens U, Poulet C, Wettwer E, et al. Atrial selectivity of antiarrhythmic drugs. J Physiol 2013; 591(17):4087–5097.

14. Ravens U. Potassium channels in atrial fibrillation: targets for atrial and pathology-specific therapy? Heart Rhythm 2008;5(5):758–9.

15. Nattel S. New ideas about atrial fibrillation 50 years on. Nature 2002;415:219–26.

16. Nattel S, Carlsson L. Innovative approaches to anti-arrhythmic drug therapy. Nat Rev Drug Discov 2006; 5(12):1034–49.

17. Bagwe S, Leonardi M, Bissett J. Novel pharmacological therapies for atrial fibrillation. Curr Opin Cardiol 2007;22:450–7.

18. Ehrlich JR, Biliczki P, Hohnloser SH, et al. Atrial-selective approaches for the treatment of atrial fibrillation. J Am Coll Cardiol 2008;51(8):787–92.

19. Amit G, Kikuchi K, Greener ID, et al. Selective molecular potassium channel blockade prevents atrial fibrillation. Circulation 2010;121(21):2263–70.

20. Larsen A, Lish P. A new bio-isostere: alkylsulphona-midophenethanolamines. Nature 1964;203:1283–4.

21. Mounsey JP, DiMarco J. Cardiovascular drugs. Dofetilide. Circulation 2000;102:2665–70.

22. Grant AO. Cardiac ion channels. Circ Arrhythm Electrophysiol 2009;2(2):185–94.

23. Sanguinetti MC, Jurkiwicz N. Two components of cardiac delayed rectifier K+ current: differential sensitivity to block by class III antiarrhythmic agents. J Gen Physiol 1990;96(1):195–215.

24. Cha Y, Wales A, Wolf P, et al. Electrophysiologic effects of the new class III antiarrhythmic drug dofetilide compared to the class IA antiarrhythmic drug quinidine in experimental canine atrial flutter. J Cardiovasc Electrophysiol 1996;7(9):809–27.

25. Kiehn J, Lacerda A, Wible B, et al. Molecular physiology and pharmacology of hERG: single-channel currents and block by dofetilide. Circulation 1996;94:2572–9.

26. Wettwer E, Hala O, Christ T, et al. Role of IKur in controlling action potential shape and contractility in the human atrium: influence of chronic atrial fibrillation. Circulation 2004;110:2299–306.

27. Carmeliet E. Voltage- and time-dependent block of the delayed K+ current in cardiac myocytes by dofetilide. J Pharmacol Exp Ther 1992;262:809–17.

28. Jaiswal A, Goldbarg S. Dofetilide induced torsade de pointes: mechanism, risk factors and management strategies. Indian Heart J 2014;66(6):640–8.

29. Frommeyer G, Eckardt L. Drug-induced proarrhythmia: risk factors and electrophysiological mechanisms. Nat Rev Cardiol 2016;13(1):36–47.

30. Hondeghem L, Snyders D. Class III antiarrhythmic agents have a lot of potential but a long way to go: reduced effectiveness and dangers of reverse use dependence. Circulation 1990;81(2):686–90.

31. Jurkiewicz N, Sanguinetti MC. Rate-dependent prolongation of cardiac action potentials by a methanesulfonanilide class III antiarrhythmic agent. Specific block of rapidly activating delayed rectifier K+ current by dofetilide. Circ Res 1993;72:75–83.

32. Colatsky T, Follmer C, Starmer CF. Channel specificity in antiarrhythmic drug action mechanism of potassium channel block and its role in suppressing and aggravating cardiac arrhythmias. Circulation 1990;82:2235–42.

33. Wang J, Feng J, Nattel S. Class III antiarrhythmic drug action in experimental atrial fibrillation. Differences in reverse use dependence and effectiveness between d-sotalol and the new antiarrhythmic drug ambasilide. Circulation 1994;90:2032–40.

34. Yang T, Roden D. Extracellular potassium modulation of drug block of IKr: implications for torsade de pointes and reverse use-dependence. Circulation 1996;93:407–11.

35. Baskin E, Lynch J. Comparative effects of increased extracellular potassium and pacing frequency on the class III activities of methanesulfonanilide IKr blockers dofetilide, D-sotalol, E-4031, and MK-499. J Cardiovasc Pharmacol 1994;24:199–208.

36. Sedgwick M, Rassmussen H, Cobbe S. Effects of the class III antiarrhythmic drug dofetilide on ventricular monophasic action potential duration and QT interval dispersion in stable angina pectoris. Am J Cardiol 1992;70:1432–7.

37. Baskin E, Lynch J. Differential atrial versus ventricular activities of class III potassium channel blockers. J Pharmacol Exp Ther 1998;285:135–42.

38. Shenasa J, Shenasa M. Insights to the electrophysiologic mechanism of sotalol, a potassium channel blocking agent in patients with ventricular tachyarrhythmias: monophasic action potential recording and response to isoproterenol. In: Vereecke J, van Bogaert PP, Verdonck F, editors. Potassium channels in normal and pathological conditions. Leuven, Belgium: Leuven University Press; 1995.

39. Dobrev D, Singh BN. Antiarrhythmic drugs. In: Saksena S, Camm AJ, editors. Electrophysiological disorders of the heart. Atlanta, GA: Elsevier; 2012. p. 1133–57.

40. Falk R, Pollak A, Singh S, et al. Intravenous dofetilide, a class III antiarrhythmic agent, for the termination of sustained atrial fibrillation or flutter. J Am Coll Cardiol 1997;29(2):385–90.

41. Li D, Benardeau A, Nattel S. Contrasting efficacy of dofetilide in differing experimental models of atrial fibrillation. Circulation 2000;102(1):104–12.

42. Greenbaum R, Campbell T, Channer K, et al. Conversion of atrial fibrillation and maintenance of sinus rhythm by dofetilide: the EMERALD (European and Australian Multicenter Evalutive Research on Atrial fibrillation Dofetilide) study. Circulation 1998; 98(Suppl I):633.

43. Campbell T, Greenbaum R, Channer K, et al. Mortality in patients with atrial fibrillation—1-year follow-up of EMERALD (European and Australian Multicenter Evaluative Research on Atrial fibrillation Dofetilide). J Am Coll Cardiol 2000;35:154A–5A.

44. Abraham JM, Saliba WI, Vekstein C, et al. Safety of oral dofetilide for rhythm control of atrial fibrillation and atrial flutter. Circ Arrhythm Electrophysiol 2015; 8(4):772–6.

45. Lauer MS. Dofetilide: is the treatment worse than the disease? J Am Coll Cardiol 2001;37(4):1106–10.

46. Singh S, Zoble R, Yellen L, et al. Efficacy and safety of oral dofetilide in converting to and maintaining sinus rhythm in patients with chronic atrial fibrillation or atrial flutter the Symptomatic Atrial Fibrillation Investigative Research on Dofetilide (SAFIRE-D) Study. Circulation 2000;102:2385–90.

47. Shenasa F. Efficacy of dofetilide in the management of patients with paroxysmal atrial fibrillation and flutter (AF/AFL): data from interrogation of rhythm management devices. J Interv Card Electrophysiol 2011;30:87–198.

48. Frost L, Mortensenb P, Tingleffc E, et al. Efficacy and safety of dofetilide, a new class III antiarrhythmic agent, in acute termination of atrial fibrillation or flutter after coronary artery bypass surgery. Int J Cardiol 1997;58:135–40.

49. Nørgaard BL, Wachtell K, Christensen PD, et al. Efficacy and safety of intravenously administered dofetilide in acute termination of atrial fibrillation and flutter: a multicenter, randomized, double-blind, placebo-controlled trial. Am Heart J 1999; 137:1062–9.

50. Suttorp MJ, Polak PE, van't Hof A, et al. Efficacy and safety of a new selective class III antiarrhythmic agent dofetilide in paroxysmal atrial fibrillation or atrial flutter. Am J Cardiol 1992;69(4):417–9.

51. Sedgwick ML, Rasmussen HS, Cobbe SM. Clinical and electrophysiologic effects of intravenous dofetilide (UK-68,798), a new class III antiarrhythmic drug, in patients with angina pectoris. Am J Cardiol 1992;69(5):513–7.

52. Brendorp B, Elming H, Kober L, et al. The prognostic value of QTc interval and QT dispersion following myocardial infarction in patients treated with or without dofetilide. Clin Cardiol 2003;26(5):219–25.

53. Mazur A, Anderson ME, Bonney S, et al. Pause-dependent polymorphic ventricular tachycardia during long-term treatment with dofetilide a placebo-controlled, implantable cardioverter-defibrillator-based evaluation. J Am Coll Cardiol 2001;37:1100–5.

54. Meijborg VM, Chauveau S, Janse MJ, et al. Interventricular dispersion in repolarization causes bifid T waves in dogs with dofetilide-induced long QT syndrome. Heart Rhythm 2015;12(6):1343–51.

55. Lehne R, Rosenthal L, editors. Pharmacology for nursing care. 8th edition. Atlanta, GA: Elsevier; 2014.

56. Saliba W. Dofetilide (Tikosyn): a new drug to control atrial fibrillation. Cleve Clin J Med 2001;68(4): 353–63.

57. Lande G, Maison-Blanche P, Fayn J, et al. Dynamic analysis of dofetilide-induced changes in ventricular repolarization. Clin Pharmacol Ther 1998;64(3):312–21.

58. Vicente J, Johannesen L, Mason JW, et al. Comprehensive T wave morphology assessment in a randomized clinical study of dofetilide, quinidine, ranolazine, and verapamil. J Am Heart Assoc 2015;4(4):e001615.

59. Sauer AJ, Kaplan R, Xue J, et al. Electrocardiographic markers of repolarization heterogeneity during dofetilid or sotalol initiation for paroxysmal atrial fibrillation. Am J Cardiol 2014;113(12):2030–5.

60. US Natl Inst Health. Current medication information for TIKOSYN (dofetilide) capsule. Revised 2013. Available at: http://www.tikosynrems.com/sites/default/files/Tikosyn%20Prescribing%20information.pdf. Accessed December 15, 2015.

61. Gordon M. Dofetilide medical review. 1999. Available at: http://www.accessdata.fda.gov/drugsatfda_docs/nda/99/20-931_Tikosyn.cfm. Accessed December 15, 2015.

62. Behr ER, Roden D. Drug-induced arrhythmia: pharmacogenomic prescribing? Eur Heart J 2013;34(2): 89–95.

63. Sugrue A, Kremen V, Qiang B, et al. Electrocardiographic predictors of torsadogenic risk during dofetilide or sotalol initiation: utility of a novel T wave analysis program. Cardiovasc Drugs Ther 2015; 29(5):433–41.

64. Pritchett ELC, Wilkinson WE. Effect of dofetilide on survival in patients with supraventricular arrhythmias. Am Heart J 1999;138(5):994–7.

65. January CT, Wann LS, Alpert JS, et al. 2014 AHA/ACC/HRS Guideline for the management of patients with atrial fibrillation: executive summary. J Am Coll Cardiol 2014;64(21): 2246–80.

66. US Natl Inst Health. TIKOSYN Treatment Guidelines. Available at: http://www.tikosynrems.com/sites/default/files/TIKOSYN_Treatment_Guidelines.pdf. Accessed December 15, 2015.

67. Chow GV, Marine JE, Fleg JL. Epidemiology of arrhythmias and conduction disorders in older adults. Clin Geriatr Med 2012;28(4):539–53.

Sotalol

John Alvin Kpaeyeh Jr, MD[a], John Marcus Wharton, MD[b],*

KEYWORDS

- Sotalol • Potassium channel blocker • Ventricular tachycardia • Atrial fibrillation
- Long QT syndrome

KEY POINTS

- Racemic sotalol is a potent competitive inhibitor of the rapid component of the delayed rectifier potassium current with significant beta-blocking properties.
- There is a near linear relationship between sotalol dosage and QT interval prolongation, with a sharp increase in the risk of proarrhythmia above a cumulative daily dosage of 320 mg.
- Sotalol is renally cleared with no significant primary drug interactions outside the risk of using concomitant agents that cause QT prolongation, bradycardia, and/or hypotension.
- Sotalol is effective for the treatment of premature ventricular contraction, atrial fibrillation, postoperative atrial fibrillation, supraventricular tachycardia, and fetal supraventricular arrhythmias and is safe to use in the setting of heart disease with the exception of uncontrolled heart failure.

INTRODUCTION

Sotalol and dofetilide are both methanesulfonanilide. Sotalol was first synthesized in 1960.[1] Shortly thereafter Singh and Vaughan-Williams (1970) demonstrated that sotalol had a unique mechanism of action, which helped lead to the development of a new category of drug, class III agents, within the Vaughan-Williams classification. Racemic, DL-sotalol was approved by the US Food and Drug Administration (FDA) for use in the treatment of ventricular tachycardia (VT) in October of 1992 and subsequently for atrial fibrillation (AF) in February of 2000. DL-sotalol was initially marketed in the United States by Berlex Laboratories under the name of Betapace or Betapace-AF, with labeling for VT and AF, respectively. Despite the differences in brand names, there was no difference in the formulation of the drug, but there were differences in labeling, dosing, and usage. Since the patent for DL-sotalol has long since expired, generic DL-sotalol preparations are now available. D- and L-stereoisomers of sotalol have been studied individually, but only DL-sotalol is commercially available. For simplicity throughout this article, sotalol will refer to DL-sotalol, while specific stereoisomers will be labeled as such (eg, D-sotalol).

PROPERTIES

Sotalol is a potent competitive inhibitor of the rapid component of the delayed rectifier potassium current, I_{Kr}. Both D- and L-stereoisomers have roughly equipotent I_{Kr}-blocking properties.[2] Sotalol does not appear to have a significant effect on the slow component of the delayed rectifier potassium current, I_{KS}.[3] Blockade of I_{Kr} by sotalol results in action potential duration (APD) and effective refractory period (ERP) prolongation in both the atria and ventricles. There is a relatively linear dose response in both atrial and ventricular APD prolongation given orally or intravenously. In the ventricle, this results in a linear response in QT prolongation with increasing serum

Disclosures: The authors have nothing to disclose.
[a] Division of Cardiology, Department of Medicine, Tourville Arrhythmia Center, Medical University of South Carolina, 114 Doughty Street, MSC 592, Charleston, SC 29425-5920, USA; [b] Cardiac Electrophysiology, Division of Cardiology, Department of Medicine, Tourville Arrhythmia Center, Medical University of South Carolina, 114 Doughty Street, BM 216, MSC 592, Charleston, SC 29425-5920, USA
* Corresponding author.
E-mail address: whartonj@musc.edu

cardiacEP.theclinics.com

concentration in both males and females, although the response is steeper in females (**Fig. 1**).[4–6]

Sotalol demonstrated reverse frequency dependence (ie, blockade of I_{Kr} is greatest at slower heart rates and less at faster heart rates)[7–9] similar to dofetilide. This reverse frequency dependence explains the higher risk of excessive QT prolongation and torsades de pointes at slower heart rates with sotalol, a fact exacerbated by the bradycardic effects of the drug. In addition, reverse frequency dependence may also explain the lower efficacy of sotalol for terminating tachycardia (because pharmacodynamic effect is decreased) despite it substantial efficacy for preventing tachycardia from basal and relatively bradycardic states (when effect is higher).[9] Of the class III drugs, their relative reverse frequency dependence may help explain their efficacy for tachycardia termination. Thus, drugs such as azimilide or ibutilide, which have little reverse frequency dependence, have greater efficacy for tachycardia termination than sotalol.[10]

The effectiveness of sotalol to prolong AERP is also attenuated by AF -nduced remodeling. In the goat model of electrically induced AF, D-sotalol increased the atrial effective refractory period (AERP) by 17% ± 6% at baseline, but by only 6% ± 5% after 2 days of AF.[11] Furthermore, D-sotalol did not decrease the inducibility of AF by single atrial extrastimuli in the electrically remodeled goat compared with control. The attenuation of persistent AF on AERP prolongation by sotalol has also been demonstrated in people.[12] The blunting of AERP prolongation by sotalol with persisting AF may be due to the relative decreased importance of I_{Kr} for repolarization and/or decreased expression of I_{Kr} in electrically remodeled atrial myocytes. The attenuation of AERP

prolongation with AF-induced remodeling may also in part explain the relative lack of efficacy of sotalol in pharmacologic conversion of AF.

The effect of sotalol on I_{Kr} may also be modulated by plasma membrane-associated proteins. In a recent study, the KCR1 membrane-associated protein significantly attenuated the effect of D-sotalol on the major pore-forming subunit of I_{Kr}.[13] It is also possible that membrane-associated proteins could increase the sensitivity of I_{Kr} to sotalol blockade and increase the risk of proarrhythmia.

Sotalol has been shown to increase the late sodium current (I_{Na-L}) in a time-dependent manner. Increase in I_{Na-L} was not seen acutely, but only after a couple of hours of exposure to sotalol or dofetilide and could result in late potentials. The effect was inhibited by ranolazine or phosphatidylinositol 3,4,5-triphophate, the latter observation suggesting modulation via the phosphoinositide 3-kinase pathway. Thus, the proarrhythmic potential of sotalol may in part be related to its ability to increase I_{Na-L} in addition to is effect on I_{Kr}.[14] Furthermore, reverse frequency dependence with sotalol has been shown to be reversed by addition of ranolazine, suggesting that I_{Na-L} may play more of a role in reverse frequency dependence than I_{Ks} (**Fig. 2**).[15]

Sotalol may block the cardiac muscarinic receptors, but does not have a significant direct effect on $I_{K,ACh}$.[16] Mori and colleagues[17] demonstrated that sotalol at concentrations of 100 μmol/L in the guinea pig atrium partially reversed carbachol-induced APD shortening. Sotalol had a concentration dependent effect on inhibiting $I_{K,ACh}$ activity during carbachol administration, but not with adenosine or GTPgammaS, suggesting that the effect of sotalol was solely through muscarinic receptor blockade.[17] Despite the demonstrated anticholinergic effect of sotalol, sufficient parasympathetic stimulation will significantly shorten D-sotalol-induced atrial APD prolongation.[18] A recent study used tracheal obstruction in the pig to create negative tracheal pressure, simulating sleep apnea. The associated increase in vagal tone shortened AERP and increased AF inducibility, which was not attenuated by sotalol.[19] These studies suggest that sotalol may be ineffective in suppressing vagally mediated AF, but clinical data supporting this assumption are not available.

Both D-sotalol and L-sotalol have roughly equipotent I_{Kr} blocking properties.[2] However, L-sotalol, but not D-sotalol, has significant nonspecific beta-adrenergic blocking properties.[20] The beta-blocking effects are typically seen when plasma concentrations are greater than 800 ng/mL.[21]

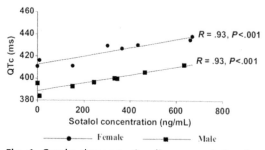

Fig. 1. Graphs demonstrating linear correlation between serum sotalol concentration and QTc interval in female and male patients, with females having an approximate 25 milliseconds longer QTc interval at all serum concentrations studied. (*From* Somberg JC, Preston RA, Ranade V, et al. Gender differences in cardiac repolarization following intravenous sotalol administration. J Cardiovasc Pharmacol 2012;17(1): 89; with permission.)

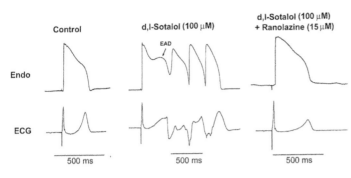

Control   d,l-Sotalol (100 µM)   d,l-Sotalol (100 µM) + Ranolazine (15 µM)

Endo   EAD

ECG

500 ms   500 ms   500 ms

Fig. 2. Transmembrane endocardial action potential (Endo) and extracellular transmural ECG signal from arterially perfused rabbit left ventricular wedge preparation in the control state and after perfusion with D,L-sotalol demonstrate the developed of early afterdepolarization (EAD) and a triggered rhythm suggestive of torsades de pointes on the extracellular recording. Addition of ranolazine to the sotalol perfusate eliminated EADs and the triggered arrhythmia. (*From* Jia S, Lian J, Guo D, et al. Modulation of late sodium current by ATX-II and ranolazine affects the reverse use-dependence and proarrhythmic liability of I_{Kr} blockade. Br J Pharmacol 2011;164(2):312; with permission.)

Sotalol has a third of the beta-blocking effect of propranolol. It has been suggested that the beta-adrenergic blocking effects of sotalol are seen at dosages as low as 25 mg, but the class III effects are not seen until higher dosages are reached above 80 mg. However, Somberg and colleagues[5] recently demonstrated linear QT responses to a single 80 mg oral dose or an intravenous 75 mg dose given over 2 hours.

The beta-blocking properties of sotalol, compared with D-sotalol, prevent isoproterenol reversal of drug-induced APD prolongation.[22] Kassotis and colleagues[23] demonstrated in the canine infarct model of epicardial VT that the combination of esmolol and D-sotalol prevented induction of VT when esmolol or D-sotalol alone did not. This was shown by mapping to be due to prolongation of induced functional lines of block to prevent induction or maintenance of induced VT. The addition of esmolol allowed significant prolongation of the ERP compared with D-sotalol alone. This beneficial effect of concomitant beta-adrenergic blockade may explain the greater safety of racemic sotalol compared with D-sotalol in high-risk patients.

AF is initiated by rapid atrial ectopics and tachycardias occurring predominantly within the pulmonary vein (PV) myocardial sleeves. In canine superfused PV sleeve preparations, sotalol in concentration of 3 to 30 µM caused small statistically insignificant increases in the APD_{85} of 10 to 15 milliseconds, without changing the ERP, Vmax, excitation threshold, or shortest drive cycle length allowing 1:1 conduction (which were all increased with vernakalant and ranolazine). Sotalol-suppressed isoproterenol plus high calcium-induced delayed after depolarization (DAD) triggered activity (**Fig. 3**), as did vernakalant and ranolazine. Because the class III effect of sotalol in the PV sleeve preparation was minimal, the authors speculated that this was mediated primarily via its antiadrenergic effect.[24] However, clinically the antiarrhythmic effects of sotalol for prevention of AF are not seen until its class III effects become manifest.

Despite having no significant antiadrenergic effect, D-sotalol decreases standing and exercise heart rate and blunts heart rate response to beta-adrenergic stimulation.[25,26] Unlike amiodarone, sotalol does not inhibit the HCN4 channel involved in the pacemaker current (I_f).[27] This suggests that the heart rate-blunting effect of D-sotalol is not mediated through suppression of I_f in the sinus node and that the effect of sotalol on decreasing heart rate is not exclusively mediated through its beta-adrenergic blocking effect. Nonetheless, heart rate slowing occurs almost immediately at the onset of a 2-hour infusion of 75 mg of sotalol, with peak slowing 1 hour into infusion and then gradual attenuation.[5,28] This suggests that the bradycardic effect of sotalol is caused dominantly by its beta-blocking properties.

PHARMACOKINETICS

Sotalol is well absorbed in the small intestine, with an oral bioavailability of 95% to 100% without hepatic first pass metabolism.[21] Peak serum concentration occurs about 2.5 to 3 hours after a single oral dosage and 2 hours after a single intravenous dosage infused over 2.5 hours.[6,29] Plasma concentrations follow linear kinetics. There is no biotransformation of sotalol and therefore no metabolites.[21] Dosing sotalol with foods decreases its bioavailability by 20%.[21] It is hydrophilic, and therefore there is limited penetration into the central nervous system.[21] Sotalol does distribute into heart, liver, and kidney tissues.[21] The volume of distribution is 1.2 to 2.4 L/kg.[21] Sotalol is predominately unchanged and renally cleared with approximately 10% to 20% being excreted fecally and unchanged. Its clearance is dependent on and

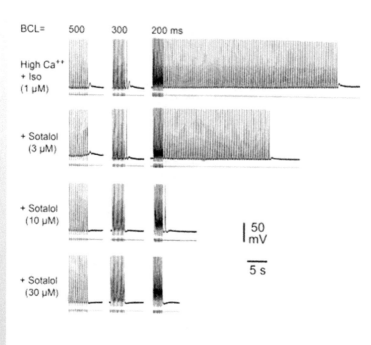

Fig. 3. Transmembrane action potential recordings from the canine pulmonary vein myocardial sleeve during superfusion with isoproterenol and high calcium concentrations demonstrate the development of delayed afterdepolarizations (DAD) after cessation of rapid pacing at basic cycle lengths (BCL) of 500 milliseconds and 300 milliseconds and DAD-induced triggered activity after pacing at 200 milliseconds (upper panel). Progressive increases in sotalol concentration in the perfusate cause increasing suppression of the amount to DAD-induced triggered activity that could be induced by rapid pacing (subsequent panels). (*From* Sicouri S, Pourrier M, Gibson JK, et al. Comparison of electrophysiological and antiarrhythmic effects of vernakalant, ranolazine, and sotalol in canine pulmonary vein sleeve preparations. Heart Rhythm 2012;9(3):426; with permission.)

therefore is proportional to renal function. In patients with normal renal function, the half-life (T1/2) is 10 to 20 hours.[21] There is thus a linear relationship of sotalol serum concentration to dosage. Sotalol does not bind significantly to plasma proteins.[21]

As sotalol is primarily renally cleared, its clearance is directly affected by renal function. In a small study by Blair and colleagues,[30] there was a linear relationship between creatinine clearance and plasma levels of sotalol. In patients with creatinine clearance greater than 39 mL/min/m², the drug's half-life was 8.1 ± 3.4 hours, with renal clearance of 46 +/- 26 mL/min/m2. With creatinine clearance between 8 and 38 mL/min/m², sotalol's half-life increased to 24.2 ± 7.5 hours, with a subsequent decrease in renal clearance down to 24 ± 7 mL/min/m². In patients on dialysis, the half-life of sotalol increased to 33.9 ± 27.1 hours. As the drug is primarily not protein bound, the elimination with hemodialysis was 5.8 ± 2.1 hours. These findings were consistent with a previous study by Tjandramaga and colleagues,[31] who also demonstrated some redistribution after hemodialysis.

In pregnancy, oral sotalol is cleared faster (half life of 10 hours).[32] This is thought to be a consequence of increased glomerular filtration rate in pregnancy. There is no change in distribution and bioavailability. Sotalol has been shown to cross the placental barrier, with a mean maternal-to-fetal ratio of 1.0 to 1.05 µg/mL.[32] In 12 hypertensive pregnant women in whom sotalol

was used for blood pressure control,[33] 2 of the 12 newborns died from severe congenital anomalies; 1 newborn suffered from neonatal hypoglycemia, and 1 newborn suffered from perinatal asphyxia. High concentrations of sotalol were found in breast milk, with a ratio of 1 to 5.4 of plasma-to-breast milk concentration in 5 of the mothers who decided to breast feed. Other studies have confirmed high levels of sotalol in breast milk. Although the safety and teratogenicity of sotalol in pregnancy and breast feeding are not known with certainty, these data suggest that use of sotalol should be avoided during pregnancy and breast feeding outside of emergency situations where the benefits outweigh the risks.

PHARMACODYNAMICS

Sotalol primarily increases the QT interval and slows the heart rate.[34,35] Effects on the PR and QRS intervals are present but minimal.[36]

The effect on the QT interval is dosage and heart rate dependent in a near linear fashion.[5,36] Because the risk of proarrhythmia and specifically torsades de pointes is QT dependent, there is a relatively close relationship of risk of torsades de pointes and sotalol dosage. The risk of torsades de pointes was 1% at daily dosages less than 320 mg bid and 5% at dosages greater than 320 mg. Although the antiarrhythmic properties of the drug increase with increasing dosage and QT prolongation, the increasing arrhythmia suppression at dosages greater than 320 mg daily has to be weighed against the increased proarrhythmic potential and risk of the arrhythmia. Although this risk–benefit analysis may be reasonable for VT (particularly if an implantable cardioverter-defibrillator (ICD) is in place for treatment of torsades de pointes if it occurs), it is more difficult to justify for nonmalignant arrhythmias such as AF or atrial flutter. It is for this reason that the US Food and Drug Administration (FDA) limited the maximum dosage of sotalol to 320 mg daily (160 mg twice daily) for treatment of AF and other atrial tachyarrhythmias. Dosages higher than 320 mg daily have been used safely in the treatment of VT, but QT interval should be monitored closely during dosing increases and during long-term follow-up, the patient should have an ICD, and addition of other drugs with QT prolonging properties should be avoided.

Women have been shown to have greater QT interval prolongation with sotalol than men.[6,29] They are also at increased risk for torsades de pointes as compared with their male counterparts.[37,38] This may in part be due to hormonal modulation of sotalol-induced QT prolongation. Although not yet evaluated with sotalol, Rodriguez and colleagues[39] demonstrated that QT prolongation with ibutilide was greater in women during menstruation and the ovulatory phase than during the luteal phase. Infants may demonstrate a higher sensitivity to QT prolongation with sotalol compared with older children.[40]

Sotalol has been shown to increase the AH, but not HV, interval. AV nodal conduction delay (AH interval) at standard doses is greatest with L-sotalol (20–60 milliseconds) and racemic sotalol (20–57 milliseconds), and least with D-sotalol (7–43 milliseconds),[20] reflecting the additional effect of concomitant beta-adrenergic blockade. Sotalol increases the ERP of the atria, ventricles, and AV nodal (AVN), as well as the functional refractory period (FRP) of the AVN. It increases the ERP anterogradely and retrogradely of accessory pathways.[41]

DRUG INTERACTIONS

Sotalol prolongs the QT interval, slows the heart rate, and lowers the blood pressure. Thus, concomitant use of drugs that affect one or more of these parameters may cause ventricular proarrhythmia, severe bradyarrhythmias, and/or hypotension. As a result, any drug that prolongs the QT interval (and the list is lengthy) can cause further increases in the QT interval in patients on sotalol and increase the risk of proarrhythmia. Thus, other QT-prolonging drugs should be avoided if possible. When not possible, strong consideration should be given for inpatient initiation for QT monitoring. There have been no reports of clinically significant pharmacokinetic drug interactions with sotalol. Because sotalol is renally cleared, drugs that decrease or enhance hepatic clearance have no effect on sotalol concentrations. Concomitant ingestion of aluminum oxide or magnesium hydroxide containing antacids within 2 hours of taking sotalol decrease sotalol bioavailability by about 20% to 25%, but have no effect if taken after 2 hours of sotalol ingestion.[42]

NEGATIVE INOTROPIC PROPERTIES

Sotalol may have negative inotropic properties and thus should be used carefully in patients with systolic heart failure, although some studies have found systolic heart function improves or remains unchanged despite its negative inotropic properties.[43–46] The negative inotropic properties are modulated primarily by the beta-adrenergic properties of sotalol, and thus concomitant beta-blockade should be stopped or decreased in patients with heart failure started on sotalol.[47] The class III effect of sotalol increases the action potential duration and the duration of the inward calcium current. This increase in intracellular calcium increases inotropy and thus to some extent counteracts the negative inotropic effects of the beta-blockade.[36,47] Thus, sotalol can be used safely in patients with severely decreased left ventricular function who have well compensated heart failure. In patients with decompensated (symptomatic) systolic dysfunction, sotalol should be avoided.

There are few data regarding the safety of sotalol in patients with diastolic dysfunction. Theoretically, the negative inotropic effects of sotalol might be useful in this situation. However, sotalol should probably be avoided in patients with significant left ventricular hypertrophy. Studies in animals with induced LVH have demonstrated an increased risk of proarrhythmia due to the effect of hypertrophy on repolarization and QT prolongation and dispersion.[48] For instance, in the study by Vos and colleagues,[10] chronic heart block-induced ventricular hypertrophy in the canine model increased the risk of d-sotalol induced torsades de pointes.

DOSING

Present sotalol initiation regimens suggest starting at a lower dosage and increasing the dosage every 3 days as tolerated symptomatically while monitoring to avoid excessive QT prolongation. However, this strategy tends to result in suboptimal dosing of sotalol, since maximizing the dosage in this manner requires protracted and expensive hospitalization. Rapid-loading regimens during hospital monitoring (analogous to dofetilide) have been recommended by some, but this should only be performed in the hospital with careful monitoring. Either 240 mg daily given as 120 mg 2 times a day or 80 mg 3 times a day or 320 mg daily given as 160 mg twice a day or 80 mg 4 times a day have been suggested as starting dosages, with each subsequent dosage decreased if needed for development of excessive QT prolongation on electrocardiograms (ECGs) 2 hours after dosing and/or significant bradycardia or other side effects. In the retrospective study by Kim and colleagues,[49] patients with atrial and ventricular arrhythmias started on 80 mg twice daily with gradual escalation upward (standard protocol) were compared with patients started on either 120 mg or 160 mg twice daily (accelerated protocol). Although the mean daily dosage was higher in the accelerated protocol, hospitalization duration was not significantly shorter, and there was a trend to higher complications rates in the accelerated protocol (6.9% vs 1.9% with the standard protocol; $P = .092$). In a small double-blind crossover trial, the targeted QT interval prolongation was reached 22.5 hours sooner in the accelerated dosing regimen compared with the conventional regimen with no adverse events in either arm during the loading phase.[50] Further randomized prospective trials of standard versus accelerated dosing regimen are needed in clinical populations to better assess the utility and safety of the accelerated sotalol dosing regimen. During sotalol initiation, ECGs should be obtained about 2 hours after each dosage at the time of peak serum concentrations and thus QT prolongation. Given the reverse use dependence of sotalol and longer QT response at slower heart rates, it is also important to measure the QT at steady state in sinus rhythm, when the ventricular rate is usually slower than during atrial tachyarrhythmias.

Beta-blockade properties are encountered even at dosages as low as 80 mg twice daily. Thus, bradycardia may be encountered with low-dose sotalol usage. For patients with significant sinus node dysfunction, sotalol should be avoided unless a pacemaker has been implanted. If a pacemaker has not been implanted, then dofetilide would be a better option, because it has minimal effect on sinus node function.

In a recent study by Weeke, 29% of 541 patients started on sotalol discontinued it for various reasons within 3 months of initiation (1% for long QT interval, 2% for bradycardia, 4.5% for adverse events, and the remainder for recurrent arrhythmia or other side effects).[51] Various factors may be predictive of developing significant complications with initiation of sotalol, including baseline long QT interval greater than 450 milliseconds, sinus bradycardia, significant sinus node dysfunction, other significant bradyarrhythmias, underlying structural heart disease, significant left ventricular hypertrophy, female gender, older age, and concomitant diuretic usage.[51] However, significant proarrhythmic and other adverse events can happen even in patients without risk factors.[52,53] Controversy thus exists as whether a low enough risk profile can be established to allow safe outpatient initiation of sotalol in selected patients. Some studies have suggested that it may be safe to start as an outpatient in carefully selected patients who are in sinus rhythm at the time of initiation.[54] However, given the potentially severe nature of adverse events, even in low risk patients, and given that none of the profiling algorithms have been systematically tested, it is not recommended that sotalol be started as an outpatient, which is how sotalol is presently labeled.

Sotalol is available in the United States in oral pill and suspension forms and as an intravenous preparation. The oral dosage in adults depends in part on the arrhythmia being treated as well as the pharmacodynamic effect. Labeling for AF indications limits maximum dosage to 160 mg twice daily (320 mg daily) in adults given the rapid increase in proarrhythmic complications beyond 320 mg daily. Higher dosages may be required for treatment of VT, but safety is abetted typically by the presence of an ICD and pacing support.

There are limited data regarding dosing in children. For children 2 years of age or younger, the initial recommended dosage is 30 mg/m^2 3 times a day (90 mg/m^2 daily) with dose increments after several days up to a maximum of 60 mg/m^2 3 times a day. For children younger than 2 years of age, dose reduction by an age-specific modifier has been recommended (see package insert). In a study by Laer and colleagues,[40] the suggested starting dose was 2 to 3 mg/kg/d in neonates, 3 to 6 mg/kg/d in infants and children younger than 6 years old, and 2 to 4 mg/kg/d in children older than 6 years.

Because the oral bioavailability of sotalol is 90% to 100%, the equivalent dosage of sotalol given intravenously is about 10% less. In the study by Somberg and colleagues,[28] sotalol 75 mg intravenously given over 2 hours had a higher Cmax than 80 mg orally, whereas sotalol 75 mg intravenously given over 5 hours had a similar Cmax and AUC as sotalol 80 mg orally. Similarly, 150 mg sotalol intravenously over 5 hours has a similar Cmax and AUC as a 160 mg dose orally.

Sotalol has been evaluated recently for intrapericardial delivery in animal models.[55] Given the relative thinness of the atria compared with the ventricles and the large atrial pericardial surface area, intrapericardial delivery has the theoretic advantage of relative selective targeting of the atria, which could lead to greater efficacy with less risk of ventricular proarrhythmia. However, in the pacing-induced AF goat model, intrapericardial sotalol only increased the epicardial AERP without altering the endocardial AERP and without increasing the AF cycle length or rate of termination compared with intravenous sotalol.[55] Further research is needed to determine if intrapericardial delivery of sotalol or other antiarrhythmic drugs will have any practical applications.

INDICATIONS
Premature Ventricular Contractions

Sotalol has been shown to be superior to placebo for suppression of premature ventricular contractions[46,56] and in one study was superior to procainamide.[57] Given the concerns about class I antiarrhythmic drugs raised by the Cardiac Arrhythmia Suppression Trial (CAST),[58] sotalol may be a reasonable option for treatment of heavily symptomatic patients with frequent ventricular ectopy. However, direct data regarding the long-term safety of sotalol for treatment of patients with high-grade ectopy are lacking. Beta-blockers have been shown to decrease mortality in high-risk, post-myocardial infarction patients. Sotalol in a non-standard dosage of 320 mg taken once daily demonstrated a nonsignificant 18% reduction in total mortality in postmyocardial infarction (post-MI) patients, but the difference did not reach statistical significance.[59] It may be that the beneficial effect of beta-blockers in this situation was attenuated by the risk of proarrhythmia by the class III effect given in a nonstandard dosage. In the Survival with Oral d-Sotalol (SWORD) Trial evaluating D-sotalol in post-MI patients, there was an increase in mortality with D-sotalol, again suggesting the beneficial effect of beta-blockade with sotalol therapy.[60]

Ventricular Tachycardia

Intravenous sotalol is an effective agent for the acute termination of hemodynamically stable VT, although data are limited.[61] In a randomized trial comparing intravenous sotalol with lidocaine in patients with hemodynamically stable VT, rates of termination were superior with sotalol (69%) compared to lidocaine (18%).[62] However, in a randomized trial of patient with ventricular fibrillation that had not responded to standard resuscitation, there was no difference in the rates of survival to hospital admission or discharge with either intravenous sotalol or lidocaine.[63] Randomized comparisons to intravenous amiodarone for either stable or unstable ventricular arrhythmias are not available.

Sotalol is an effective agent for chronic treatment of VT.[64–66] Sotalol has been shown to be superior to placebo for suppression of VT.[64] More importantly, sotalol is more effective for suppression of VT than the class I antiarrhythmic drugs. In the pivotal Electrophysiologic Study Versus Electrocardiographic Monitoring (ESVEM) Trial,[67] patients with ventricular tachyarrhythmias were randomized to undergo serial drug testing either by electrophysiologic (EP) testing or Holter monitoring with exercise testing.[67] Seven different antiarrhythmic drugs were randomly tested, including the class I antiarrhythmic drugs imipramine, mexiletine, pirmenol, procainamide, propafenone, and quinidine and the sole class III drug, DL-sotalol. Sotalol was superior for arrhythmia suppression compared with each of the class I agents individually. Pooling the data from the class I drugs together, sotalol was superior in terms of arrhythmia recurrence, all-cause mortality, cardiovascular mortality, and arrhythmic mortality (Fig. 4). Efficacy was higher with sotalol compared with the class I antiarrhythmic drugs, whether efficacy was assessed by EP testing or Holter monitoring. Limited data have suggested that sotalol and amiodarone are equally effective in treating VT in patients with both ischemic and nonischemic cardiomyopathy.[44,68]

The impact on cardiovascular and arrhythmic mortality may be due in part to the beta-blocking properties of DL-sotalol. In a post-hoc analysis of the ESVEM trial, arrhythmia recurrence on sotalol was lower over long-term follow-up than that with a class I drug with or without concomitant use of a beta-blocker.[69] However, mortality with a class 1 agent with beta-blockade was similar to sotalol, but both were lower than a class I agent without concomitant beta-blockade (although the difference in mortality between patients on class I drugs with and without beta-blockade did not reach statistical significance). Although the data are intriguing and suggest that it is more than the beta-blocking properties of sotalol that enhance its efficacy for suppressing VT, the number of patients and the retrospective study design leave this question unanswered.

ATRIAL FIBRILLATION
Acute Pharmacologic Cardioversion

Sotalol has been shown to be mildly effective for acute pharmacologic cardioversion of AF.[70,71]

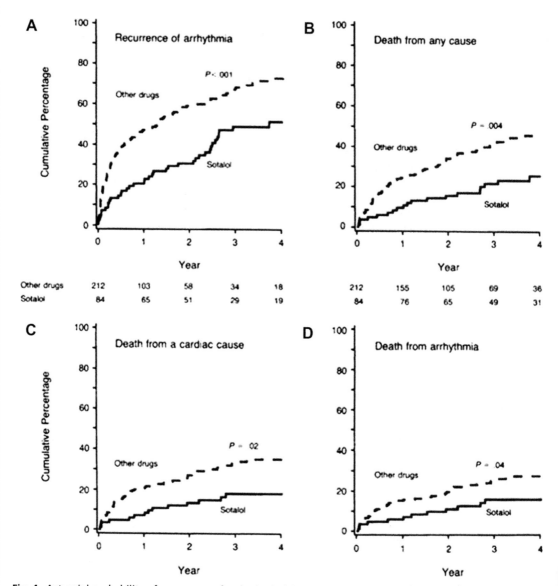

Fig. 4. Actuarial probability of recurrence of arrhythmia (A), death from any cause (B), death from cardiac cause (C), and death from arrhythmia (D) in the ESVEM Trial demonstrate the greater efficacy and safety of sotalol to the 6 other class I antiarrhythmic drugs (other drugs). (*From* Mason JW. A comparison of seven antiarrhythmic drugs in patients with ventricular tachyarrhythmias. Electrophysiologic Study vs Electrocardiographic Monitoring Investigators. N Engl J Med 1993;329(7):456; with permission.)

Rates of pharmacologic cardioversion range from 24% to 30% depending on various clinical factors.[70] Sotalol is less effective for pharmacologic cardioversion than quinidine, flecainide, and propafenone.[10,72] Sotalol is as effective for acute pharmacologic cardioversion as amiodarone.[70] In a randomized trial of single-dose intravenous sotalol, amiodarone, or digoxin followed by oral dosing in patients with AF of less than 24 hours duration, there was a significant reduction in the time to resumption of sinus rhythm with sotalol

(13.0 ± 2.5 hours) and amiodarone (18.1 ± 2.9 hours) compared with digoxin (26.9 ± 3.4 hours).[73] Sinus rhythm was established in 88%, 77%, and 58% at 48 hours, respectively. In a comparison to ibutilide, intravenous sotalol was less effective for either AF or atrial flutter and had a higher incidence of adverse effects of bradycardia and hypotension.[10] In a meta-analysis of trials evaluating the efficacy of antiarrhythmic drugs for acute termination of AF, dofetilide and ibutilide were also more effective than sotalol.[71] Thus, given the presently available data, sotalol has a limited role in the acute pharmacologic management of AF.

Maintenance of Sinus Rhythm

Sotalol is an effective agent for maintenance of sinus rhythm in patients with paroxysmal and persistent AF.[70] However, an appropriate dosage must be used. In the dose-ranging study by Benditt and colleagues,[74] sotalol 80 mg twice daily was no more effective in maintenance of sinus rhythm than placebo. However, both sotalol 120 mg twice daily and 160 mg twice daily were more effective than placebo for maintenance of sinus rhythm. There was a suggestion in this study that 120 mg twice daily may be safer than 160 mg twice daily based on a risk and benefit comparison. However, as with all antiarrhythmic drugs, sotalol should be dosed in the individual based upon the pharmacodynamic response to the drug, with careful monitoring of the QT interval and heart rate. In a randomized comparison of low-dose sotalol (mean daily dosage of 167 ± 66 mg) to atenolol (62 ± 26 mg) and metoprolol (104 ± 47 mg daily), there was no difference in arrhythmia recurrence, cardioversion, or hospitalization between groups in patients with tachycardia–bradycardia syndrome and implanted antitachycardia pacemakers.[75] Thus, for sotalol to be effective in AF suppression, it must be used in higher dosages in most patients with normal renal function.

Sotalol has been shown to have a similar efficacy and safety profile for maintenance of sinus rhythm compared with quinidine, propafenone, and flecainide.[76–79] In the Canadian Trial of Atrial Fibrillation (CTAF), sotalol was equally effective for maintaining sinus rhythm compared with propafenone, but less effective than amiodarone[80] (**Fig. 5**). The mean follow-up in that study was 16 months, and at that point, the rate of discontinuation for adverse events while taking amiodarone as compared with either sotalol or propafenone was bordering on statistical significance (0.06).[80]

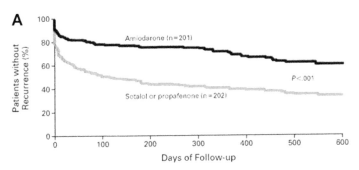

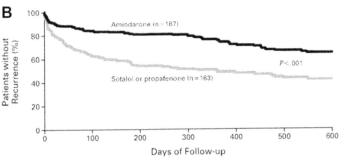

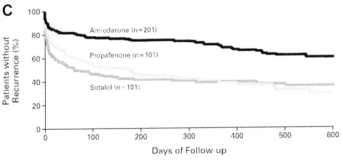

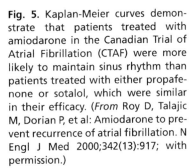

Fig. 5. Kaplan-Meier curves demonstrate that patients treated with amiodarone in the Canadian Trial of Atrial Fibrillation (CTAF) were more likely to maintain sinus rhythm than patients treated with either propafenone or sotalol, which were similar in their efficacy. (*From* Roy D, Talajic M, Dorian P, et al: Amiodarone to prevent recurrence of atrial fibrillation. N Engl J Med 2000;342(13):917; with permission.)

In the Sotalol Amiodarone Atrial Fibrillation Efficacy Trial (SAFE-T), patients with persistent AF were randomized to sotalol, amiodarone, or placebo.[70] Amiodarone was superior at maintaining sinus rhythm.[70] Of note, in a subanalysis of SAFE-T, neither sotalol nor amiodarone increased exercise relative to placebo in patients maintaining sinus rhythm.[81]

The Atrial Fibrillation Follow-Up Investigation of Rhythm Management (AFFIRM) Trial in patients with AF and one or more stroke risk factors raised concerns about the potential long-term risks of antiarrhythmic drugs in these patients. A recent subanalysis of the data from AFFIRM revealed that sotalol had a similar effect to amiodarone and the class IC agents of increasing the primary endpoint of mortality and first cardiovascular hospitalization compared with rate control only

(Fig. 6). However, unlike amiodarone, which increased mortality, there was no difference in mortality between sotalol and rate control arms.[82] The difference between sotalol and rate control in the primary endpoint was driven solely by an increase in first cardiovascular hospitalization. In an analysis of all patients with AF treated without antiarrhythmic drug therapy or treated with flecainide, propafenone, sotalol, or amiodarone between 1995 and 2004 in Denmark (n = 141,500 patients), there was no increase in mortality with any of the antiarrhythmic drug. Specifically, for sotalol, the hazard ratio for Cox analysis with time-dependent variables was 0.65 (95% confidence interval [CI] 0.63–0.68) compared with no therapy.[83] However, flecainide and propafenone, but not amiodarone, were also associated with decreased hazard ratios. Because

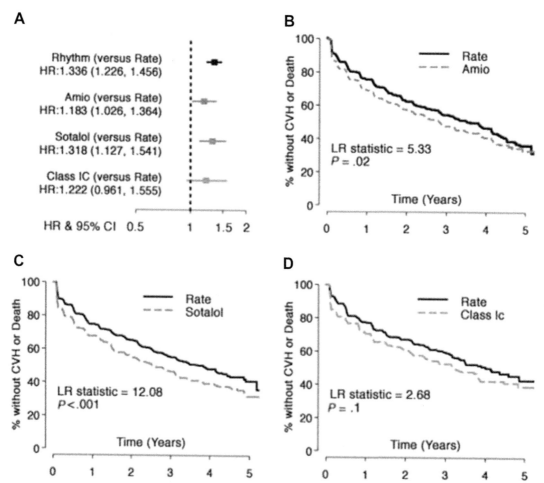

Fig. 6. HR (A) and Kaplan-Meier curves for amiodarone (B), sotalol (C), and class IC drugs (D) in the AFFIRM trial demonstrate similar primary outcome of time to first cardiovascular hospitalization or death compared with matched rate control cohort. (*From* Saksena S, Slee A, Waldo AL, et al. Cardiovascular outcomes in the AFFIRM Trial (Atrial Fibrillation Follow-Up Investigation of Rhythm Management): an assessment of individual antiarrhythmic drug therapies compared with rate control with propensity score-matched analyses. J Am Coll Cardiol 2011;58(19):1980; with permission.)

the data are not randomized, it cannot be inferred that sotalol decreases mortality from this study. Nonetheless, the AFFIRM subanalysis and Danish data suggest that long-term sotalol usage in AF populations does not increase mortality as long as patients are appropriately followed.

Postoperative Atrial Fibrillation

Multiple studies have shown that sotalol is effective for prevention of AF occurring after open heart surgery[84–88] (**Fig. 7**). These studies have generally shown that sotalol is superior to placebo, but some controversy remains as to whether it is superior to beta-blockers.[88,89] Some of the controversy is due to the use of low sotalol dosages in some of these trials, which, as mentioned previously, is no more effective than a beta-blocker.[74] A recent meta-analysis revealed significant reductions in postoperative atrial tachyarrhythmias with sotalol compared to placebo (45%), no therapy (69%), and beta-blocker (50%).[85] There was not a significant difference between sotalol and amiodarone. In the placebo-controlled trials, there was not a significant difference in complications between sotalol (4.9%) and placebo (3.6%), and rates of discontinuation compared with beta-blockers were also not significantly different.[85] The risk of ventricular proarrhythmia appears to be small in the postoperative state (0.14%), mortality was not changed, and hospital stay was decreased by a half a day.[85] Thus, sotalol is a reasonable option for prevention or treatment of AF.

SUPRAVENTRICULAR TACHYCARDIA

Intravenous sotalol has been shown to be effective in terminating supraventricular tachycardia (SVT). In a randomized, placebo-controlled crossover trial, intravenous sotalol given as 1.5 mg/kg over 10 minutes) terminated 83% of SVTs compared with 16% with placebo, with the most common adverse effect being hypotension.[90] Because sotalol increases the ERP of the atria, ventricles, AV node, and accessory pathways, it should be effective for acute termination of all mechanisms of SVT. However, some studies have suggested that intravenous sotalol may be less effective for terminating AV reciprocating tachycardia.[91] There are few data evaluating the utility and safety of single-dose oral sotalol for acute termination of SVT.[92] However, given the potential risks including proarrhythmia of acutely administered sotalol and given the high efficacy of intravenous adenosine for AV nodal-dependent and focal atrial tachycardias, there is little role for intravenous sotalol except for termination of macroreentrant atrial tachycardias.

Oral sotalol is also effective for prevention of recurrent paroxysmal SVT, but it is rarely used for that situation given the safety and reasonable efficacy of AV nodal-blocking agents and the efficacy and safety of catheter ablation. Sotalol has also been shown to be effective for prevention of macroreentrant atrial tachycardias and other SVTs in the setting of repair of congenital heart disease.[93]

FETAL SUPRAVENTRICULAR ARRHYTHMIAS

Sotalol has been shown to be effective for the transplacental treatment of fetal SVT or AF.[94–96] In a retrospective analysis of 159 cases of fetal supraventricular arrhythmias (114 with SVT), sotalol was associated with higher rates of prenatal AF termination than digoxin or flecainide, although the latter 2 agents were more effective in terminating fetal SVT (**Fig. 8**). At day 5 of treatment, 29% of fetuses with AF were in sinus rhythm compared to 13% with digoxin and 21% with flecainide. However, if AF persisted beyond 5 days, ventricular rates during SVT or AF were lower with flecainide or digoxin compared with sotalol.[94]

PACING AND DEFIBRILLATION THRESHOLDS

In patients with pacemakers and defibrillators, sotalol clinically has little effect on pacing threshold.[75,97] Similarly, sotalol may have no effect or actually decrease defibrillation thresholds (DFTs) in the atria and ventricles. In a canine model of vagally mediated AF, the DFT with intracardiac

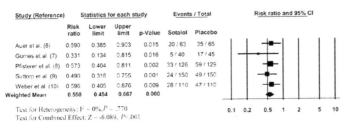

Study (Reference)	Statistics for each study				Events / Total		Risk ratio and 95% CI
	Risk ratio	Lower limit	Upper limit	p-Value	Sotalol	Placebo	
Auer et al. (6)	0.590	0.385	0.903	0.015	20 / 63	35 / 65	
Gomes et al. (7)	0.331	0.134	0.815	0.016	5 / 40	17 / 45	
Pfisterer et al. (8)	0.573	0.404	0.811	0.002	33 / 126	59 / 129	
Suttorp et al. (9)	0.490	0.318	0.755	0.001	24 / 150	49 / 150	
Weber et al. (10)	0.596	0.405	0.876	0.009	28 / 110	47 / 110	
Weighted Mean	0.550	0.454	0.667	0.000			

Test for Heterogeneity: I² = 0%, P = .770
Test for Combined Effect: Z = -6.089, P<.001

0.1   0.2   0.5   1   2   5   10

Favours Sotalol   Favours Placebo

Fig. 7. Meta-analysis of trials evaluating the effect of sotalol for prevention of postoperative SVTs demonstrates a significant suppressive effect of sotalol in all trials. (*From* Kerin NZ, Jacob S. The efficacy of sotalol in preventing postoperative atrial fibrillation: a meta-analysis. Am J Med 2011;124(9):875.e4; with permission.)

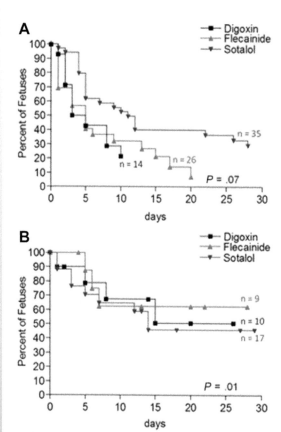

A

B

Fig. 8. Graphs demonstrate freedom from prenatal termination of SVT (*A*) and atrial flutter (*B*) with treatment with digoxin, flecainide, and sotalol. Digoxin and flecainide were superior to sotalol for termination of SVT, but sotalol was superior to digoxin or flecainide for termination of atrial flutter. (*From* Jaeggi ET, Carvalho JS, De Groot E, et al. Comparison of transplacental treatment of fetal supraventricular tachyarrhythmias with digoxin, flecainide, and sotalol: results of a non-randomized multicenter study. Circulation 2011;124(16):1751; with permission.)

AF was decrease from 1.72 ± 1.12 J to 0.59 ± 0.60 J after 5 mg/kg of intravenous D-sotalol.[98] In patients with acute AF, atrial DFT was reduced with intravenous sotalol, but not in patients with chronic AF.[99] In a randomized trial of ICD patients, orally administered sotalol decreased the ventricular DFT from 8.09 ± 4.81 J to 7.20 ± 5.30 J, but this was not statistically significant.[100] In the study by Dorian and colleagues,[101] the ventricular DFT was reduced from 12.4 ± 5.0 J to 8.4 ± 4.0 J after administering intravenous D-sotalol, which also increased induced VF cycle length and made induced VF more likely to spontaneously terminate.

There have been 3 randomized trials evaluating the effect of sotalol on the frequency of ICD shocks. In one small study, the effect of sotalol on the risk of subsequent ICD shocks was less than beta-blockers.[102] In the larger d,l-Sotalol Implantable Cardioverter-Defibrillator Study, sotalol decreased the frequency of inappropriate and appropriate ICD shocks.[102] In the Optimal Pharmacologic Therapy in Cardioverter Defibrillator Patients (OPTIC) study, patients with ICDs were randomized to beta-blocker, sotalol, and low-dose amiodarone plus beta-blocker.[103] There was a trend for sotalol to reduce the risk of ICD shocks compared with beta-blockers alone (hazard ratio [HR] = 0.61; 95% CI 0.37–1.10; $P = .055$), but amiodarone was more effective than either sotalol or beta-blockers (**Fig. 9**). Despite the fact that relatively low-dose sotalol was used (mean dosage 190 mg/d), discontinuation after 1 year of follow-up was higher for sotalol (23.5%) than amiodarone (18.2%) and beta-blockers (5.3%).[103] Given these results, routine use of sotalol prophylactically in patients with ICDs is

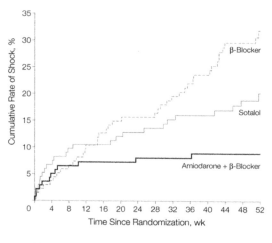

Fig. 9. Kaplan-Meier curves from the Optimal Pharmacologic Therapy in Cardioverter Defibrillator Patients (OPTIC) Study demonstrate that sotalol was superior to beta-blockers alone for prevention of ICD shocks but was not as effective as amiodarone with beta-blocker. (*From* Connelly SJ, Dorian P, Roberts RS, et al. Comparison of beta-blockers, amiodarone plus beta-blockers, or sotalol for prevention of shocks from implantable cardioverter defibrillators: the OPTIC study: a randomized trial. JAMA 2006;295(2):168; with permission.)

No. at Risk					
β-Blocker	138	119	109	91	42
Sotalol	134	118	108	94	35
Amiodarone + β-Blocker	140	124	115	106	56

probably not advisable, but it remains an excellent option in patients with recurrent AF and/or VT.

REFERENCES

1. Larsen AA, Lish PM. A new bio-isostere: alkylsulphonamidophenethanolamines. Nature 1964;203:1283–4.
2. Kato R, Ikeda N, Yabek SM, et al. Electrophysiologic effects of the levo- and dextrorotatory isomers of sotalol in isolated cardiac muscle and their in vivo pharmacokinetics. J Am Coll Cardiol 1986;7(1):116–25.
3. Sanguinetti MC, Jurkiewicz NK. Two components of cardiac delayed rectifier K^+ current. Differential sensitivity to block by class III antiarrhythmic agents. J Gen Physiol 1990;96(1):195–215.
4. Wyse KR, Ye V, Campbell TJ. Action potential prolongation exhibits simple dose-dependence for sotalol, but reverse dose-dependence for quinidine and disopyramide: implications for proarrhythmia due to triggered activity. J Cardiovasc Pharmacol 1993;21(2):316–22.
5. Somberg JC, Preston RA, Ranade V, et al. QT prolongation and serum sotalol concentration are highly correlated following intravenous and oral sotalol. Cardiology 2010;116(3):219–25.
6. Darpo B, Karnad DR, Badilini F, et al. Are women more susceptible than men to drug-induced QT prolongation? concentration-QTc modelling in a phase 1 study with oral rac-sotalol. Br J Clin Pharmacol 2014;77(3):522–31.
7. Schmitt C, Brachmann J, Karch M, et al. Reverse use-dependent effects of sotalol demonstrated by recording monophasic action potentials of the right ventricle. Am J Cardiol 1991;68(11):1183–7.
8. Marschang H, Beyer T, Karolyi L, et al. Differential rate and potassium-dependent effects of the class III agents d-sotalol and dofetilide on guinea pig papillary muscle. Cardiovasc Drugs Ther 1998;12(6):573–83.
9. Nattel S, Bourne G, Talajic M. Insights into mechanisms of antiarrhythmic drug action from experimental models of atrial fibrillation. J Cardiovasc Electrophysiol 1997;8(4):469–80.
10. Vos MA, Golitsyn SR, Stangl K, et al. Superiority of ibutilide (a new class III agent) over DL-sotalol in converting atrial flutter and atrial fibrillation. The ibutilide/sotalol comparator study group. Heart 1998;79(6):568–75.
11. Duytschaever M, Blaauw Y, Allessie M. Consequences of atrial electrical remodeling for the anti-arrhythmic action of class IC and class III drugs. Cardiovasc Res 2005;67(1):69–76.
12. Tse HF, Lau CP. Electrophysiologic actions of dl-sotalol in patients with persistent atrial fibrillation. J Am Coll Cardiol 2002;40(12):2150–5.
13. Kupershmidt S, Yang IC, Hayashi K, et al. The IKr drug response is modulated by KCR1 in transfected cardiac and noncardiac cell lines. FASEB J 2003;17(15):2263–5.
14. Yang T, Chun YW, Stroud DM, et al. Screening for acute IKr block is insufficient to detect torsades de pointes liability: role of late sodium current. Circulation 2014;130(3):224–34.
15. Jia S, Lian J, Guo D, et al. Modulation of the late sodium current by ATX-II and ranolazine affects reverse use-dependence and proarrhythmic liability of IKr blockade. Br J Pharmacol 2011;164(2):308–16.
16. Zaza A, Malfatto G, Schwartz PJ. Effects on atrial repolarization of the interaction between K+ channel blockers and muscarinic receptor stimulation. J Pharmacol Exp Ther 1995;273(3):1095–104.
17. Mori K, Hara Y, Saito T, et al. Anticholinergic effects of class III antiarrhythmic drugs in guinea pig atrial cells. Different molecular mechanisms. Circulation 1995;91(11):2834–43.
18. Wang J, Feng J, Nattel S. Class III antiarrhythmic drug action in experimental atrial fibrillation. Differences in reverse use dependence and effectiveness between d-sotalol and the new antiarrhythmic drug ambasilide. Circulation 1994;90(4):2032–40.
19. Linz D, Schotten U, Neuberger HR, et al. Combined blockade of early and late activated atrial potassium currents suppresses atrial fibrillation in a pig model of obstructive apnea. Heart Rhythm 2011;8(12):1933–9.
20. Gomoll AW, Bartek MJ. Comparative beta-blocking activities and electrophysiologic actions of racemic sotalol and its optical isomers in anesthetized dogs. Eur J Pharmacol 1986;132(2–3):123–35.
21. Hanyok JJ. Clinical pharmacokinetics of sotalol. Am J Cardiol 1993;72(4):19A–26A.
22. Groh WJ, Gibson KJ, McAnulty JH, et al. Beta-adrenergic blocking property of dl-sotalol maintains class III efficacy in guinea pig ventricular muscle after isoproterenol. Circulation 1995;91(2):262–4.
23. Kassotis J, Sauberman RB, Cabo C, et al. Beta receptor blockade potentiates the antiarrhythmic actions of d-sotalol on reentrant ventricular tachycardia in a canine model of myocardial infarction. J Cardiovasc Electrophysiol 2003;14(11):1233–44.
24. Sicouri S, Pourrier M, Gibson JK, et al. Comparison of electrophysiological and antiarrhythmic effects of vernakalant, ranolazine, and sotalol in canine pulmonary vein sleeve preparations. Heart Rhythm 2012;9(3):422–9.
25. Funck-Brentano C, Silberstein DJ, Roden DM, et al. A mechanism of D-(+)-sotalol effects on heart rate not related to beta-adrenoceptor antagonism. Br J Clin Pharmacol 1990;30(2):195–202.
26. Yasuda SU, Barbey JT, Funck-Brentano C, et al. D-sotalol reduces heart rate in vivo through a

beta-adrenergic receptor-independent mechanism. Clin Pharmacol Ther 1993;53(4):436–42.

27. Tamura A, Ogura T, Uemura H, et al. Effects of anti-arrhythmic drugs on the hyperpolarization-activated cyclic nucleotide-gated channel current. J Pharmacol Sci 2009;110(2):150–9.

28. Somberg JC, Preston RA, Ranade V, et al. Developing a safe intravenous sotalol dosing regimen. Am J Ther 2010;17(4):365–72.

29. Somberg JC, Preston RA, Ranade V, et al. Gender differences in cardiac repolarization following intravenous sotalol administration. J Cardiovasc Pharmacol Ther 2012;17(1):86–92.

30. Blair AD, Burgess ED, Maxwell BM, et al. Sotalol kinetics in renal insufficiency. Clin Pharmacol Ther 1981;29(4):457–63.

31. Tjandramaga TB, Verbeeck R, Thomas J, et al. The effect of end-stage renal failure and haemodialysis on the elimination kinetics of sotalol. Br J Clin Pharmacol 1976;3(2):259–65.

32. O'Hare MF, Leahey W, Murnaghan GA, et al. Pharmacokinetics of sotalol during pregnancy. Eur J Clin Pharmacol 1983;24(4):521–4.

33. O'Hare MF, Murnaghan GA, Russell CJ, et al. Sotalol as a hypotensive agent in pregnancy. Br J Obstet Gynaecol 1980;87(9):814–20.

34. Singh BN, Vaughan Williams EM. A third class of anti-arrhythmic action. Effects on atrial and ventricular intracellular potentials, and other pharmacological actions on cardiac muscle, of MJ 1999 and AH 3474. Br J Pharmacol 1970;39(4):675–87.

35. Manoach M, Tribulova N. Sotalol: the mechanism of its antiarrhythmic-defibrillating effect. Cardiovasc Drug Rev 2001;19(2):172–82.

36. Hohnloser SH, Woosley RL. Sotalol. N Engl J Med 1994;331(1):31–8.

37. Lehmann MH, Hardy S, Archibald D, et al. Sex difference in risk of torsade de pointes with d,l-sotalol. Circulation 1996;94(10):2535–41.

38. Lehmann MH, Hardy S, Archibald D, et al. JTc prolongation with d,l-sotalol in women versus men. Am J Cardiol 1999;83(3):354–9.

39. Rodriguez I, Kilborn MJ, Liu XK, et al. Drug-induced QT prolongation in women during the menstrual cycle. JAMA 2001;285(10):1322–6.

40. Laer S, Elshoff JP, Meibohm B, et al. Development of a safe and effective pediatric dosing regimen for sotalol based on population pharmacokinetics and pharmacodynamics in children with supraventricular tachycardia. J Am Coll Cardiol 2005;46(7):1322–30.

41. Nathan AW, Hellestrand KJ, Bexton RS, et al. Electrophysiological effects of sotalol–just another beta blocker? Br Heart J 1982;47(6):515–20.

42. Laer S, Neumann J, Scholz H. Interaction between sotalol and an antacid preparation. Br J Clin Pharmacol 1997;43(3):269–72.

43. Mahmarian JJ, Verani MS, Hohmann T, et al. The hemodynamic effects of sotalol and quinidine: analysis by use of rest and exercise gated radionuclide angiography. Circulation 1987;76(2):324–31.

44. Multicentre randomized trial of sotalol vs amiodarone for chronic malignant ventricular tachyarrhythmias. Amiodarone vs sotalol study group. Eur Heart J 1989;10(8):685–94.

45. Nademanee K, Feld G, Hendrickson J, et al. Electrophysiologic and antiarrhythmic effects of sotalol in patients with life-threatening ventricular tachyarrhythmias. Circulation 1985;72(3):555–64.

46. Anderson JL, Askins JC, Gilbert EM, et al. Multicenter trial of sotalol for suppression of frequent, complex ventricular arrhythmias: a double-blind, randomized, placebo-controlled evaluation of two doses. J Am Coll Cardiol 1986;8(4):752–62.

47. Holubarsch C, Schneider R, Pieske B, et al. Positive and negative inotropic effects of DL-sotalol and D-sotalol in failing and nonfailing human myocardium under physiological experimental conditions. Circulation 1995;92(10):2904–10.

48. Kaufman ES, Zimmermann PA, Wang T, et al. Risk of proarrhythmic events in the atrial fibrillation follow-up investigation of rhythm management (AFFIRM) study: a multivariate analysis. J Am Coll Cardiol 2004;44(6):1276–82.

49. Kim RJ, Juriansz GJ, Jones DR, et al. Comparison of a standard versus accelerated dosing regimen for D,L-sotalol for the treatment of atrial and ventricular dysrhythmias. Pacing Clin Electrophysiol 2006;29(11):1219–25.

50. Barbey JT, Sale ME, Woosley RL, et al. Pharmacokinetic, pharmacodynamic, and safety evaluation of an accelerated dose titration regimen of sotalol in healthy middle-aged subjects. Clin Pharmacol Ther 1999;66(1):91–9.

51. Weeke P, Delaney J, Mosley JD, et al. QT variability during initial exposure to sotalol: experience based on a large electronic medical record. Europace 2013;15(12):1791–7.

52. Chung MK, Schweikert RA, Wilkoff BL, et al. Is hospital admission for initiation of antiarrhythmic therapy with sotalol for atrial arrhythmias required? Yield of in-hospital monitoring and prediction of risk for significant arrhythmia complications. J Am Coll Cardiol 1998;32(1):169–76.

53. Agusala K, Oesterle A, Kulkarni C, et al. Risk prediction for adverse events during initiation of sotalol and dofetilide for the treatment of atrial fibrillation. Pacing Clin Electrophysiol 2015;38(4):490–8.

54. Reiffel JA. Inpatient versus outpatient antiarrhythmic drug initiation: safety and cost-effectiveness issues. Curr Opin Cardiol 2000;15(1):7–11.

55. van Brakel TJ, Hermans JJ, Accord RE, et al. Effects of intrapericardial sotalol and flecainide on transmural atrial electrophysiology and atrial

fibrillation. J Cardiovasc Electrophysiol 2009;20(2):207–15.

56. Anastasiou-Nana MI, Gilbert EM, Miller RH, et al. Usefulness of d, l sotalol for suppression of chronic ventricular arrhythmias. Am J Cardiol 1991;67(6):511–6.

57. Lidell C, Rehnqvist N, Sjogren A, et al. Comparative efficacy of oral sotalol and procainamide in patients with chronic ventricular arrhythmias: a multicenter study. Am Heart J 1985;109(5 Pt 1):970–5.

58. Preliminary report: effect of encainide and flecainide on mortality in a randomized trial of arrhythmia suppression after myocardial infarction. The cardiac arrhythmia suppression trial (CAST) investigators. N Engl J Med 1989;321(6):406–12.

59. Julian DG, Prescott RJ, Jackson FS, et al. Controlled trial of sotalol for one year after myocardial infarction. Lancet 1982;1(8282):1142–7.

60. Waldo AL, Camm AJ, deRuyter H, et al. Effect of d-sotalol on mortality in patients with left ventricular dysfunction after recent and remote myocardial infarction. The SWORD Investigators. Survival With Oral d-Sotalol. Lancet 1996;348(9019):7–12.

61. deSouza IS, Martindale JL, Sinert R. Antidysrhythmic drug therapy for the termination of stable, monomorphic ventricular tachycardia: a systematic review. Emerg Med J 2015;32(2):161–7.

62. Ho DS, Zecchin RP, Richards DA, et al. Double-blind trial of lignocaine versus sotalol for acute termination of spontaneous sustained ventricular tachycardia. Lancet 1994;344(8914):18–23.

63. Kovoor P, Love A, Hall J, et al. Randomized double-blind trial of sotalol versus lignocaine in out-of-hospital refractory cardiac arrest due to ventricular tachyarrhythmia. Intern Med J 2005;35(9):518–25.

64. Kuhlkamp V, Mewis C, Mermi J, et al. Suppression of sustained ventricular tachyarrhythmias: a comparison of d,l-sotalol with no antiarrhythmic drug treatment. J Am Coll Cardiol 1999;33(1):46–52.

65. Haverkamp W, Martinez-Rubio A, Hief C, et al. Efficacy and safety of d,l-sotalol in patients with ventricular tachycardia and in survivors of cardiac arrest. J Am Coll Cardiol 1997;30(2):487–95.

66. Antz M, Cappato R, Kuck KH. Metoprolol versus sotalol in the treatment of sustained ventricular tachycardia. J Cardiovasc Pharmacol 1995;26(4):627–35.

67. Mason JW. A comparison of seven antiarrhythmic drugs in patients with ventricular tachyarrhythmias. Electrophysiologic study versus electrocardiographic monitoring investigators. N Engl J Med 1993;329(7):452–8.

68. Man KC, Williamson BD, Niebauer M, et al. Electrophysiologic effects of sotalol and amiodarone in patients with sustained monomorphic ventricular tachycardia. Am J Cardiol 1994;74(11):1119–23.

69. Reiffel JA, Hahn E, Hartz V, et al. Sotalol for ventricular tachyarrhythmias: beta-blocking and class III contributions, and relative efficacy versus class I drugs after prior drug failure. ESVEM investigators. Electrophysiologic study versus electrocardiographic monitoring. Am J Cardiol 1997;79(8):1048–53.

70. Singh BN, Singh SN, Reda DJ, et al. Amiodarone versus sotalol for atrial fibrillation. N Engl J Med 2005;352(18):1861–72.

71. McNamara RL, Tamariz LJ, Segal JB, et al. Management of atrial fibrillation: review of the evidence for the role of pharmacologic therapy, electrical cardioversion, and echocardiography. Ann Intern Med 2003;139(12):1018–33.

72. Reisinger J, Gatterer E, Heinze G, et al. Prospective comparison of flecainide versus sotalol for immediate cardioversion of atrial fibrillation. Am J Cardiol 1998;81(12):1450–4.

73. Joseph AP, Ward MR. A prospective, randomized controlled trial comparing the efficacy and safety of sotalol, amiodarone, and digoxin for the reversion of new-onset atrial fibrillation. Ann Emerg Med 2000;36(1):1–9.

74. Benditt DG, Williams JH, Jin J, et al. Maintenance of sinus rhythm with oral d,l-sotalol therapy in patients with symptomatic atrial fibrillation and/or atrial flutter. d,l-sotalol atrial fibrillation/flutter study group. Am J Cardiol 1999;84(3):270–7.

75. Capucci A, Botto G, Molon G, et al. The drug and pace health cliNical evaluation (DAPHNE) study: a randomized trial comparing sotalol versus beta-blockers to treat symptomatic atrial fibrillation in patients with brady-tachycardia syndrome implanted with an antitachycardia pacemaker. Am Heart J 2008;156(2):373.e1–8.

76. Carunchio A, Fera MS, Mazza A, et al. A comparison between flecainide and sotalol in the prevention of recurrences of paroxysmal atrial fibrillation. G Ital Cardiol 1995;25(1):51–68.

77. Reimold SC, Cantillon CO, Friedman PL, et al. Propafenone versus sotalol for suppression of recurrent symptomatic atrial fibrillation. Am J Cardiol 1993;71(7):558–63.

78. Kochiadakis GE, Marketou ME, Igoumenidis NE, et al. Amiodarone, sotalol, or propafenone in atrial fibrillation: which is preferred to maintain normal sinus rhythm? Pacing Clin Electrophysiol 2000;23(11 Pt 2):1883–7.

79. Patten M, Maas R, Bauer P, et al. Suppression of paroxysmal atrial tachyarrhythmias–results of the SOPAT trial. Eur Heart J 2004;25(16):1395–404.

80. Roy D, Talajic M, Dorian P, et al. Amiodarone to prevent recurrence of atrial fibrillation. Canadian trial of atrial fibrillation investigators. N Engl J Med 2000;342(13):913–20.

81. Atwood JE, Myers JN, Tang XC, et al. Exercise capacity in atrial fibrillation: a substudy of the

sotalol-amiodarone atrial fibrillation efficacy trial (SAFE-T). Am Heart J 2007;153(4):566–72.

82. Saksena S, Slee A, Waldo AL, et al. Cardiovascular outcomes in the AFFIRM trial (atrial fibrillation follow-up investigation of rhythm management). An assessment of individual antiarrhythmic drug therapies compared with rate control with propensity score-matched analyses. J Am Coll Cardiol 2011;58(19):1975–85.

83. Andersen SS, Hansen ML, Gislason GH, et al. Antiarrhythmic therapy and risk of death in patients with atrial fibrillation: a nationwide study. Europace 2009;11(7):886–91.

84. Gomes JA, Ip J, Santoni-Rugiu F, et al. Oral d,l sotalol reduces the incidence of postoperative atrial fibrillation in coronary artery bypass surgery patients: a randomized, double-blind, placebo-controlled study. J Am Coll Cardiol 1999;34(2):334–9.

85. Kerin NZ, Jacob S. The efficacy of sotalol in preventing postoperative atrial fibrillation: a meta-analysis. Am J Med 2011;124(9):875.e1–9.

86. Parikka H, Toivonen L, Heikkila L, et al. Comparison of sotalol and metoprolol in the prevention of atrial fibrillation after coronary artery bypass surgery. J Cardiovasc Pharmacol 1998;31(1):67–73.

87. Aerra V, Kuduvalli M, Moloto AN, et al. Does prophylactic sotalol and magnesium decrease the incidence of atrial fibrillation following coronary artery bypass surgery: a propensity-matched analysis. J Cardiothorac Surg 2006;1:6.

88. Patel A, Dunning J. Is sotalol more effective than standard beta-blockers for the prophylaxis of atrial fibrillation during cardiac surgery. Interact Cardiovasc Thorac Surg 2005;4(2):147–50.

89. Arsenault KA, Yusuf AM, Crystal E, et al. Interventions for preventing post-operative atrial fibrillation in patients undergoing heart surgery. Cochrane Database Syst Rev 2013;(1):CD003611.

90. Jordaens L, Gorgels A, Stroobandt R, et al. Efficacy and safety of intravenous sotalol for termination of paroxysmal supraventricular tachycardia. The sotalol versus placebo multicenter study group. Am J Cardiol 1991;68(1):35–40.

91. Huikuri HV, Koistinen MJ, Takkunen JT. Efficacy of intravenous sotalol for suppressing inducibility of supraventricular tachycardias at rest and during isometric exercise. Am J Cardiol 1992;69(5):498–502.

92. Hamer AW, Strathmore N, Vohra JK, et al. Oral flecainide, sotalol, and verapamil for the termination of paroxysmal supraventricular tachycardia. Pacing Clin Electrophysiol 1993;16(7 Pt 1):1394–400.

93. Koyak Z, Kroon B, de Groot JR, et al. Efficacy of antiarrhythmic drugs in adults with congenital heart disease and supraventricular tachycardias. Am J Cardiol 2013;112(9):1461–7.

94. Jaeggi ET, Carvalho JS, De Groot E, et al. Comparison of transplacental treatment of fetal supraventricular tachyarrhythmias with digoxin, flecainide, and sotalol: results of a nonrandomized multicenter study. Circulation 2011;124(16):1747–54.

95. Shah A, Moon-Grady A, Bhogal N, et al. Effectiveness of sotalol as first-line therapy for fetal supraventricular tachyarrhythmias. Am J Cardiol 2012; 109(11):1614–8.

96. van der Heijden LB, Oudijk MA, Manten GT, et al. Sotalol as first-line treatment for fetal tachycardia and neonatal follow-up. Ultrasound Obstet Gynecol 2013;42(3):285–93.

97. Kuhlkamp V, Mewis C, Suchalla R, et al. Effect of amiodarone and sotalol on the defibrillation threshold in comparison to patients without antiarrhythmic drug treatment. Int J Cardiol 1999;69(3): 271–9.

98. Iskos D, Lurie KG, Adler SW, et al. Effect of parenteral d-sotalol on transvenous atrial defibrillation threshold in a canine model of atrial fibrillation. Am Heart J 1996;132(1 Pt 1):116–9.

99. Lau CP, Lok NS. A comparison of transvenous atrial defibrillation of acute and chronic atrial fibrillation and the effect of intravenous sotalol on human atrial defibrillation threshold. Pacing Clin Electrophysiol 1997;20(10 Pt 1):2442–52.

100. Hohnloser SH, Dorian P, Roberts R, et al. Effect of amiodarone and sotalol on ventricular defibrillation threshold: the optimal pharmacological therapy in cardioverter defibrillator patients (OPTIC) trial. Circulation 2006;114(2):104–9.

101. Dorian P, Newman D, Sheahan R, et al. D-sotalol decreases defibrillation energy requirements in humans: a novel indication for drug therapy. J Cardiovasc Electrophysiol 1996;7(10):952–61.

102. Seidl K, Hauer B, Schwick NG, et al. Comparison of metoprolol and sotalol in preventing ventricular tachyarrhythmias after the implantation of a cardioverter/defibrillator. Am J Cardiol 1998;82(6): 744–8.

103. Connolly SJ, Dorian P, Roberts RS, et al. Comparison of beta-blockers, amiodarone plus beta-blockers, or sotalol for prevention of shocks from implantable cardioverter defibrillators: the OPTIC study: a randomized trial. JAMA 2006; 295(2):165–71.

Dronedarone
Basic Pharmacology and Clinical Use

Rafik Tadros, MD[a], Stanley Nattel, MD[a], Jason G. Andrade, MD[a,b,*]

KEYWORDS

- Dronedarone • Atrial fibrillation • Rhythm control • Antiarrhythmic drug

KEY POINTS

- Dronedarone is an amiodarone derivative shown to moderately reduce arrhythmia recurrence, decrease ventricular rate, and prevent hospitalizations in patients with nonpermanent atrial fibrillation (AF).
- In contrast, it increases all-cause mortality in patients with permanent AF and those with moderate to severe heart failure.
- Through CYP3A4 and P-glycoprotein inhibition, dronedarone has numerous drug interactions. Its use in combination with digoxin should be avoided or carefully monitored.
- Dronedarone is less effective than amiodarone, but has less thyroid and neurologic toxicity; direct comparison with other antiarrhythmic drugs and AF ablation is limited.
- Low-dose dronedarone with ranolazine seems to be promising for rhythm control, but a larger clinical trial is needed to assess its effect on cardiovascular outcomes.

INTRODUCTION

Atrial fibrillation (AF) is a highly prevalent arrhythmia with substantial morbidity and associated costs.[1] Drug therapy remains the cornerstone of AF management for the majority of patients and consists of anticoagulation and arrhythmia management (rate with or without rhythm control). In contrast with the approval and widespread clinical use of several novel anticoagulants for AF in the last decade, antiarrhythmic drug (AAD) development has been much less fruitful. Challenges facing AAD development in AF include (1) the complexity of AF pathophysiology, including multiple electrical and structural determinants,[2] (2) the lack of any clear-cut clinical benefit associated with a strategy of rhythm control when compared with the simpler approach of ventricular rate control,[3,4] (3) the toxicities associated with AADs, including ventricular proarrhythmia,[5] and (4) the "competition" with the rapid development of AF ablation.[6] Only a single new AAD has obtained approval by the US Food and Drug Administration (FDA) since 2000. Dronedarone was developed as an amiodarone derivative with less toxicity. Like amiodarone, dronedarone is a multichannel blocker. Randomized controlled trials (RCTs) of dronedarone involving nearly 10,000 patients have established the usefulness of the drug in AF but also highlighted its dangers in certain patient populations. Postapproval studies reiterate the benefits and risks of dronedarone use in "real life." This review summarizes the available pharmacologic and clinical data on dronedarone and discusses its place in the AF rhythm management armamentarium.

Disclosures: None (R. Tadros and S. Nattel); J.G. Andrade is supported by a Michael Smith Foundation Clinical Scholar award (Award No: 5963).
[a] Department of Medicine, Université de Montréal and Montreal Heart Institute, 5000 Rue Belanger, Montreal, Québec H1T 1C8, Canada; [b] Heart Rhythm Services, Department of Medicine, University of British Columbia, 2775 Laurel Street, Vancouver, British Columbia V5Z 1M9, Canada
* Corresponding author. Department of Medicine, University of British Columbia, 2775 Laurel Street, Vancouver, British Columbia V5Z 1M9, Canada.
E-mail address: Jason.guy.andrade@umontreal.ca

cardiacEP.theclinics.com

BASIC PHARMACOLOGY
Molecular Structure: An Amiodarone Derivative

Dronedarone was designed based on the structure of amiodarone, with the objective of reducing side effects and decreasing its elimination half-life (**Fig. 1**).[7] Thyroid toxicity was eliminated by the removal of the 2 iodine atoms from amiodarone, and the reduction of half-life was accomplished by reducing lipophilicity through the addition of a methylsulfonamide group.

Pharmacokinetics

Peak dronedarone concentration is reached within approximately 4 hours of oral administration.[8] Although its absorption is good when taken with food, the oral bioavailability is only approximately 15% because of first-pass metabolism. Plasma protein binding exceeds 98%. Plasma steady state is reached within 7 days of oral administration of 400 mg twice daily (BID). Dronedarone elimination is predominantly through fecal excretion of metabolites formed by the cytochrome P450 CYP3A4. In contrast with amiodarone's long elimination half-life (several weeks), the lower lipophilicity of dronedarone reduces its half-life to approximately 24 hours.

Pharmacodynamics: Ion Channel Blockade

Similar to amiodarone, dronedarone is a multichannel blocker, which explains the broad range of its electrophysiologic effects. At progressively higher concentrations, it blocks the L-type calcium current (I_{CaL}), the rapid then slow components of the delayed rectifier potassium current (I_{Kr}, I_{Ks}), and the inward rectifier potassium current (I_{K1}).[9] Dronedarone also effectively blocks the cardiac sodium current (I_{Na}) in isolated human atrial myocytes, with minimal effects on its kinetics.[10] Bogdan and colleagues[11] demonstrate that I_{Na} and I_{CaL} blockade increases with a less polarized (less negative) holding potential. Such state-dependent block possibly contributes to dronedarone's atrial-selective properties, because atrial myocytes are less polarized at

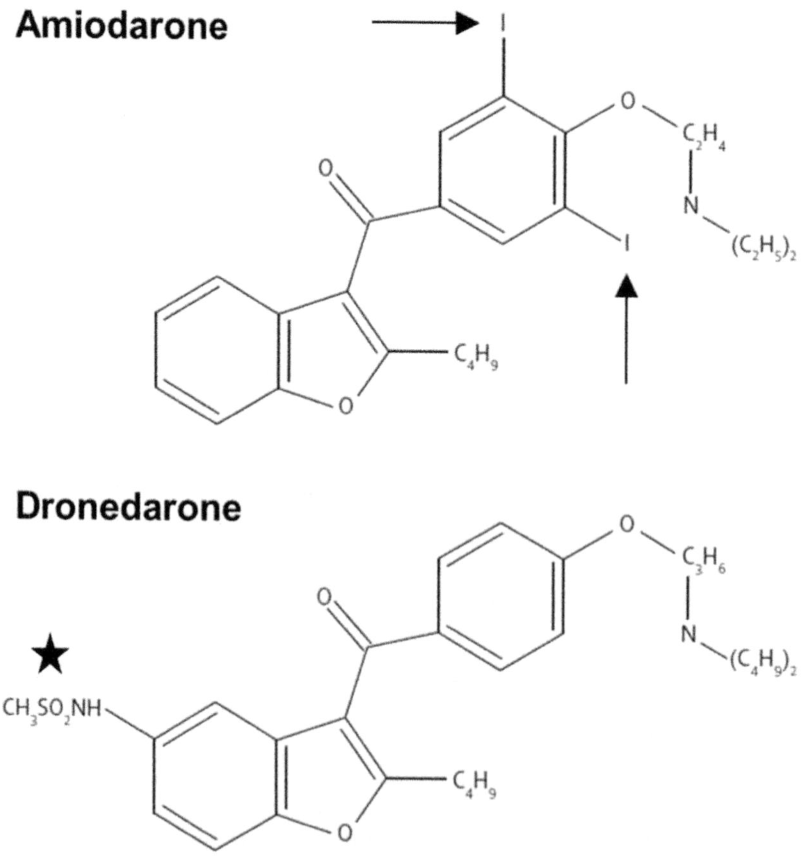

Fig. 1. Molecular structure of amiodarone and dronedarone. Dronedarone is derived from amiodarone by removing the iodine atoms (*arrows*) and adding a methylsulfonamide moiety (*star*). (*Adapted from* Dobrev D, Nattel S. New antiarrhythmic drugs for treatment of atrial fibrillation. Lancet 2010;375:1214; with permission.)

rest than ventricular myocytes. Another mechanism that may provide atrial-selective properties to dronedarone is the muscarinic receptor-independent blockade of the acetylcholine-dependent potassium current ($I_{K,Ach}$) at low concentrations.[12,13] Finally, Bogdan and colleagues[11] also showed that moderate concentrations of dronedarone block the pacemaker current (I_f) in *HCN4*-transfected cells.[11]

Pharmacodynamics: Cellular and Global Effects

Negative chronotropy
Dronedarone decreases automaticity in isolated sinus node cells.[14] In vivo, it reduces sinus rhythm heart rate without affecting isoproterenol-induced heart rate increase or verapamil-induced heart rate decrease.[15] The addition of ivabradine does not further decrease heart rate, suggesting that the negative chronotropic response to dronedarone is mainly related to I_f inhibition rather than adrenergic or I_{CaL} blockade.

Negative dromotropy
In anesthetized pigs, dronedarone prolongs the PR interval and decreases the ventricular rate during AF, but has no effect when added to ivabradine.[16] This would suggest that dronedarone's negative dromotropic effect might be mediated by I_f inhibition, although the role of I_f in atrioventricular conduction is unclear. Clinically, the AV blocking effect of dronedarone provides it with a beneficial rate control effect during AF.[17]

Negative inotropy
Dronedarone decreases systolic intracellular calcium concentration, cell shortening, and ventricular contractility.[9] This negative inotropic effect likely underlies the increased mortality associated with dronedarone in patients with severe heart failure (HF) with systolic dysfunction.[18]

Ventricular effects
Dronedarone prolongs the QT and QTc intervals, ventricular action potential duration and refractory periods in chronic animal studies.[14] Like amiodarone (but unlike sotalol), it does not increase repolarization dispersion and has minimal reverse use dependence and might thus be less arrhythmogenic.[14,19] Dronedarone also decreases ventricular action potential upstroke dV/Dt[14] and conduction velocity.[9]

Atrial effects
Chronic dronedarone prolongs the action potential duration and refractory period of isolated atrial myocytes.[20] In contrast, acute administration of dronedarone decreases the action potential duration. Both acute and chronic dronedarone decrease upstroke velocity (dV/dt). Dronedarone decreases pulmonary vein spontaneous and hydrogen peroxide–induced firing.[21] The combination of decreased pulmonary vein firing, increased refractoriness and reduced conduction velocity (dV/dt) underlies the anti-AF effect of dronedarone.[22]

CLINICAL TRIAL DATA

Several RCTs assessed the efficacy and safety of dronedarone in patients with nonpermanent AF, permanent AF, and HF (**Table 1**).

Dronedarone Reduces Recurrence of Atrial Fibrillation

The efficacy of dronedarone in maintaining sinus rhythm after conversion from AF was assessed in 3 trials: Dronedarone Atrial FibrillatioN study after Electrical Cardioversion (DAFNE),[23] American-Australian-African Trial With Dronedarone in Patients With Atrial Fibrillation or Atrial Flutter for the Maintenance of Sinus Rhythm (ADONIS),[24] and EURopean Trial In Atrial Fibrillation (AF) or Flutter (AFL) Patients Receiving Dronedarone for the maIntenance of Sinus Rhythm (EURIDIS).[24] The DAFNE study assessed whether dronedarone in 3 different doses (400, 600, or 800 mg BID) versus placebo reduced AF recurrence after chemical or electrical cardioversion from persistent AF (defined as an AF episode lasting 72 hours to 12 months).[23] At 6 months of follow-up, dronedarone 400 mg BID reduced AF recurrence by 55% versus placebo (95% CI, 72%–28%; $P = .001$). The risk reduction for higher doses was not statistically significant. Drug discontinuation, mainly owing to gastrointestinal (GI) side effects, occurred in 3.9% of subjects at the lowest dose (vs none in the placebo group). Subsequently, ADONIS and EURIDIS,[24] 2 trials with identical designs, assessed the efficacy of dronedarone in maintaining sinus rhythm in larger cohorts of patients with paroxysmal or persistent AF after spontaneous, chemical, or electrical conversion. In total, 409 and 828 patients were respectively randomized to placebo or dronedarone 400 mg BID, and followed for 12 months with periodic clinical visits and transtelephonic electrocardiogram transmission. In the combined analysis, 75% and 62% of patients on placebo and dronedarone, respectively, reached the primary endpoint of AF recurrence (hazard ratio [HR], 0.75; 95% CI, 0.65–0.87; $P <.001$). Dronedarone also significantly reduced the secondary

Table 1
Summary of main randomized clinical trials of dronedarone

Study	n	Population	Study Groups	Primary Endpoint	Follow-up (mo)	Main Result	Comments
Nonpermanent AF trials							
DAFNE[23]	270	PersAF (72 h–12 mo) with planned cardioversion.	Dron (400, 600, or 800 BID) or Plac	Time to first AF recurrence after conversion (n = 199) (transtelephonic monitor)	6	Only Dron 400 BID significantly increased time to first AF recurrence vs Plac (60 vs 5.3 d; $P = .001$).	Recurrence rates at 6 mo: Dron 65% vs Plac 90%. High Dron doses were not more effective but were associated with more adverse effects.
ADONIS[24]	625	ParoxAF or PersAF converted in preceding 3 mo	Dron 400 BID or Plac	Time to first AF recurrence (transtelephonic monitor)	12	Median time to AF recurrence: Dron 158 d vs Plac 59 d ($P = .002$).	Recurrence rate at 12 mo: Dron 61% vs Plac 73%. Dron decreased ventricular rate during AF.
EURIDIS[24]	612	ParoxAF or PersAF converted in preceding 3 mo	Dron 400 BID or Plac	Time to first AF recurrence (transtelephonic monitor)	12	Median time to AF recurrence: Dron 96 d vs Plac 41 d ($P = .01$).	Recurrence rate at 12 mo: Dron 67% vs Plac 78%. Dron decreased ventricular rate during AF. Dron decreased hospitalization or death.
ATHENA[26]	4628	ParoxAF or PersAF in preceding 6 mo with additional risk factors.	Dron 400 BID or Plac	First CV hospitalization or death from any cause	Median 22 Min 12	Dron decreased the primary endpoint (32% vs 39%, P <.001)	Dron decreased CV death and hospitalization for AF and for ACS. *Risk profile:* Mean age 72; HF 21% (mainly NYHA II); LVEF <35% 4%; CAD 30%; HTN 86%; DM NR; Dig 14%.
DIONYSOS[47]	504	PersAF (>72 h) with planned cardioversion.	Dron 400 BID or Amiodaone 600 × 28 d then 200	AF recurrence or nonconversion (12-lead ECG) or study drug discontinuation	Median 7	The primary endpoint occurred in 75% and 59% of patients on dron or amiodarone, respectively (P <.0001).	Dron associated with more AF recurrence, more GI adverse effects but fewer non-GI adverse effects including thyroid and neurologic toxicities.

Trial	N	Population	Drug groups	Primary endpoint	Duration (mo)	Results	Comments / Risk profile
HARMONY[77]	134	AF with duration <7 d and burden 2%–70% on dual-chamber pacemaker interrogation	Ranol 750, Dron 225, Ranol 750 + Dron 150, Ranol 750 + Dron 225, or Plac[b]	AF burden over 12 wk (absolute and percent change from baseline)	3	Ranol 750 + Dron 150 was the only group associated with decreased AF burden vs Plac (P = .008).	Drug combination was associated with higher rates of adverse events but comparable rates of adverse events leading to drug discontinuation as either drug alone.
Permanent AF trials							
ERATO[43]	174	PermAF ≥6 mo with ventricular rate ≥80 bpm	Dron 400 BID or Plac	Change in mean ventricular rate on a 24-h Holter monitoring at day 14 vs 0	4	At 14 d, Dron decreased mean ventricular rate by 11.7 bpm vs 0.7 bpm increase for Plac (P <.0001).	Rate reduction was sustained at 4 mo. Peak heart rate during exercise was also reduced vs Plac (P <.0001) without changes in exercise tolerance.
PALLAS[44a]	3236	PermAF ≥6 mo and age ≥65 with an additional risk factor	Dron 400 BID or Plac	Coprimary endpoints: (1) stroke, MI, systemic embolism or CV death; (2) CV hospitalization or death from any cause	Median 3.5	Both primary endpoints occurred more in Dron. First coprimary endpoint: HR, 2.29, P = .002. Second coprimary endpoint: HR, 1.95, P <.001.	Dronedarone increased all-cause mortality (HR, 1.94, P = .049). *Risk profile:* Mean age 75; HF 68%; LVEF <40% 21%; CAD 41%; HTN 84%; DM 36%; Dig 33%.
Heart failure trial							
ANDROMEDA[18a]	627	New or worsening HF with LV systolic dysfunction (LVEF ≈ 35% or less).	Dron 400 BID or Plac	Death from any cause or hospitalization for worsening HF	Median 2	Study prematurely terminated because of increased all-cause mortality in the Dron group (8.1% vs 3.8% in Plac; P = .03).	Main causes of death: HF and arrhythmia or sudden death. *Risk profile:* Mean age 72; HF 100%; LVEF <35% 100%; CAD 65%; HTN 37%; DM 22%; AF 38%; Dig 31%.

Abbreviations: ACS, acute coronary syndrome; AF, atrial fibrillation; BID, twice daily; bpm, beats per minute; CAD, coronary artery disease; CV, cardiovascular; Dig, digoxin; DM, diabetes mellitus; Dron, dronedarone; GI, gastrointestinal; h, hours; HF, heart failure; HR, hazard ratio; HTN, hypertension; LV, left ventricular; LVEF, left ventricular ejection fraction; mo, months; NR, not reported; NYHA, New York Heart Association class; ParoxAF, paroxysmal AF; PermAF, permanent AF; PersAF, persistent AF; Plac, placebo; Ranol, ranolazine.

[a] Prematurely terminated because of increased events in the dronedarone group.

[b] All drugs given BID at the doses shown.

Data from Refs. 18,23,24,26,43,44,47,77

endpoints of ventricular rate at first AF recurrence (117 vs 103 beats/min), symptomatic AF recurrence (HR, 0.71) and hospitalization or death (HR, 0.73). With the exception of a higher incidence of creatinine increase in the dronedarone group, no difference in rates of adverse events between groups was observed. Study drug was discontinued in 15% and 18% of patients in the placebo and dronedarone groups, respectively. Overall, dronedarone moderately reduces both overall and symptomatic AF recurrences, with a good tolerability profile compared with placebo.

Dronedarone Reduces Hospitalizations in Nonpermanent Atrial Fibrillation

A Trial With Dronedarone to Prevent Hospitalization or Death in Patients With Atrial Fibrillation (ATHENA), the largest completed dronedarone trial, was designed to assess whether dronedarone reduces cardiovascular events in AF patients, as compared with placebo.[25,26] A total of 4628 patients with paroxysmal or persistent AF and 1 or more risk factors were randomized to receive dronedarone 400 mg BID or placebo and followed for 21 ± 5 months. The primary endpoint was cardiovascular hospitalization or death from any cause. A primary outcome event occurred in 32% and 39% of patients in the dronedarone and placebo groups, respectively (HR, 0.79; 95% CI, 0.69–0.84; P <.001). Dronedarone also significantly decreased the secondary outcomes of cardiovascular death (HR, 0.71) and death from cardiac arrhythmia (HR, 0.55). A post hoc analysis of hospitalizations in ATHENA showed that the beneficial effect of dronedarone is mainly driven by decreased AF-related hospitalizations but also hospitalizations for acute coronary syndrome (P = .03).[27] Length of hospitalization was also reduced. The benefit of dronedarone did not depend on prespecified baseline characteristics, including left ventricular ejection fraction and HF.[26,28] A metaanalysis combining patients with lone AF from EURIDIS, ADNONIS, and ATHENA showed that dronedarone also reduces hospitalizations in this low-risk group.[29]

In ATHENA,[26] dronedarone was associated with increased risk of total adverse events (predominantly GI, skin related, and creatinine increase), but a similar risk of serious adverse events. Premature discontinuation of study drug because of an adverse event occurred in 13% of patients in the dronedarone group and 8% of patients in the placebo group (P <.001). Rates of abnormal liver function tests were similar (approximately 0.5%), but routine liver function tests were not performed.

The rhythm and rate control effects of dronedarone were further characterized in a post hoc analysis.[17] This study showed that dronedarone delayed and decreased the likelihood of AF recurrence in patients with sinus rhythm at baseline (HR, 0.75), decreased the need for cardioversion (HR, 0.68), and prevented progression to permanent AF (8% for dronedarone, 13% for placebo groups; P <.001). Dronedarone was associated with a lower mean heart rate than placebo in first arrhythmia recurrence (85.3 vs 95.5 bpm) and in sinus rhythm (61.5 vs 65.0 bpm).

A post hoc analysis of ATHENA showed that dronedarone reduced the risk of stroke from 1.8% per year to 1.2% per year (HR, 0.66; 95% CI, 0.46–0.96; P = .027).[30] The effect on stroke risk might be related to reduction in AF burden; such benefit has never been shown for a strategy of pharmacologic rhythm control.[31] Alternate explanations include a pleiotropic effect of dronedarone, based on a rat model in which dronedarone reduced infarct size and improved neurologic outcome after middle cerebral artery occlusion.[32] Unexpectedly, the drug reduced the incidence of a first acute coronary syndrome in ATHENA.[33] Postulated mechanisms include improvement of coronary microcirculation through modulation of gene expression,[34] antithrombotic effects[35] or simply the benefit of heart rate reduction.

The ATHENA trial showed that dronedarone reduced cardiovascular hospitalizations, was generally well tolerated and safe in patients with coronary artery disease (CAD). The drug also seemed to be cost effective in preventing death or hospitalizations (CAD $7560 per quality-adjusted life-year).[36]

Dronedarone Increases Mortality in Heart Failure

HF with systolic dysfunction is frequently complicated by atrial and ventricular arrhythmias, which confer significant morbidity and mortality. Several AADs have previously been evaluated in the HF population, showing either lack of benefit[37–39] or increased mortality.[40] The Antiarrhythmic trial with DROnedarone in Moderate to severe congestive heart failure Evaluating morbidity DecreAse (ANDROMEDA) trial[18] assessed whether dronedarone could reduce cardiovascular morbidity and mortality in patients hospitalized for worsened HF and severe systolic dysfunction. A total of 627 patients were randomized to dronedarone 400 mg BID or placebo. The trial was terminated prematurely after a median follow-up of 2 months because of increased mortality in the dronedarone group (8.1%) versus placebo (3.8%; HR, 2.13;

95% CI, 1.07–4.25; P = .03). The excess mortality in the dronedarone group was attributable to cardiovascular death (7.7% vs 2.8%), mainly owing to worsened HF (3.2% vs 0.6%) and documented arrhythmia (1.9% vs 0.6%). Based on these results, dronedarone should not be used in patients with HF and/or severe systolic dysfunction, although the exact recommendations vary among cardiovascular societies,[1,41,42] as discussed.

Dronedarone Increases Mortality in Permanent Atrial Fibrillation

In follow-up of ATHENA[26] and European Study of Dronedarone in Atrial Fibrillation (ERATO)[43] (a small trial that showed decreased heart rate with dronedarone in permanent AF), the Permanent Atrial fibriLLAtion Outcome Study Using Dronedarone on Top of Standard Therapy (PALLAS) trial[44] was designed to test whether dronedarone could reduce major cardiovascular events in high-risk patients with permanent AF. The study included patients 65 years or older with cardiovascular risk factors in whom a rate control strategy had been chosen for persistent AF/flutter of greater than 6 months' duration. A total of 3236 patients were randomized to either dronedarone or placebo. The first coprimary endpoint was a composite of stroke, myocardial infarction, systemic embolism, and cardiovascular death. The second coprimary endpoint was cardiovascular hospitalization or death. After a median follow-up of 3.5 months, the study was terminated prematurely because of an excess of events in the dronedarone group (first coprimary endpoint: HR, 2.29; 95% CI, 1.34–3.94; P = .002; second coprimary endpoint: HR, 1.95; 95% CI, 1.45–2.62; P <.001). There were 25 deaths in the dronedarone group versus 13 in the placebo group (P = .049). Dronedarone also increased cardiovascular death, and death from arrhythmia, stroke, cardiovascular hospitalization, and HF. The exact underlying mechanism by which dronedarone increases cardiovascular events in PALLAS, but decreased them in ATHENA, is not entirely understood.[45] Patients in PALLAS had more HF than in ATHENA, which might in part account for the increased adverse events. Moreover, PALLAS patients were more likely to be cotreated with digoxin, which interacts with dronedarone, as discussed elsewhere in this paper.[46] Dronedarone is now contraindicated in patients with permanent AF.[1,41,42]

Dronedarone Versus Amiodarone

Dronedarone was developed to be an amiodarone derivative with fewer adverse effects. Consequently, comparing these drugs for efficacy in maintaining sinus rhythm and tolerability is highly informative. This was attempted in the Efficacy & Safety of Dronedarone Versus Amiodarone for the Maintenance of Sinus Rhythm in Patients With Atrial Fibrillation (DIONYSOS) trial,[47] which randomized 504 patients with AF of greater than 72 hours in whom a rhythm control strategy was selected, to either dronedarone (400 mg BID) or amiodarone (600 mg daily for 28 days, then 200 mg daily). The primary endpoint was a composite of AF recurrence or study drug discontinuation for inefficacy or intolerance. After a median treatment duration of 7 months, the primary endpoint occurred in 75% and 59% of patients in the dronedarone and amiodarone groups, respectively (HR, 1.59; 95% CI, 1.28–1.98; P <.0001). AF recurrence occurred in 64% versus 42% and drug discontinuation occurred in 10% versus 13% of patients in the dronedarone and amiodarone groups, respectively, highlighting the much lower efficacy but somewhat better tolerability of dronedarone. Overall, 39% versus 45% of patients on dronedarone and amiodarone groups, respectively, had an adverse event (HR, 0.80; 95% CI, 0.60–1.07; P = .129). Dronedarone was associated with lower thyroid and neurologic (tremor or sleep disorder) toxicities but more GI side effects (diarrhea and nausea), compared with amiodarone. Liver enzyme elevation occurred in similar proportions of patients. Dronedarone-treated patients had lower rates of bradycardia (heart rate ≤50/min) and QTc prolongation (≥500 ms), and fewer supratherapeutic International Normalized Ratio (>4.5) and hemorrhagic events than amiodarone-treated patients.

Data from DIONYSOS demonstrate the lower efficacy and higher GI adverse events of dronedarone compared with its parent drug amiodarone. Conversely, it is associated with less thyroid and neurologic toxicity, and less warfarin interaction. Of note, the trial was not designed to compare efficacy with regard to other clinical endpoints, such as hospitalization and mortality, as was the ATHENA trial. These results are consistent with a prior metaanalysis, which suggested that dronedarone is less effective to maintain sinus rhythm and but with fewer adverse effects than amiodarone.[48] This study also showed a trend toward greater mortality with amiodarone (odds ratio [OR], 1.61; 95% CI, 0.97–2.68; P = .066).[48]

Systematic Reviews and Metaanalysis

Lafuente-Lafuente and colleagues[49] recently published a Cochrane systematic review of clinical trials of AAD for maintenance of sinus rhythm after conversion from AF. Their metaanalysis of 4 placebo-controlled dronedarone studies (DAFNE, EURIDIS, ADONIS, and ATHENA) showed that dronedarone was significantly associated with lower AF recurrence (OR, 0.59), less stroke (OR, 0.66), more proarrhythmia (OR, 2.5), and more drug withdrawals because of adverse effects (OR, 1.6). There was no difference in overall mortality.

Another metaanalysis included 9664 patients from all AF placebo-controlled trials including PALLAS, ERATO, and patients with AF from ANDROMEDA.[50] Despite adjustment, the significant interstudy heterogeneity of dronedarone effects on clinical outcomes complicates interpretation. In the permanent AF subgroup, dronedarone increases cardiovascular mortality (HR, 2.32; 95% CI, 1.13–4.75). In contrast, dronedarone decreases cardiovascular hospitalization (HR, 0.751; 95% CI, 0.68–0.83) in the nonpermanent AF subgroup. Dronedarone also showed a trend toward more cardiovascular mortality in the subgroup of patients on digoxin (HR, 2.16; 95% CI, 0.91–6.54). Dronedarone effects in other subgroups (HF, CAD) were either inconclusive because of study interaction or nonsignificant.

A mixed treatment comparison metaanalysis of RCTs involving different AADs in AF suggested that dronedarone is the least effective in maintaining sinus rhythm.[51] In contrast, it is the only AAD that decreases the risk of stroke, and it had the lowest rate of proarrhythmic events including bradycardia. Sotalol and possibly amiodarone increase mortality, while dronedarone does not. Of note, neither ANDROMEDA (which is not an AF trial) nor PALLAS (not yet published at the time) were included in the analysis.

REAL-WORLD EXPERIENCE
Large Cohort Studies

The largest real-world safety data comes from a Swedish registry including 4856 AF patients receiving dronedarone and 170,139 AF patients not receiving the drug.[52] In accordance with clinical recommendations, dronedarone was prescribed to patients with fewer comorbidities. Compared with other AADs, dronedarone and flecainide had the lowest unadjusted mortality rates. After propensity score matching the association with lower mortality remained. The results of this study should be interpreted as a reassurance regarding the safety of dronedarone when used in otherwise healthy AF patients. Whether dronedarone is indeed superior is uncertain. Allen Lapointe and colleagues[53] recently compared the efficacy of dronedarone and other AADs by

retrospectively assessing the time from first AAD prescription to first hospitalization for AF in 8562 patients without CAD or HF. Dronedarone was associated with an increased risk of AF hospitalization compared with amiodarone (HR, 2.6), sotalol (HR, 1.7), and class IC AAD (HR, 1.6). Recognizing the inherent limitations of retrospective studies, these data suggest that dronedarone may be less effective than other AADs, which was suggested in the mixed treatment comparison metaanalysis.[51]

Postapproval Reports of Adverse Events

Since dronedarone's approval, several cases of ventricular proarrhythmia have been reported in the literature[54,55] and in the FDA's adverse event reporting system.[56] In the 2-year period after dronedarone approval by the FDA, there were 138 cases of ventricular arrhythmia (37 torsades des pointes) reported in association with dronedarone versus 113 cases (29 torsades des pointes) for amiodarone.[56] Although this observation raises concern for potential increased proarrhythmic effects of dronedarone, the significance of the comparison must be tempered by the inherent bias associated with adverse event reporting rates being preferentially higher for newer drugs. On the other hand, the total number of patients receiving amiodarone was likely much higher.

Cases of lung toxicity[57–59] and severe hepatitis and liver failure[60,61] have also been reported. Accordingly, dronedarone should not be used in patients with previous lung or hepatic toxicity from amiodarone. It should also be avoided in patients with underlying hepatic disease. Liver function tests should be periodically performed for at least the first 6 months of therapy to detect preclinical hepatic injury. Severe cutaneous hypersensitivity reactions have also been reported.[62,63]

USE FOR OTHER INDICATIONS

Dronedarone is only approved for maintenance of sinus rhythm after conversion from AF. Some clinicians also reported effective treatment of ventricular tachycardia in nonischemic cardiomyopathy with dronedarone.[64–67] In contrast, animal studies suggest that dronedarone is associated with decreased survival in cardiac arrest, but does not seem to increase defibrillation threshold as seen with amiodarone.[68,69] Based on results from ANDROMEDA, dronedarone is contraindicated in patients with moderate to severe HF. Its use in less severe HF or in systolic dysfunction without HF is strongly discouraged. A potential use of dronedarone has been suggested in

Chagas disease cardiomyopathy, through antiparasitic and antiarrhythmic effects, also reported for amiodarone.[70]

DRUG INTERACTIONS

Dronedarone is metabolized by, and is a moderate inhibitor of, CYP3A4. It is also a potent P-glycoprotein inhibitor. Correspondingly, it is associated with many drug interactions.[8] The most clinically important ones are discussed.

Strong CYP3A4 Inhibitors

Dronedarone should not be used in combination with potent CYP3A4 inhibitors, because of the risk of dronedarone intoxication. Strong CYP3A4 inhibitors include antifungal agents such as ketoconazole, the macrolide antibiotic clarithromycin, and protease inhibitors like ritonavir.

Digoxin

By blocking P-glycoprotein, dronedarone increases digoxin plasma levels. In a post hoc analysis of PALLAS, Hohnloser and colleagues[46] assessed the interaction of digoxin and dronedarone use on mortality outcomes. Patients randomized to dronedarone had significantly higher digoxin plasma concentrations at day 7 compared with those randomized to placebo (median, 1.1 vs 0.7 ng/mL; P <.0001). Among patients on digoxin at baseline, dronedarone was associated with an increased all-cause mortality (HR, 5.5; P <.01). In contrast, mortality was unchanged by dronedarone in patients without digoxin (HR, 0.82; P = NS; interaction P = .02). Similar results were observed for CV and arrhythmic mortality, but not for HF events. The authors speculate that the dronedarone-related increase in mortality is, at least in part, mediated by an interaction with digoxin. The mechanism is most likely pharmacokinetic, that is, dronedarone produces increased digoxin concentrations, which are associated with increased mortality, as shown in a post hoc analysis of the Digitalis Investigation Group (DIG) trial.[71] Alternatively, it is possible that the combination of digoxin and dronedarone itself is proarrhythmic. Acute ouabain exposure is associated with increased VF inducibility in dronedarone-treated explanted rabbit hearts animals compared with nondronedarone treated controls.[72]

Based on these data, concurrent use of dronedarone and digoxin should avoided. If prescribed, digoxin dose reduction (approximately 50%) is recommended. Plasma digoxin levels should be less than 0.8 ng/mL (1 nmol/L).

Pharmacokinetic Interactions with Other Cardiovascular Drugs

P-glycoprotein and CYP3A4 inhibition by dronedarone increases plasma concentrations of novel oral anticoagulants.[73] Dose adjustment should be considered, depending on the specific drug and patient characteristics like thromboembolic versus hemorrhagic risks and renal function. Dronedarone can also increase the International Normalized Ratio in warfarin users,[74] and plasma levels of calcium channel blockers. Concurrent use of dronedarone and nondihydropyridine calcium channel blockers (verapamil or diltiazem) should be avoided, or if used carefully monitored for signs of toxicity. Finally, dronedarone can increase plasma levels of statins, so patients on both should avoid high statin doses and be monitored for muscle toxicity.

QT-Prolonging Drugs

Although the proarrhythmic risk with dronedarone is low, its concurrent use with other QT-prolonging drug should be avoided because of the increased potential for torsades des pointes.

RECOMMENDATIONS FOR CONTEMPORARY USE
Clinical Practice Guidelines

Cardiovascular societies from Canada (Canadian Cardiovascular Society [CCS][42]), Europe (European Cardiovascular Society [ESC][41]) and the United States (American Heart Association [AHA]/American College of Cardiology [ACC]/Heart Rhythm Society [HRS][1]) recently published updated guidelines for the management of AF, integrating results from all RCTs discussed.

When should dronedarone be used?

In patients without structural heart disease, all 3 guidelines consider dronedarone one of the first-line drug therapies for the maintenance of sinus rhythm after conversion from AF. In the AHA/ACC/HRS and CCS guidelines, this also applies to patients with CAD without HF. In contrast, the ESC guidelines recommend sotalol as the first-line AAD in CAD, with dronedarone reserved as a second choice. The AHA/ACC/HRS and ESC also recommend dronedarone as the only first-line agent for patients with left ventricular hypertrophy.

When should dronedarone not be used?

Based on PALLAS, all 3 guidelines recommend that dronedarone should not be used for rate control in permanent AF. Based on results from ANDROMEDA, dronedarone should not be used in patients with HF. The AHA/ACC/HRS state that dronedarone should not be used in patients with New York Heart Association (NYHA) class III and IV patients who have had an episode of decompensated HF in the past 4 weeks, in accordance with the inclusion criteria of ANDROMEDA. The ESC guidelines state that dronedarone should not be used in patients with moderate to severe HF and should be avoided in those with less severe HF, if alternatives exist. In contrast, the CCS extends the recommendation by stating that dronedarone should not be used in any patient with a history of HF or an left ventricular ejection fraction of 40% or less. This recommendation is based on the ANDROMEDA study but also considers the higher rate of baseline HF in PALLAS versus ATHENA as a possible mechanism for dronedarone harm in PALLAS versus its benefit in ATHENA.[45]

Practical Aspects

Dronedarone seems less effective in maintaining sinus rhythm, but may be superior in other aspects, such as stroke reduction and less risk for proarrhythmia and mortality, compared with other rhythm control drugs.[48,51–53] One practical advantage of using dronedarone is its combined rate and rhythm control effects, which reduce the need to add a second drug. If dronedarone is used, concurrent drug use should be examined at baseline and periodically thereafter to identify drug interactions. Liver function testing should be performed before drug initiation, repeated at least once in the first 6 months, and then yearly. A clinical evaluation with an electrocardiogram should be performed at least every year to detect AF, or electrophysiologic toxicity (important QT prolongation or bradycardia). In patients who progress to permanent AF or those who develop HF, dronedarone should be stopped.

FUTURE DIRECTIONS: ANTIARRHYTHMIC DRUG COMBINATION

Based on basic electrophysiology and animal models, the combination of ranolazine and dronedarone has been suggested to increase efficacy at lower doses and thereby reduce adverse effects. Reduced dose dronedarone/ranolazine combinations decreased AF inducibility in both isolated canine preparations[75] and an acute-ischemia pig model.[76] A clinical follow-up, the Study to Evaluate the Effect of Ranolazine and Dronedarone When Given Alone and in Combination in Patients With Paroxysmal Atrial Fibrillation (HARMONY), was performed and recently published.[77] HARMONY compared the efficacy of placebo, ranolazine

alone (750 mg BID), dronedarone alone (225 mg BID), and 2 combinations of ranolazine (750 mg BID) and dronedarone (150 or 225 mg BID) on AF burden in 134 patients with paroxysmal AF implanted with pacemakers. At baseline, mean AF burden was 17.4% (range, 2%–72%). The combination of ranolazine and dronedarone 225 mg BID was the only group with significant reduction of AF burden from baseline versus placebo (-57%; $P = .008$). Of the 20 patients in this group, 9 experienced a 70% or greater reduction in AF burden, and 4 had an increased AF burden. Although the drug combination was associated with higher overall rates of adverse events than either drug alone, the rates of adverse events requiring drug discontinuation were similar in all drug groups. Although these data are promising, a larger clinical trial is warranted before a ranolazine/dronedarone combination can be recommended for clinical use in AF rhythm control.

REFERENCES

1. January CT, Wann LS, Alpert JS, et al. 2014 AHA/ACC/HRS guideline for the management of patients with atrial fibrillation: a report of the American College of Cardiology/American Heart Association Task Force on Practice Guidelines and the Heart Rhythm Society. J Am Coll Cardiol 2014;64:e1–76.
2. Andrade J, Khairy P, Dobrev D, et al. The clinical profile and pathophysiology of atrial fibrillation: relationships among clinical features, epidemiology, and mechanisms. Circ Res 2014;114:1453–68.
3. Gillis AM, Verma A, Talajic M, et al. Canadian Cardiovascular Society atrial fibrillation guidelines 2010: rate and rhythm management. Can J Cardiol 2011;27:47–59.
4. Tadros R, Khairy P, Rouleau JL, et al. Atrial fibrillation in heart failure: drug therapies for rate and rhythm control. Heart Fail Rev 2014;19:315–24.
5. Ehrlich JR, Biliczki P, Hohnloser SH, et al. Atrial-selective approaches for the treatment of atrial fibrillation. J Am Coll Cardiol 2008;51:787–92.
6. Nishida K, Datino T, Macle L, et al. Atrial fibrillation ablation: translating basic mechanistic insights to the patient. J Am Coll Cardiol 2014;64:823–31.
7. Heijman J, Heusch G, Dobrev D. Pleiotropic effects of antiarrhythmic agents: dronedarone in the treatment of atrial fibrillation. Clin Med Insights Cardiol 2013;7:127–40.
8. Sanofi-Aventis. Multaq product monograph. 2014.
9. Gautier P, Guillemare E, Marion A, et al. Electrophysiologic characterization of dronedarone in guinea pig ventricular cells. J Cardiovasc Pharmacol 2003;41:191–202.
10. Lalevee N, Nargeot J, Barrere-Lemaire S, et al. Effects of amiodarone and dronedarone on voltage-dependent

sodium current in human cardiomyocytes. J Cardiovasc Electrophysiol 2003;14:885–90.

11. Bogdan R, Goegelein H, Ruetten H. Effect of drone-darone on Na+, Ca2+ and HCN channels. Naunyn Schmiedebergs Arch Pharmacol 2011;383:347–56.

12. Altomare C, Barbuti A, Viscomi C, et al. Effects of dronedarone on acetylcholine-activated current in rabbit SAN cells. Br J Pharmacol 2000;130:1315–20.

13. Guillemare E, Marion A, Nisato D, et al. Inhibitory effects of dronedarone on muscarinic K+ current in guinea pig atrial cells. J Cardiovasc Pharmacol 2000;36:802–5.

14. Sun W, Sarma JS, Singh BN. Electrophysiological effects of dronedarone (SR33589), a noniodinated benzofuran derivative, in the rabbit heart: comparison with amiodarone. Circulation 1999;100:2276–81.

15. Sobrado LF, Varone BB, Machado AD, et al. Dronedarone's inhibition of If current is the primary mechanism responsible for its bradycardic effect. J Cardiovasc Electrophysiol 2013;24:914–8.

16. Verrier RL, Sobrado MF, Pagotto VP, et al. Inhibition of I(f) in the atrioventricular node as a mechanism for dronedarone's reduction in ventricular rate during atrial fibrillation. Heart Rhythm 2013;10:1692–7.

17. Page RL, Connolly SJ, Crijns HJ, et al. Rhythm- and rate-controlling effects of dronedarone in patients with atrial fibrillation (from the ATHENA trial). Am J Cardiol 2011;107:1019–22.

18. Kober L, Torp-Pedersen C, McMurray JJ, et al. Increased mortality after dronedarone therapy for severe heart failure. N Engl J Med 2008;358:2678–87.

19. Milberg P, Frommeyer G, Uphaus T, et al. Electrophysiologic profile of dronedarone on the ventricular level: beneficial effect on postrepolarization refractoriness in the presence of rapid phase 3 repolarization. J Cardiovasc Pharmacol 2012;59:92–100.

20. Sun W, Sarma JS, Singh BN. Chronic and acute effects of dronedarone on the action potential of rabbit atrial muscle preparations: comparison with amiodarone. J Cardiovasc Pharmacol 2002;39:677–84.

21. Hanafy DA, Chen YC, Chang SL, et al. Different effects of dronedarone and amiodarone on pulmonary vein electrophysiology, mechanical properties and H2O2-induced arrhythmogenicity. Eur J Pharmacol 2013;702:103–8.

22. Dobrev D, Nattel S. New antiarrhythmic drugs for treatment of atrial fibrillation. Lancet 2010;375:1212–23.

23. Touboul P, Brugada J, Capucci A, et al. Dronedarone for prevention of atrial fibrillation: a dose-ranging study. Eur Heart J 2003;24:1481–7.

24. Singh BN, Connolly SJ, Crijns HJ, et al. Dronedarone for maintenance of sinus rhythm in atrial fibrillation or flutter. N Engl J Med 2007;357:987–99.

25. Hohnloser SH, Connolly SJ, Crijns HJ, et al. Rationale and design of ATHENA: a placebo-controlled, double-blind, parallel arm Trial to assess the efficacy of dronedarone 400 mg bid for the prevention of cardiovascular Hospitalization or death from any cause in patiENts with Atrial fibrillation/atrial flutter. J Cardiovasc Electrophysiol 2008;19:69–73.

26. Hohnloser SH, Crijns HJ, van Eickels M, et al. Effect of dronedarone on cardiovascular events in atrial fibrillation. N Engl J Med 2009;360:668–78.

27. Torp-Pedersen C, Crijns HJ, Gaudin C, et al. Impact of dronedarone on hospitalization burden in patients with atrial fibrillation: results from the ATHENA study. Europace 2011;13:1118–26.

28. Hohnloser SH, Crijns HJ, van Eickels M, et al. Dronedarone in patients with congestive heart failure: insights from ATHENA. Eur Heart J 2010;31:1717–21.

29. Duray GZ, Torp-Pedersen C, Connolly SJ, et al. Effects of dronedarone on clinical outcomes in patients with lone atrial fibrillation: pooled post hoc analysis from the ATHENA/EURIDIS/ADONIS studies. J Cardiovasc Electrophysiol 2011;22:770–6.

30. Connolly SJ, Crijns HJ, Torp-Pedersen C, et al. Analysis of stroke in ATHENA: a placebo-controlled, double-blind, parallel-arm trial to assess the efficacy of dronedarone 400 mg BID for the prevention of cardiovascular hospitalization or death from any cause in patients with atrial fibrillation/atrial flutter. Circulation 2009;120:1174–80.

31. Wyse DG, Waldo AL, DiMarco JP, et al. A comparison of rate control and rhythm control in patients with atrial fibrillation. N Engl J Med 2002;347:1825–33.

32. Engelhorn T, Schwarz MA, Heusch G, et al. Reduction of cerebral infarct size by dronedarone. Cardiovasc Drugs Ther 2011;25:523–9.

33. Pisters R, Hohnloser SH, Connolly SJ, et al. Effect of dronedarone on clinical end points in patients with atrial fibrillation and coronary heart disease: insights from the ATHENA trial. Europace 2014;16:174–81.

34. Bukowska A, Hammwohner M, Sixdorf A, et al. Dronedarone prevents microcirculatory abnormalities in the left ventricle during atrial tachypacing in pigs. Br J Pharmacol 2012;166:964–80.

35. Breitenstein A, Sluka SH, Akhmedov A, et al. Dronedarone reduces arterial thrombus formation. Basic Res Cardiol 2012;107:302.

36. Berg J, Sauriol L, Connolly S, et al. Cost-effectiveness of dronedarone in patients with atrial fibrillation in the ATHENA trial. Can J Cardiol 2013;29:1249–55.

37. Torp-Pedersen C, Moller M, Bloch-Thomsen PE, et al. Dofetilide in patients with congestive heart failure and left ventricular dysfunction. Danish Investigations of Arrhythmia and Mortality on Dofetilide Study Group. N Engl J Med 1999;341:857–65.

38. Singh SN, Fletcher RD, Fisher SG, et al. Amiodarone in patients with congestive heart failure and asymptomatic ventricular arrhythmia. Survival trial of

antiarrhythmic therapy in congestive heart failure. N Engl J Med 1995;333:77–82.

39. Bardy GH, Lee KL, Mark DB, et al. Amiodarone or an implantable cardioverter-defibrillator for congestive heart failure. N Engl J Med 2005;352:225–37.

40. Waldo AL, Camm AJ, deRuyter H, et al. Effect of d-sotalol on mortality in patients with left ventricular dysfunction after recent and remote myocardial infarction. The SWORD Investigators. Survival with Oral d-Sotalol. Lancet 1996;348:7–12.

41. Camm AJ, Lip GY, De Caterina R, et al. 2012 focused update of the ESC Guidelines for the management of atrial fibrillation: an update of the 2010 ESC Guidelines for the management of atrial fibrillation. Developed with the special contribution of the European Heart Rhythm Association. Eur Heart J 2012;33:2719–47.

42. Skanes AC, Healey JS, Cairns JA, et al. Focused 2012 update of the Canadian Cardiovascular Society atrial fibrillation guidelines: recommendations for stroke prevention and rate/rhythm control. Can J Cardiol 2012;28:125–36.

43. Davy JM, Herold M, Hoglund C, et al. Dronedarone for the control of ventricular rate in permanent atrial fibrillation: the Efficacy and safety of dRonedArone for the cOntrol of ventricular rate during atrial fibrillation (ERATO) study. Am Heart J 2008;156(527):e1–9.

44. Connolly SJ, Camm AJ, Halperin JL, et al. Dronedarone in high-risk permanent atrial fibrillation. N Engl J Med 2011;365:2268–76.

45. Nattel S. Dronedarone in atrial fibrillation–Jekyll and Hyde? N Engl J Med 2011;365:2321–2.

46. Hohnloser SH, Halperin JL, Camm AJ, et al. Interaction between digoxin and dronedarone in the PALLAS trial. Circ Arrhythm Electrophysiol 2014;7: 1019–25.

47. Le Heuzey JY, De Ferrari GM, Radzik D, et al. A short-term, randomized, double-blind, parallel-group study to evaluate the efficacy and safety of dronedarone versus amiodarone in patients with persistent atrial fibrillation: the DIONYSOS study. J Cardiovasc Electrophysiol 2010;21:597–605.

48. Piccini JP, Hasselblad V, Peterson ED, et al. Comparative efficacy of dronedarone and amiodarone for the maintenance of sinus rhythm in patients with atrial fibrillation. J Am Coll Cardiol 2009;54: 1089–95.

49. Lafuente-Lafuente C, Valembois L, Bergmann JF, et al. Antiarrhythmics for maintaining sinus rhythm after cardioversion of atrial fibrillation. Cochrane Database Syst Rev 2015;(3):CD005049.

50. Hohnloser SH, Connolly SJ, John Camm A, et al. An individual patient-based meta-analysis of the effects of dronedarone in patients with atrial fibrillation. Europace 2014;16:1117–24.

51. Freemantle N, Lafuente-Lafuente C, Mitchell S, et al. Mixed treatment comparison of dronedarone,

amiodarone, sotalol, flecainide, and propafenone, for the management of atrial fibrillation. Europace 2011;13:329–45.

52. Friberg L. Safety of dronedarone in routine clinical care. J Am Coll Cardiol 2014;63:2376–84.

53. Allen LaPointe NM, Dai D, Thomas L, et al. Comparisons of hospitalization rates among younger atrial fibrillation patients receiving different antiarrhythmic drugs. Circ Cardiovasc Qual Outcomes 2015;8:292–300.

54. Gonzalez JE, Sauer WH, Krantz MJ. Ventricular ectopy and QTc-interval prolongation associated with dronedarone therapy. Pharmacotherapy 2013;33: e179–81.

55. Huemer M, Sarganas G, Bronder E, et al. Torsade de pointes tachycardia in a patient on dronedarone therapy. Pharmacotherapy 2015;35(5):e61–5.

56. Kao DP, Hiatt WR, Krantz MJ. Proarrhythmic potential of dronedarone: emerging evidence from spontaneous adverse event reporting. Pharmacotherapy 2012;32:767–71.

57. Stack S, Nguyen DV, Casto A, et al. Diffuse alveolar damage in a patient receiving dronedarone. Chest 2015;147:e131–3.

58. Siu CW, Wong MP, Ho CM, et al. Fatal lung toxic effects related to dronedarone use. Arch Intern Med 2012;172:516–7.

59. Hernandez Voth AR, Catalan JS, Benavides Manas PD, et al. A 73-year-old man with interstitial lung disease due to dronedarone. Am J Respir Crit Care Med 2012;186:201–2.

60. Jahn S, Zollner G, Lackner C, et al. Severe toxic hepatitis associated with dronedarone. Curr Drug Saf 2013;8:201–2.

61. Joghetaei N, Weirich G, Huber W, et al. Acute liver failure associated with dronedarone. Circ Arrhythm Electrophysiol 2011;4:592–3.

62. Gecks T, Prochnau D, Franz M, et al. Toxic epidermal necrolysis during dronedarone treatment: first report of a severe serious adverse event of a new antiarrhythmic drug. Cardiovasc Toxicol 2015; 15(4):399–401.

63. Smith SM, Al-Bataineh M, Iorfido SB, et al. A case report: Multaq-induced leukocytoclastic vasculitis. Am J Ther 2014;21:e69–70.

64. Shaaraoui M, Freudenberger R, Levin V, et al. Suppression of ventricular tachycardia with dronedarone: a case report. J Cardiovasc Electrophysiol 2011;22:201–2.

65. Nanda S, Levin V, Martinez MW. Ventricular tachycardia in "end stage" hypertrophic cardiomyopathy: a role of dronedarone. Minerva Cardioangiol 2012; 60:637–42.

66. Exposito V, Rodriguez-Entem F, Gonzalez-Enriquez S, et al. Dronedarone for recurrent ventricular tachycardia: a real alternative? Indian Pacing Electrophysiol J 2012;12:73–6.

67. Fink A, Duray GZ, Hohnloser SH. A patient with recurrent atrial fibrillation and monomorphic ventricular tachycardia treated successfully with dronedarone. Europace 2011;13:284–5.

68. Chevalier P, Timour Q, Morel E, et al. Chronic oral amiodarone but not dronedarone therapy increases ventricular defibrillation threshold during acute myocardial ischemia in a closed-chest animal model. J Cardiovasc Pharmacol 2012;59:523–8.

69. Glover BM, Hu X, Aves T, et al. Dronedarone and Captisol-enabled amiodarone in an experimental cardiac arrest. J Cardiovasc Pharmacol 2013;61:385–90.

70. Benaim G, Paniz Mondolfi AE. The emerging role of amiodarone and dronedarone in Chagas disease. Nat Rev Cardiol 2012;9:605–9.

71. Rathore SS, Curtis JP, Wang Y, et al. Association of serum digoxin concentration and outcomes in patients with heart failure. JAMA 2003;289:871–8.

72. Frommeyer G, Milberg P, Schulze Grotthoff J, et al. Dronedarone and digitalis: individually reduced post-repolarization refractoriness enhances life-threatening arrhythmias. Europace 2015;17(8):1300–8.

73. Mochalina N, Juhlin T, Platonov PG, et al. Concomitant use of dronedarone with dabigatran in patients with atrial fibrillation in clinical practice. Thromb Res 2015;135(6):1070–4.

74. Pogge EK, Haber SL. Elevated international normalized ratio associated with use of dronedarone and warfarin. Ann Pharmacother 2011;45:e46.

75. Burashnikov A, Sicouri S, Di Diego JM, et al. Synergistic effect of the combination of ranolazine and dronedarone to suppress atrial fibrillation. J Am Coll Cardiol 2010;56:1216–24.

76. Verrier RL, Pagotto VP, Kanas AF, et al. Low doses of ranolazine and dronedarone in combination exert potent protection against atrial fibrillation and vulnerability to ventricular arrhythmias during acute myocardial ischemia. Heart Rhythm 2013; 10:121–7.

77. Reiffel JA, Camm AJ, Belardinelli L, et al. The HARMONY trial: combined ranolazine and dronedarone in the management of paroxysmal atrial fibrillation: mechanistic and therapeutic synergism. Circ Arrhythm Electrophysiol 2015;8(5):1048–56.

Ranolazine: Electrophysiologic Effect, Efficacy, and Safety in Patients with Cardiac Arrhythmias

Mohammad Shenasa, MD*, Hamid Assadi, MD,
Shahriar Heidary, MD, Hossein Shenasa, MD

KEYWORDS

- Antiarrhythmic drug therapy • Atrial fibrillation • Late sodium current channel blocker • Ranolazine
- Ventricular arrhythmias

KEY POINTS

- Ranolazine is currently approved as an antianginal agent in patients with chronic angina (class IIA).
- Ranolazine exhibits antiarrhythmic effects that are related to its multichannel blocking effect, predominantly inhibition of late sodium (late I_{Na}) current and the rapid potassium rectifier current (I_{Kr}), as well as I_{Ca}, late I_{Ca}, and I_{Na-Ca}. It also suppresses the early and delayed afterdepolarizations.
- Ranolazine is effective in the suppression of atrial and ventricular arrhythmias (off-label use) without significant proarrhythmic effect.
- Currently, ongoing trials are evaluating the efficacy and safety of ranolazine in patients with cardiac arrhythmias; preliminary results suggest that ranolazine, when used alone or in combination with dronedarone, is safe and effective in reducing atrial fibrillation.
- Ranolazine is not currently approved by the US Food and Drug Administration as an antiarrhythmic agent.

INTRODUCTION

Ranolazine, a piperazine derivative, was initially introduced as an antianginal/anti-ischemic agent.[1–8] The mechanism(s) of anti-ischemic effects assumed to be related to the shifting of the myocardial adenosine triphosphate (ATP) production from the fatty acid metabolism to an oxygen-efficient carbohydrate oxidation and reduction in oxygen consumption.[1] In general, myocardial ischemia disrupts the oxygen supply and demand process. As a result, ischemia produces intercellular Na^+ and Ca^{2+} overload. In this process, most of the Na^+ influx due to the ischemia enters the cells via the cardiac Na^+ channels. This increase in intracellular Na^+ causes activation of voltage-gated L-type Ca^{2+} influx. Furthermore, as a result of ischemia, late opening of I_{Na} (sodium current) occurs in early phase of repolarization.[9] Ranolazine was later found to have a cardiac multichannel blocking property, specifically a blockade of the late sodium current (late I_{Na}) and of the rapid delayed-rectifier potassium current (I_{Kr}). It also exhibits minor effects on other cardiac channels, such as I_{Ca} (calcium current), late I_{Ca}, and I_{Na-Ca} (sodium-calcium current).[7,8,10–19] More recently, ranolazine was found to exhibit the mechanosensitive property of I_{Na} current. Unlike potassium-activated stress channels, this effect is less explored

Conflict of Interest and Disclosures: None.
Heart and Rhythm Medical Group, Department of Cardiovascular Services, O'Connor Hospital, 105 North Bascom Avenue, San Jose, CA 95128, USA
* Corresponding author.
E-mail address: Mohammad.shenasa@gmail.com

cardiacEP.theclinics.com

on Na$^+$ currents.[20-22] Studies on the isolated ischemic myocytes suggest that ranolazine reduces Ca^{2+} overload through inhibition of the late I$_{Na}$.[1] For full detail on the mechanism of anti-ischemic effect of ranolazine, see Ref.[1]

In a large randomized trial, the Metabolic Efficiency with Ranolazine for Less Ischemia in Non-ST-Elevation acute coronary syndrome (MERLIN)-Thrombolysis In Myocardial Infarction (TIMI) 36 (MERLIN-TIMI 36), effect of ranolazine was evaluated in patients with non-ST-segment elevation acute coronary syndrome and found that ranolazine prescribed in the first week after admission for acute coronary syndrome was also effective in reducing atrial and ventricular arrhythmias.[7,8,11]

Several recent reports evaluated the electrophysiologic effects, safety, and efficacy of ranolazine in patients with cardiac arrhythmias. In this review, we discuss the electrophysiologic effects and safety profile of ranolazine based on the current data from the available trials.

ELECTROPHYSIOLOGIC EFFECTS OF THE LATE SODIUM CURRENT

The sodium current has 2 components[8,10,12–15,17,23–26]:

1. Peak I$_{Na}$ occurs at phase zero of action potential (AP) and has a rapid inward current in approximately 1 to 2 ms.
2. The late I$_{Na}$ takes place in phase 2 and early phase 3 of AP and lasts approximately 100 to 300 ms. Increase in late I$_{Na}$ prolongs action potential duration (APD) and blockade of it shortens APD. Most sodium channel blockers exhibit both early and late I$_{Na}$ block effect; however, at different magnitudes. Ranolazine, for example, exerts 9 to 5 times higher late than early Na$^+$ blocking effect.[12]

Although I$_{Na}$ occurs during phase zero (upstroke) of AP, late I$_{Na}$ operates during phase 2 and early phase 3 of AP. Thus, any enhancement of late I$_{Na}$ prolongs APD. On the other hand, agents that block the late I$_{Na}$ current shorten the APD.[12]

In general, atrial AP is shorter in the atrium than the ventricle and becomes significantly shorter in remodeled atria, such as atrial fibrillation (AF). It has been shown that late I$_{Na}$ and its blocking agent, such as ranolazine, respond in a concentration, voltage, and rate-dependent (use-dependent) fashion.[8,12,23,27] Interestingly, the effect of shortening the APD in late I$_{Na}$ blockades is more prominent in healthy than remodeled atrial cells.[12] The role of late I$_{Na}$ in the genesis of arrhythmias is well described in a review by Shryock and colleagues.[28] Augmentation of late I$_{Na}$ has an arrhythmogenic effect that induces a variety of arrhythmias, summarized in **Fig. 1**.

Compared with early I$_{Na}$, late I$_{Na}$ dissociates faster from Na$^+$ channels. This effect has important electrophysiological significance, in which the latter has less proarrhythmic effect. In clinical scenario, the early Na$^+$ channel blockers had a significant proarrhythmic effect that is less commonly used.[8]

Augmentation of the late I$_{Na}$ induces early (EAD) and delayed afterdepolarization (DAD). They play as a trigger for induction of sustained arrhythmias.[8,29] It is therefore conceivable that blockade of the late I$_{Na}$ would eliminate both EAD and DAD.

Interestingly, the 2 major I$_{Na}$ and I$_{Kr}$ blocking properties have a contrasting effect; that is, late I$_{Na}$ causes prolongation of APD, whereas I$_{Kr}$ shortens APD. Furthermore, ranolazine has a diverse and differential effect of different areas of the myocardium; that is, atrial, myocardial, and Purkinje fibers. Ranolazine also exhibits different magnitude of effect on the epicardium and endocardium.[8,23]

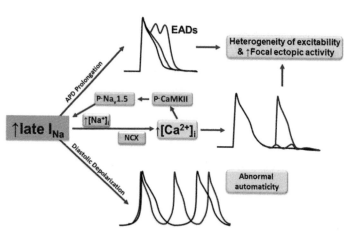

Fig. 1. Mechanisms of late I$_{Na}$-induced arrhythmia. ↑, increase. (*From* Shryock JC, Song Y, Rajamani S, et al. The arrhythmogenic consequences of increasing late INa in the cardiomyocyte. Cardiovasc Res 2013;99(4):603; with permission.)

ELECTROPHYSIOLOGIC EFFECTS OF RANOLAZINE

Ranolazine inhibits late I_{Na}, I_{Kr}, I_{Ca}, late I_{Ca}, and I_{Na-Ca} with little to no effect on I_{to}, I_{K1}, and IKs.[8]

Ranolazine thus, by blocking the late I_{Na}, produces prolongation of both atrial and ventricular effective refractory period (ERP). This effect is more pronounced in the atria than ventricles.[8,23] As mentioned earlier, augmentation of late I_{Na} causes intracellular cardiac overload. By blocking the late I_{Na} current, ranolazine also reverses the accumulation of I_{Na} as well as overload over I_{Ca} in myocardial cells. This reduction of intracellular Na^+ and Ca^{2+} overload has an antiarrhythmic effect.[23,24]

Experimental studies have demonstrated that late I_{Na} blocking agents, such as ranolazine, suppress induction of AF as well as terminate electrically induced AF.[12,23,24]

Unlike the peak I_{Na} current blocking agent, the late I_{Na} blocking agents, such as ranolazine and amiodarone, dissociate (unbind) rapidly from I_{Na}. This is probably why late I_{Na} blockers exert less proarrhythmic effects.[30] Studies by Burashnikov and Antzelevitch[12] have demonstrated that ranolazine has atrial selectivity properties. As said before, this effect is more pronounced in healthy atrial myocytes than diseased (remodeled) cells.[12]

Late I_{Na} blocking agents, such as ranolazine, are also effective in suppressing both EAD and DAD triggered activity (see **Fig. 1**).[12,24,31]

EVALUATION OF RANOLAZINE ON EXPERIMENTAL MODELS OF ARRHYTHMIAS

Kumar and colleagues[32] examined the effect of ranolazine on atrial and ventricular electrophysiological properties in a pig model of induced arrhythmias. In this model, ranolazine increased atrial ERP to a greater extent than ventricular ERP. Also, the duration of induced AF was significantly reduced after ranolazine.

Bhimani and colleagues[33] investigated the effect of ranolazine in a dog model of sterile pericarditis in which AF and atrial flutter (AFL) were induced. The finding of this study revealed that ranolazine significantly prolonged the AFL cycle length and also terminated AF and AFL. Similar to previous study, ranolazine also prolonged the atrial ERP. It is conceivable that the electrophysiologic effect of ranolazine in this animal model is the result of direct effect rather than antiischemic effect of ranolazine that is seen in clinical trials.

Sicouri and colleagues[34] showed that ranolazine significantly prolonged the ERP, conduction slowing, and suppression of late phase III EAD and DAD-mediated triggered activity in canine pulmonary veins.

Kloner and colleagues[35] compared electrophysiological effects of ranolazine with sotalol, lidocaine, and placebo in an ischemia/reperfusion rate model. In this head-to-head comparison of ranolazine with lidocaine and sotalol, ranolazine was as effective and was not inferior to the other 2 agents in reducing the ischemia reperfusion-induced ventricular tachyarrhythmias.

Milberg and colleagues,[36] using a Langendorff-perfused, isolated rabbit heart, evaluated the efficacy of ranolazine, sotalol, and flecainide in a stretch-induced AF model. The study found that all 3 drugs increased interatrial ERP and atrial post-repolarization refractoriness. In this model, sotalol increased the APD. Ranolazine and flecainide significantly decreased acute atrial dilatation-induced AF (stretch-induced AF).

Alves Bento and colleagues[37] evaluated the effect of ranolazine on catecholamine-induced ventricular tachycardia (VT) and T-wave alternans in an intact porcine model. In this model, ranolazine significantly reduced catecholamine-induced VT and abolished T-wave alternans.

Verrier and colleagues[11] reviewed the mechanisms of ranolazine in different animal models of various arrhythmias.

Interestingly, ranolazine was found to have a protective effect during cardioplegia in a Langendorff-perfused rat model. In this model, ranolazine improved diastolic function that was imposed during cardioplagia. This may have clinical implications in patients with left ventricular (LV) systolic dysfunction who are undergoing cardioplegia; however, further investigation to confirm this effect is warranted.[38]

ANTIARRHYTHMIC EFFECTS OF RANOLAZINE

The antiarrhythmic effects of ranolazine were first described in the MERLIN-TIMI 36 trial. The treatment with ranolazine in high-risk groups, that is, non-ST-segment elevation and acute coronary syndrome, had significantly reduced the episodes of VT lasting more than 8 beats as well as supraventricular tachycardias and specifically new-onset AF.[5,6]

Ranolazine, like ibutilide, also facilitates electrical conversion of AF to sinus rhythm.[39] Murdock and colleagues[40] reported on the efficacy of ranolazine in 25 patients who failed direct cardioversion and were subsequently treated with ranolazine. Cardioversion successfully terminated AF in 19 (76%) of 25 patients. The remaining 6 patients sustained permanent AF.

CLINICAL TRIALS OF RANOLAZINE

The major trials on antiarrhythmic effect of ranolazine are summarized in **Table 1**.

Metabolic Efficiency with Ranolazine for Less Ischemia in Non-ST-Elevation Acute Coronary Syndrome–Thrombolysis in Myocardial Infarction Trial

The MERLIN-TIMI 36 Trial evaluated the safety of ranolazine in patients with non–ST-elevation acute coronary syndromes[5,6] (see **Table 1**). This trial was a double-blind, randomized (1:1), placebo-controlled, multinational trial that included 6560 patients within 48 hours of onset of acute coronary symptoms. Patients received intravenous (IV) ranolazine followed by either oral extended release of ranolazine (1000 mg twice a day in 3279 patients) or placebo (3281 patients).

Primary endpoints of this trial were cardiovascular death, recurrent ischemia, myocardial infarction, or documented arrhythmias.[1] All patients also received the standard treatment for acute coronary syndromes per the guidelines.[5,6] The results of this trial revealed that addition of ranolazine to standard treatment of acute coronary syndrome did not reduce major cardiovascular events or all-cause mortality. However, ranolazine did not adversely affect all-cause death or symptomatic documented arrhythmias.[5]

This trial showed ranolazine was effective as an antianginal agent in a high-risk patient group.[5,6] Subsidiary analysis of this trial also showed that ranolazine did not pose any proarrhythmic effect and reduced the incidence of AF recurrence up to a 1-year follow-up.[6,41–43]

Ranolazine in Atrial Fibrillation Following an Electrical Cardioversion Trial

The Ranolazine in Atrial Fibrillation Following An ELectricaL cardioversion (RAFFAELLO) trial was designed as a prospective, multicenter, double-blind randomized, placebo-controlled (phase 2 dose-ranging) trial and examined the safety and efficacy of ranolazine in preventing the recurrences of AF after successful cardioversion[44] (see **Table 1**). In this trial, 238 patients were randomized into 4 groups: ranolazine 375 mg (65 patients), 500 mg (60 patients), 750 mg (58 patients) twice a day, respectively. Each dose was compared against placebo (55 patients). The primary endpoint of this trial was time to recurrence of AF after successful cardioversion. The conclusion of the RAFFAELLO trial was that ranolazine was safe in all 3 doses, although none of the individual doses significantly prolonged time to

recurrence of AF after successful cardioversion. However, the 500-mg and 750-mg groups combined reduced AF recurrences. Importantly, ranolazine did not prolong the QTc interval. There were no proarrhythmic effects in the ranolazine-treated groups.[44]

HARMONY Trial

The HARMONY Trial (Effect of Ranolazine and Dronedarone When Given Alone and in Combination on Atrial Fibrillation Burden in Subjects with Paroxysmal Atrial Fibrillation) was a phase 2 randomized, parallel, placebo-controlled trial designed to compare the effectiveness of ranolazine and dronedarone, alone or in combination, on AF burden in patients with paroxysmal AF[45] (see **Table 1**). The HARMONY trial included 134 patients, randomized into 5 arms of the study. Patients were randomized to ranolazine 750 mg (19 of 26 patients completed), ranolazine 750 mg plus dronedarone 150 mg (21 of 26 patients completed), ranolazine 750 mg plus dronedarone 225 mg (20 of 27 patients completed), dronedarone in 225 mg (22 of 26 patients completed), and placebo (17 of 26 patients completed). However, the hypothesis of this study was based on the results of experiments that showed the combination of ranolazine and dronedarone.[41,46] Patients included in this study were those with implanted cardiac pacemakers with atrial arrhythmia detection algorithms who had documented paroxysmal AF. The primary endpoint of this study was a presented decrease in AF burden over 12 weeks. Other endpoints included a change in AF burden at each study visit and a change in the number and duration of AF episodes. It is conceivable that because both ranolazine and dronedarone are multi-ion channel blockers, that the combination of the 2 agents would be more effective. The results of this trial showed that the combination of ranolazine and dronedarone was more effective than placebo and each drug (ranolazine 750 mg or dronedarone 225 mg) alone in reducing AF burden.[41] No significant adverse effects including proarrhythmic events were reported.

The synergistic and electrophysiologic effects of ranolazine and dronedarone on atrial and ventricular arrhythmias are well described by Burashnikov and colleagues.[46]

Ranolazine Implantable Cardioverter-Defibrillator Trial

The Ranolazine Implantable Cardioverter-defibrillator trial (RAID) was a double-blind, randomized, placebo-controlled, phase III trial[47] (see **Table 1**). The purpose was to evaluate the

Table 1
Clinical trials on ranolazine

Trial Name	Type	No. of Patients	Dosage	Endpoints	Results
MERLIN-TIMI 36[5,6] 2007	Multinational, double-blind, randomized, placebo-controlled, parallel-group clinical trial	6560	*Ranolazine IV +* *Oral extended release: 1000 mg* twice a day (3279 patients) OR *Placebo* (3281 patients)	*Primary endpoint:* Cardiovascular death, recurrent ischemia, myocardial infarction, or documented arrhythmias	Additional ranolazine to standard treatment of ACS did not reduce major cardiovascular events or all-cause mortality; ranolazine did not adversely affect all-cause death or symptomatic documented arrhythmias; ranolazine was effective as an antianginal agent in a high-risk patient group; ranolazine did not pose any proarrhythmic effect; ranolazine significantly reduced episodes of VT, SVT, and new-onset AF
RAFFAELLO[44] 2015	Double-blind, randomized, double-dummy, placebo-controlled, dose-ranging phase II study	238	*Ranolazine: 375 mg* (65 patients), 500 mg (60 patients), 750 mg (58 patients) *Placebo* (55 patients)	*Primary endpoint:* Time to recurrence after successful cardioversion	Ranolazine was safe in all 3 doses; 500-mg and 750-mg groups combined reduced AF recurrences; ranolazine did not prolong the QTc interval; no proarrhythmic effects in the ranolazine-treated groups
HARMONY[45] 2015	Double-blind, randomized, placebo-controlled, parallel-group study	134	*Ranolazine: 750 mg* (19 patients) *Ranolazine + Dronedarone:* 750 mg + 150 mg (21 patients) *Ranolazine + Dronedarone:* 750 mg + 225 mg (20 patients) *Dronedarone: 225 mg* (22 patients) *Placebo* (17 patients)	*Primary endpoint:* Presented decrease in AF burden over 12 wk *Other endpoints:* Change in AF burden at each study visit, change in the number and duration of AF episodes	Combination of ranolazine and dronedarone was more effective than placebo and each drug (ranolazine 750 mg or dronedarone 225 mg) alone in reducing AF burden; No significant adverse effects including proarrhythmic events were reported

(continued on next page)

Table 1
(continued)

Trial Name	Type	No. of Patients	Dosage	Endpoints	Results
RAID In progress	Double-blind, randomized, placebo-controlled, phase III study	Currently Recruiting (est. 1440)	*Ranolazine:* 500 mg BID for 1 wk and then increase to 1000 mg BID *Placebo*	*Primary endpoint:* Reduction in ventricular tachycardia or fibrillation requiring ICD interventions (ie, antitachycardia pacing therapy, ICD shocks, or death)	In progress
Ranolazine New Onset AF in Post-OP Cardiac Surgery	Double-blind, randomized, placebo-controlled, 1:1	54	*Ranolazine:* 1000 mg BID *Placebo*	*Primary endpoint:* AF up to 14 d postoperatively *Secondary endpoint:* Readmission 30 d postoperatively	38% reduction in the incidence of postoperative AF compared with 30% on placebo
Heart & Rhythm Medical Group 2014	Retrospective observational study	31	*Ranolazine:* 500 mg BID *Placebo*	Incidence, duration of AF/AFL, number of PAC/PVC couples, and VT	Ranolazine at 500 mg BID significantly reduced atrial and ventricular arrhythmias; no significant change in ECG interval; no proarrhythmic effects

Abbreviations: ACS, acute coronary syndrome; AF, atrial fibrillation; AFL, atrial flutter; BID, twice a day; ECG, electrocardiogram; ICD, implantable cardioverter-defibrillators; PAC, premature atrial contraction; PVC, premature ventricular contraction; SVT, supraventricular tachycardia; VT, ventricular tachycardia.

effectiveness of ranolazine in reducing ventricular arrhythmias and death in patients with implantable cardioverter-defibrillators (ICDs). The drug was tested in patients with ischemic cardiomyopathy, nonischemic cardiomyopathy, and heart failure (HF). The primary endpoint of the study is reduction in VT or ventricular fibrillation requiring ICD interventions; that is, antitachycardia pacing therapy, ICD shocks, or death. This trial is currently ongoing and has completed patient recruitment of 1440 patients. Patients will be randomized to ranolazine 500 mg twice a day for 1 week and then increased to 1000 mg twice a day compared with placebo. The study is expected to be completed by February 2017.[47]

Ranolazine for Incomplete Vessel Revascularization Percutaneous Coronary Intervention Trial

Recently, the Ranolazine for Incomplete Vessel Revascularization Percutaneous Coronary Intervention (RIVER-PCI) trial investigated the effect of ranolazine on angina and quality of life after percutaneous coronary interventions with incomplete revascularization.[2] It was a randomized, one-to-one, placebo-controlled trial comparing ranolazine with placebo. A total of 2389 patients were included in this trial. This trial was not designed to evaluate the role of ranolazine in arrhythmias. The endpoints of this trial were recurrence of angina and quality of life at 6 months, especially in patients with diabetes. The results of this trial revealed that patients enrolled on ranolazine arm of the trial had significantly lower episodes of angina; however, those effects were not maintained at 12 months.[2]

Ranolazine in Patients with New-Onset Atrial Fibrillation in Postoperative Cardiac Surgery

In this single-center, double-blind, randomized (1:1) study of ranolazine 1000 mg twice a day compared with placebo showed that there was a 38% reduction in the incidence of AF on ranolazine compared with 30% on placebo[48] (see **Table 1**). The difference did not reach statistical significance probably due to the high spontaneous conversion of AF after cardiac surgery.[48]

Heart and Rhythm Medical Group

Antiarrhythmic effect of ranolazine was evaluated retrospectively in 31 patients (49% men; mean age 80 ± 8 years) who were treated with ranolazine 500 mg BID for chronic angina control[49,50] (see **Table 1**; **Tables 2–4**). The patients underwent electrocardiogram (ECG), echocardiogram, and 24-hour Holter monitoring before and 2 weeks

Table 2
Effect of ranolazine on the electrocardiogram

	Heart rate, beats per min	PR, ms	QRS	QT	QTc
Before	67.3	178.7	98.8	412.9	433.6
After	66.2	182.1	99.9	412.7	432.2
P	.269	.203	.312	.482	.379

after ranolazine. The frequency of atrial extrasystoles, couples, and tachycardia, as well as the rate and duration of AF were analyzed before and after ranolazine. Similarly, the frequency of premature ventricular contractions (PVCs), couples, and nonsustained ventricular arrhythmias were analyzed. The results of this retrospective, observational study revealed the following:

1. There were no significant changes in the ECG interval during sinus rhythm (see **Table 2**).
2. Both atrial and ventricular arrhythmias decreased significantly (see **Table 3**).
3. AF was present in 7 patients, and was abolished in 6.
4. Nonsustained VT, that is, more than 8 beats, was present in 5 patients and was abolished in all.
5. There were no proarrhythmic effects at this dosage of ranolazine.
6. Importantly, the echocardiogram results revealed that ranolazine significantly reduced the left atrial dimensions and increased LV ejection fraction from 43 ± 7 to 64 ± 8 (P>.008) (see **Table 4**).
7. Indices of diastolic dysfunction, that is, mitral E/A ratio did not significantly change; however, E/E′ ratio (mitral annular velocities) increased from 7.1 to 9.3 (P>.019).

To our knowledge, this is the first study that explored the effect of ranolazine on LV performance. This improvement may, in part, play a role in anti-ischemic and antiarrhythmic properties of ranolazine.[49,50]

EFFECT OF RANOLAZINE IN EXPERIMENTAL AND CLINICAL LONG-QT SYNDROME

Two experimental studies evaluated the effect of ranolazine on the model of long-QT syndrome and showed that ranolazine had suppressed the EADs and decreased intracellular (Na^+ and Ca^{2+}) overload and prevented prolongation of QT interval and induction of Torsades de Pointes (TdP).[10,51]

Moss and colleagues[52] evaluated the effect of IV ranolazine (45 mg per hour for 3 hours followed by 90 mg per hour for 5 hours) on ventricular

Table 3
Effect of ranolazine on ventricular and supraventricular arrhythmias

	Total	PAC	Pair	SVT	Longest SVT, beats	Fastest SVT, beats per min	AF
					Atrial		
Before	660	149	8	7.3	5.5	134	.14
After	65.5	42	1.3	0.9	1.5	105	0
P	.008	.04	.005	.01	.014	.015	.1

Abbreviations: AF, atrial fibrillation; PAC, atrial contraction; SVT, supraventricular tachycardia.

repolarization in 5 patients with long-QT 3 syndrome. In this patient series, ranolazine significantly decreased the QTc in a concentration-dependent manner, as well as shortened LV isovolumic relaxation time and other LV diastolic indices. Further studies are warranted to examine the effect of ranolazine in a larger patient population at risk of ventricular tachyarrhythmias, TdP, and sudden cardiac death. It is assumed that in long-QT syndrome the mechanism of ventricular arrhythmias is related to an increase in late I_{Na} and ranolazine. By suppressing this effect, the QT interval is shortened against ventricular arrhythmias and TdP.

EFFECT OF RANOLAZINE IN PATIENTS WITH ATRIAL FIBRILLATION

Subsidiary analysis of MERLIN-TIMI 36 revealed that ranolazine significantly reduced AF episodes and AF burden.[41] Furthermore, other studies have demonstrated that ranolazine is effective in reducing AF burden in patients with paroxysmal and persistent AF. Studies also reported that ranolazine is effective in reducing postoperative atrial arrhythmias alone and in combination with amiodarone.[40,53–55] For further discussion regarding AF, see the section Clinical Trials of Ranolazine (see **Table 1**).

EFFECT OF RANOLAZINE IN PATIENTS WITH VENTRICULAR TACHYCARDIA

Limited data are available on the efficacy and safety of ranolazine in patients with ventricular tachyarrhythmias.[54,56] Data from the MERLIN trial suggested ranolazine significantly reduced the incidence of ventricular arrhythmias and sudden cardiac death.[6,7] This effect is probably related to the modification of the substrate or blockade of the late I_{Na} by ranolazine or other electrophysiologic effects such as modifying the occurrence EADs and DADs.

Fig. 2 compares the effect of ranolazine with placebo in patients who have nonsustained VT ($\geq$8 beats) in the incidence of sudden cardiac death.

Yeung and colleagues[57] reported on the effect of ranolazine in 8 patients. In the 6 patients with PVCs, all had a PVC burden of greater than 10%. In the same patients with PVCs, 2 of the 6 had PVC-induced cardiomyopathy, which was normalized after treatment with ranolazine (PVC burden decreased by 60.2% [P = .06]). In the other 2 patients with incessant VT, despite class II antiarrhythmic therapy, ranolazine eliminated ventricular arrhythmias and prevented recurrent ICD therapies. Ranolazine doses ranged from 500 mg to 1000 mg BID. Ranolazine completely abolished VTs and there were no further ICD therapies in these 2 patients despite previously failed class III antiarrhythmic agents. Most patients in this study had moderate to severe LV systolic dysfunction. The effect of ranolazine was more pronounced in patients with reduced LV systolic function compared with those with preserved LV systolic function.[57]

RANOLAZINE IN PATIENTS WITH HEART FAILURE

The effect of ranolazine on animal models of HF showed that ranolazine significantly improved LV

Table 4
Effect of ranolazine on the echocardiographic indices

	LAD, mm	LVEF, %	LVID Diastole, mm	LVID Systole, mm	Mitral E/A	E/E'
Baseline	46 ± 6	60 ± 9	44.6 (31–56)	26.9 (16–36)	1.21 ± 0.7	7.14 ± 1.4
Ranolazine	43 ± 7	64 ± 8	44.2 (34–55)	27.3 (20–39)	0.92 ± 0.3	9.36 ± 1.1
P	.01	.008	.319	.359	.16	.019

Abbreviations: LAD, left atrial dimension; LVEF, left ventricular ejection fraction; LVID, left ventricular internal dimension.

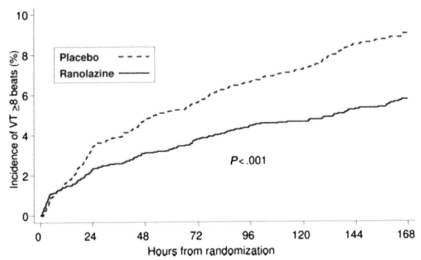

Fig. 2. The effect of Ranolazine compared with placebo on ventricular tachycardia last ≥ 8 beats. (*From* Scirica BM, Morrow DA, Hod H, et al. Effect of ranolazine, an antianginal agent with novel electrophysiological properties, on the incidence of arrhythmias in patients with non ST-segment elevation acute coronary syndrome: results from the metabolic efficiency with ranolazine for less ischemia in non ST-elevation acute coronary syndrome thrombolysis in myocardial infarction 36 (MERLIN-TIMI 36) randomized controlled trial. Circulation 2007;116(15):1650; with permission.)

performance after IV administration of 0.5 mg/kg followed by a continued infusion of 1.0 mg/kg per hour. Furthermore, ranolazine decreased LV end-diastolic pressure and increased LV ejection fraction. Ranolazine did not exhibit any significant hemodynamic adverse effects such as hypotension. Similarly, IV ranolazine in patients with systolic HF showed that there was significant improvement in LV ejection fraction.[1,58] Preliminary data from our laboratory has also shown that oral ranolazine at 500 mg twice a day has significantly improved LV ejection fraction as well as diastolic function indices (see **Table 4**).[49,50] The pathophysiological pathways on the role of late I_{Na} and its inhibition in HF is complex and is beyond the scope of this review and is well discussed by Horvath and Bers.[25]

EFFECT OF RANOLAZINE ON THE ELECTROCARDIOGRAM AND ECHOCARDIOGRAM

Ranolazine did not significantly change the heart rate nor significantly prolong the PR interval, QRS duration, or QT interval in our series (see **Tables 2** and **4**).[49,50] The effect of ranolazine on the ECG was evaluated in the CARISA (Combination Assessment of Ranolazine In Stable Angina) trial and showed that ranolazine prolonged the QTc interval by an average of 2 to 5 ms.[1] Although this effect did not reach a statistical significance, it was recommended that

ranolazine is contraindicated in patients with preexisting QT prolongation of those who exhibit QT prolongation during ranolazine treatment and those with hepatic impairment.[59]

COMBINATION OF RANOLAZINE WITH OTHER ANTIARRHYTHMIC AGENTS

Several studies and trials have compared ranolazine alone or in a combination of ranolazine with dronedarone (HARMONY) or amiodarone.[45]

Burashnikov and colleagues[46] examined the synergistic effect of ranolazine plus amiodarone therapy in an isolated coronary-perfused right, left atrial pulmonary vein and LV preparation canine model and was compared with ranolazine and amiodarone alone. In this model, each drug alone had a weak electrophysiologic effect; however, the combination of the 2 compounds had significant synergic properties. Furthermore, this combination was effective in preventing the induction of AF.

On the clinical side, Fragakis and colleagues[55] compared the effectiveness of ranolazine with ranolazine plus amiodarone for conversion of recent-onset AF (less than 48-hour duration) in 51 patients. The study compared IV amiodarone for 24 hours or IV amiodarone plus ranolazine (1500 mg) at time of randomization. The primary endpoint of the study was conversion of AF to sinus rhythm at the randomization. This study found the time to conversion from AF to sinus rhythm was shorter in patients who received IV amiodarone plus oral ranolazine. There was no proarrhythmic effect noted in this study.

Similarly, Koskinas and colleagues[60] reported the combination of ranolazine with amiodarone improves conversion of recent-onset AF to sinus rhythm. The study comprised 121 patients with recent-onset (less than 48-hour duration) AF. The patients received loading dose of IV amiodarone of 5 mg/kg followed by a maintenance dose of 50 mg per hour plus a single dose of 1500 mg of ranolazine. This combination was compared with amiodarone alone (same dose). The results revealed that combination of the 2 agents was superior (87%) compared with amiodarone alone (17%) in converting AF to sinus rhythm (P<.024). There was no significant proarrhythmic effect.

The HARMONY trial, which also compared ranolazine alone with the combination of ranolazine and dronedarone in a randomized, placebo-controlled study was discussed previously.[45]

PHARMACOKINETICS OF RANOLAZINE

Ranolazine has mostly renal excretion; however, it has extensive liver metabolism through cytochrome (CYP) 450, CYP3A4, and the CYPD26 enzyme.[61] Ranolazine has a largely variable absorption rate and has an approximately 76% bioavailability after oral administration.[62] Peak plasma concentration is at 2 to 5 hours after oral administration.[62] The half-life of ranolazine is calculated at 6 to 22 hours, and has approximately 62% protein binding.[62] Ranolazine is mostly metabolized through the liver via the CYP3A4 pathway and has less than 5% renal excretion; therefore, ranolazine in contraindicated in patients with hepatic impairment.[59] The maximum recommended dosage is 1000 mg twice a day. Steady state is achieved within 3 days of twice-daily dosing. Ranolazine has multiple metabolites, and at least 11 metabolites have been identified.[1]

DRUG INTERACTIONS WITH RANOLAZINE

Pharmacologic agents that have a reversal inhibition CYP3A4 enzyme increase the blood plasma level of ranolazine on an average of 2.5 to 4.5; therefore, pharmacologic agents that inhibit the CYP3A4 enzymatic pathways will interact and increase the ranolazine blood plasma level and should be avoided.[63] Currently, more than 200 pharmacologic agents are reported to interact with ranolazine.[64] Other agents, such as ketoconazole, diltiazem, and some statins, such as simvastatin and atorvastatin, may interact with ranolazine and increase its blood plasma

level.[54,60,65] Importantly, ranolazine has been reported to increase digoxin concentrations.[60]

RANOLAZINE IN PREGNANCY

Currently there are no data regarding the safety of ranolazine in pregnancy and breastfeeding; however, the FDA has classified it as category C.

ADVERSE EFFECTS OF RANOLAZINE

Ranolazine at the recommendation dosage does not pose a risk of TdP or proarrhythmia. Other noncardiac adverse effects include abdominal pain, asthenia, constipation, dizziness, headache, and nausea.[1] The overall incidence of noncardiac side effects is less than 7%.[1]

DISCUSSION

Ranolazine is a unique compound with an anti-ischemic effect and significant multichannel ion-blocking property, which exhibits antiarrhythmic effects. Due to its selective late I_{Na} and I_{Kr} blocking effect, it is effective against atrial and ventricular arrhythmias of diverse mechanism.[54] Importantly, ranolazine was effective in reducing ventricular tachyarrhythmias in this high-risk phase; that is, acute coronary syndrome. Furthermore, ranolazine did not increase all-cause mortality or sudden cardiac death.[5,6,41]

Due to Na^+ and K^+ channel selectivity and because ranolazine has fast unbinding property from the Na channel despite modest prolongation of the QT interval, ranolazine has no significant proarrhythmia, specifically TdP reported by Saad and colleagues.[54] Although ranolazine exhibits direct antiarrhythmic property, its anti-ischemic effect and improvement in LV performance (ie, increase in LV systolic and diastolic function) may play an important role in efficacy and safety of ranolazine. This, of course needs further experimental and clinical studies.[50] Although ranolazine is not currently approved as an antiarrhythmic, the ongoing trials may provide evidence for the use of ranolazine alone or in combination.

GUIDELINES

Because ranolazine is not FDA approved as an antiarrhythmic agent, there is no guideline regarding its use. Hopefully with the completion of ongoing trials, ranolazine will be included in future guidelines.

SUMMARY

- Ranolazine is currently approved as an antianginal agent in patients with recurrent angina.

- Ranolazine exhibits significant multichannel blocker effect, mostly late I_{Na} and I_{Kr}, which has a potential significant antiarrhythmic effect; that is, both for atrial and ventricular arrhythmias.
- Ranolazine has a 90% liver metabolism and should not be used in patients with impaired liver function.
- Ranolazine is an effective agent in patients with atrial and ventricular arrhythmias without significant QT prolongation or proarrhythmic effect.
- Ranolazine is not yet FDA approved as an antiarrhythmic agent.

ACKNOWLEDGMENTS

The authors thank Mariah Smith for her superb assistance in preparation of this article.

REFERENCES

1. Chaitman BR. Ranolazine for the treatment of chronic angina and potential use in other cardiovascular conditions. Circulation 2006;113(20):2462–72.
2. Alexander KP, Weisz G, Prather K, et al. Effects of ranolazine on angina and quality of life after percutaneous coronary intervention with incomplete revascularization: results from the Ranolazine for Incomplete Vessel Revascularization (RIVER-PCI) trial. Circulation 2015;133(1):39–47.
3. Morrow DA, Scirica BM, Karwatowska-Prokopczuk E, et al. Evaluation of a novel antiischemic agent in acute coronary syndromes: design and rationale for the Metabolic Efficiency with Ranolazine for Less Ischemia in Non-ST-elevation acute coronary syndromes (MERLIN)-TIMI 36 trial. Am Heart J 2006;151(6):1186.e1–9.
4. Page RLI, Ghushchyan V, Read RA, et al. Comparative effectiveness of ranolazine versus traditional therapies in chronic stable angina pectoris and concomitant diabetes mellitus and impact on health care resource utilization and cardiac interventions. Am J Cardiol 2015;116(9):1321–8.
5. Morrow DA, Scirica BM, Karwatowska-Prokopczuk E, et al. Effects of ranolazine on recurrent cardiovascular events in patients with non–ST-elevation acute coronary syndromes: the MERLIN-TIMI 36 randomized trial. JAMA 2007;297:1775–83.
6. Scirica BM, Morrow DA, Hod H, et al. Effect of ranolazine, an antianginal agent with novel electrophysiological properties, on the incidence of arrhythmias in patients with non ST-segment elevation acute coronary syndrome: results from the metabolic efficiency with ranolazine for less ischemia in non ST-elevation acute coronary syndrome thrombolysis in myocardial infarction 36 (MERLIN-TIMI 36) randomized controlled trial. Circulation 2007;116(15):1647–52.
7. Scirica BM, Braunwald E, Belardinelli L, et al. Relationship between nonsustained ventricular tachycardia after non-ST-elevation acute coronary syndrome and sudden cardiac death: observations from the metabolic efficiency with ranolazine for less ischemia in non-ST-elevation acute coronary syndrome-thrombolysis in myocardial infarction 36 (MERLIN-TIMI 36) randomized controlled trial. Circulation 2010;122(5):455–62.
8. Antzelevitch C, Belardinelli L, Zygmunt AC, et al. Electrophysiological effects of ranolazine, a novel antianginal agent with antiarrhythmic properties. Circulation 2004;110(8):904–10.
9. Chaitman BR, Skettino SL, Parker JO, et al. Anti-ischemic effects and long-term survival during ranolazine monotherapy in patients with chronic severe angina. J Am Coll Cardiol 2004;43(8):1375–82.
10. Wu L, Shryock JC, Song Y, et al. Antiarrhythmic effects of ranolazine in a guinea pig in vitro model of long-QT syndrome. J Pharmacol Exp Ther 2004; 310(2):599–605.
11. Verrier RL, Kumar K, Nieminen T, et al. Mechanisms of ranolazine's dual protection against atrial and ventricular fibrillation. Europace 2013;15(3):317–24.
12. Burashnikov A, Antzelevitch C. Role of late sodium channel current block in the management of atrial fibrillation. Cardiovasc Drugs Ther 2013; 27(1):79–89.
13. Belardinelli L, Shryock JC, Fraser H. Inhibition of the late sodium current as a potential cardioprotective principle: effects of the late sodium current inhibitor ranolazine. Heart 2006;92(Suppl 4):iv6–14.
14. Noble D, Noble PJ. Late sodium current in the pathophysiology of cardiovascular disease: consequences of sodium-calcium overload. Heart 2006; 92(Suppl 4):iv1–5.
15. Maltsev VA, Kyle JW, Undrovinas A. Late Na+ current produced by human cardiac Na+ channel isoform Nav1.5 is modulated by its beta1 subunit. J Physiol Sci 2009;59(3):217–25.
16. Grant AO. Cardiac ion channels. Circ Arrhythm Electrophysiol 2009;2(2):185–94.
17. Rook MB, Evers MM, Vos MA, et al. Biology of cardiac sodium channel Nav1.5 expression. Cardiovasc Res 2012;93(1):12–23.
18. Chaitman B, Pepine CJ, Parker JO, et al. Effects of ranolazine with atenolol, amlodipine, or diltiazem on exercise tolerance and angina frequency in patients with severe chronic angina: a randomized controlled trial. JAMA 2004;291:309–16.
19. Pepine CJ, Wolff AA. A controlled trial with a novel anti-ischemic agent, ranolazine, in chronic stable angina pectoris that is responsive to conventional antianginal agents. Am J Cardiol 1999; 84(1):46–50.
20. Morris CE. Voltage-gated channel mechanosensitivity: fact or friction? Front Physiol 2011;2:25.

21. Beyder A, Strege PR, Reyes S, et al. Ranolazine decreases mechanosensitivity of the voltage-gated sodium ion channel Na(v)1.5: a novel mechanism of drug action. Circulation 2012;125(22): 2698–706.

22. Abriel H. Cardiac sodium channel Na(v)1.5 mechanosensitivity is inhibited by ranolazine. Circulation 2012;125(22):2681–3.

23. Antzelevitch C, Burashnikov A, Sicouri S, et al. Electrophysiologic basis for the antiarrhythmic actions of ranolazine. Heart Rhythm 2011;8(8):1281–90.

24. Gupta T, Khera S, Kolte D, et al. Antiarrhythmic properties of ranolazine: a review of the current evidence. Int J Cardiol 2015;187:66–74.

25. Horvath B, Bers DM. The late sodium current in heart failure: pathophysiology and clinical relevance. ESC Heart Fail 2014;1(1):26–40.

26. Hasenfuss G, Maier LS. Mechanism of action of the new anti-ischemia drug ranolazine. Clin Res Cardiol 2008;97(4):222–6.

27. Rajamani S, El-Bizri N, Shryock JC, et al. Use-dependent block of cardiac late Na(+) current by ranolazine. Heart Rhythm 2009;6(11):1625–31.

28. Shryock JC, Song Y, Rajamani S, et al. The arrhythmogenic consequences of increasing late INa in the cardiomyocyte. Cardiovasc Res 2013;99(4):600–11.

29. Song Y, Shryock JC, Belardinelli L. An increase of late sodium current induces delayed afterdepolarizations and sustained triggered activity in atrial myocytes. Am J Physiol Heart Circ Physiol 2008;294(5): H2031–9.

30. Comtois P, Sakabe M, Vigmond EJ, et al. Mechanisms of atrial fibrillation termination by rapidly unbinding Na+ channel blockers: insights from mathematical models and experimental correlates. Am J Physiol Heart Circ Physiol 2008;295(4): H1489–504.

31. Moreno JD, Clancy CE. Pathophysiology of the cardiac late Na current and its potential as a drug target. J Mol Cell Cardiol 2012;52(3):608–19.

32. Kumar K, Nearing BD, Carvas M, et al. Ranolazine exerts potent effects on atrial electrical properties and abbreviates atrial fibrillation duration in the intact porcine heart. J Cardiovasc Electrophysiol 2009;20(7):796–802.

33. Bhimani AA, Yasuda T, Sadrpour SA, et al. Ranolazine terminates atrial flutter and fibrillation in a canine model. Heart Rhythm 2014;11(9):1592–9.

34. Sicouri S, Glass A, Belardinelli L, et al. Antiarrhythmic effects of ranolazine in canine pulmonary vein sleeve preparations. Heart Rhythm 2008;5(7): 1019–26.

35. Kloner RA, Dow JS, Bhandari A. First direct comparison of the late sodium current blocker ranolazine to established antiarrhythmic agents in an ischemia/reperfusion model. J Cardiovasc Pharmacol Ther 2011;16(2):192–6.

36. Milberg P, Frommeyer G, Ghezelbash S, et al. Sodium channel block by ranolazine in an experimental model of stretch-related atrial fibrillation: prolongation of interatrial conduction time and increase in post-repolarization refractoriness. Europace 2013; 15(5):761–9.

37. Alves Bento AS, Bacic D, Saran Carneiro J, et al. Selective late INa inhibition by GS-458967 exerts parallel suppression of catecholamine-induced hemodynamically significant ventricular tachycardia and T-wave alternans in an intact porcine model. Heart Rhythm 2015;12(12):2508–14.

38. Hwang H, Arcidi JM Jr, Hale SL, et al. Ranolazine as a cardioplegia additive improves recovery of diastolic function in isolated rat hearts. Circulation 2009;120(11 Suppl):S16–21.

39. Hongo RH, Themistoclakis S, Raviele A, et al. Use of ibutilide in cardioversion of patients with atrial fibrillation or atrial flutter treated with class IC agents. J Am Coll Cardiol 2004;44(4):864–8.

40. Murdock DK, Kaliebe J, Larrain G. The use of ranolazine to facilitate electrical cardioversion in cardioversion-resistant patients: a case series. Pacing Clin Electrophysiol 2012;35(3):302–7.

41. Scirica BM, Belardinelli L, Chaitman BR, et al. Effect of ranolazine on atrial fibrillation in patients with non-ST elevation acute coronary syndromes: observations from the MERLIN-TIMI 36 trial. Europace 2015;17(1):32–7.

42. Stone PH, Gratsiansky NA, Blokhin A, et al. Antianginal efficacy of ranolazine when added to treatment with amlodipine: the ERICA (Efficacy of Ranolazine in Chronic Angina) trial. J Am Coll Cardiol 2006; 48(3):566–75.

43. Wilson SR, Scirica BM, Braunwald E, et al. Efficacy of ranolazine in patients with chronic angina observations from the randomized, double-blind, placebo-controlled MERLIN-TIMI (Metabolic Efficiency With Ranolazine for Less Ischemia in Non-ST-Segment Elevation Acute Coronary Syndromes) 36 trial. J Am Coll Cardiol 2009;53(17): 1510–6.

44. De Ferrari GM, Maier LS, Mont L, et al. Ranolazine in the treatment of atrial fibrillation: results of the dose-ranging RAFFAELLO (Ranolazine in Atrial Fibrillation Following An ELectricaL CardiOversion) study. Heart Rhythm 2015;12(5):872–8.

45. Reiffel JA, Camm AJ, Belardinelli L, et al. The HARMONY Trial: combined ranolazine and dronedarone in the management of paroxysmal atrial fibrillation: mechanistic and therapeutic synergism. Circ Arrhythm Electrophysiol 2015;8: 1048–56.

46. Burashnikov A, Sicouri S, Di Diego JM, et al. Synergistic effect of the combination of ranolazine and dronedarone to suppress atrial fibrillation. J Am Coll Cardiol 2010;56(15):1216–24.

47. Ranolazine Implantable Cardioverter-Defibrillator Trial (RAID). Available at: https://clinicaltrials.gov/ct2/show/NCT01215253. Accessed January 15, 2016.

48. Bekheit S, Asti D, Meghani M, et al. Effect of ranolazine on the incidence of atrial fibrillation following cardiac surgery Staten Island University Hospital. Circulation 2015;132:A13387.

49. Assadi H, Shenasa H, Heidary S, et al. Antiarrhythmic effects of ranolazine in patients with cardiac arrhythmias. J Am Coll Cardiol 2014;63(12):A336.

50. Assadi H, Shenasa H, Heidary S, et al. Improvement in diastolic indices by ranolazine: a potential mechanism for its anti-ischemic and antiarrhythmic effects. J Am Coll Cardiol 2015;65(10):A385.

51. Parikh A, Mantravadi R, Kozhevnikov D, et al. Ranolazine stabilizes cardiac ryanodine receptors: a novel mechanism for the suppression of early afterdepolarization and torsades de pointes in long QT type 2. Heart Rhythm 2012;9(6):953–60.

52. Moss AJ, Zareba W, Schwarz KQ, et al. Ranolazine shortens repolarization in patients with sustained inward sodium current due to type-3 long-QT syndrome. J Cardiovasc Electrophysiol 2008;19(12):1289–93.

53. Simopoulos V, Tagarakis GI, Daskalopoulou SS, et al. Ranolazine enhances the antiarrhythmic activity of amiodarone by accelerating conversion of new-onset atrial fibrillation after cardiac surgery. Angiology 2014;65(4):294–7.

54. Saad M, Mahmoud A, Elgendy IY, et al. Ranolazine in cardiac arrhythmia. Clin Cardiol 2015. [Epub ahead of print].

55. Fragakis N, Koskinas KC, Katritsis DG, et al. Comparison of effectiveness of ranolazine plus amiodarone versus amiodarone alone for conversion of recent-onset atrial fibrillation. Am J Cardiol 2012;110(5):673–7.

56. Bunch TJ, Mahapatra S, Murdock D, et al. Ranolazine reduces ventricular tachycardia burden and ICD shocks in patients with drug-refractory ICD shocks. Pacing Clin Electrophysiol 2011;34(12):1600–6.

57. Yeung E, Krantz MJ, Schuller JL, et al. Ranolazine for the suppression of ventricular arrhythmia: a case series. Ann Noninvasive Electrocardiol 2014;19(4):345–50.

58. Hayashida W, Eyll C, Rousseau MF, et al. Effects of ranolazine on left ventricular regional diastolic function in patients with ischemic heart disease. Cardiovasc Drugs Ther 1994;8(5):741–7.

59. Abdallah H, Jerling M. Effect of hepatic impairment on the multiple-dose pharmacokinetics of ranolazine sustained-release tablets. J Clin Pharmacol 2005;45(7):802–9.

60. Koskinas KC, Fragakis N, Katritsis D, et al. Ranolazine enhances the efficacy of amiodarone for conversion of recent-onset atrial fibrillation. Europace 2014;16(7):973–9.

61. CV Therapeutics. FDA briefing document for the Cardiovascular and Renal Drugs Advisory Committee: Ranexa (ranolazine), extended-release tablets. Available at: http://www.fda.gov/ohrms/dockets/ac/03/briefing/4012B2_15_CV-Therapeutics-RANEXA.pdf. Accessed January 25, 2016.

62. RANEXA Gilead Sciences Guidelines. 2016. Available at: http://www.gilead.com/~/media/files/pdfs/medicines/cardiovascular/ranexa/ranexa_pi.pdf. Accessed January 26, 2016.

63. Jerling M, Huan B-L, Leung K, et al. Studies to investigate the pharmacokinetic interactions between ranolazine and ketoconazole, diltiazem, or simvastatin during combined administration in healthy subjects. J Clin Pharmacol 2005;45(4):422–33.

64. Ranolazine drug interactions. Available at: http://www.drugs.com/drug-interactions/ranolazine.html. Accessed January 30, 2016.

65. Correa D, Landaeu M. Ranolazine-induced myopathy in a patient on chronic statin therapy. J Clin Neuromuscul Dis 2013;14:114–6.

Proarrhythmic and Torsadogenic Effects of Potassium Channel Blockers in Patients

Mark McCauley, MD, PhD, Sharath Vallabhajosyula, MD,
Dawood Darbar, MD*

KEYWORDS

- Arrhythmia • Potassium channel blocker • Torsades de pointes

KEY POINTS

- The most common arrhythmia requiring antiarrhythmic drugs is atrial fibrillation.
- Many antiarrhythmic drugs used to treat atrial fibrillation block the rapid delayed rectifier K^+ current (I_{Kr}), and marked QT prolongation and torsades de pointes are major class toxicities.
- Risk factors associated with drug-induced QT prolongation and risk of torsades de pointes include female gender, bradycardia, electrolyte disturbances, recent conversion from atrial fibrillation to sinus rhythm, variations in drug distribution, and subclinical congenital long QT syndrome.
- Incorporating data from the clinical and basic realms will improve the understanding of the underlying mechanisms by which potassium-channel blocking drugs mediate QT prolongation and increase susceptibility to torsades de pointes.
- Bridging this gap will not only help prevent drug-induced torsades de pointes but also fulfill the promise of predictive and precision medicine.

INTRODUCTION

Vaughn Williams' class III antiarrhythmic drugs (AAD), of which blockers of the rapid component of the delayed rectifier potassium current, I_{Kr}, are most prevalent, are known to cause QT interval prolongation on the electrocardiogram (ECG) and have been well described to predispose patients to ventricular arrhythmias.[1–3] Drug-induced long QT syndrome (diLQTS) is now a well-characterized mechanism whereby patients develop torsades de pointes (TdP) and risk for arrhythmic death.[4] Mechanistic details of the underlying genetic and pharmacologic risk factors for ventricular arrhythmias are discussed elsewhere in this series. However, many patient-related risk factors for the development of TdP have been identified, including female gender, bradycardia, electrolyte disturbances, recent conversion from atrial fibrillation (AF) to sinus rhythm, variations in drug distribution, and subclinical forms of the congenital long QT syndrome (LQTS), all of which are important for modifying ventricular arrhythmia risk (**Table 1**). In this review, the history and mechanisms of risk factors for diLQTS and TdP are discussed, and recent advances in patient clinical characteristics and the complex interplay of how these patient-related clinical risk factors

Funding Sources: This work was in part supported by the National Institutes of Health grants R01 HL092217, R01HL124935, and R01HL085690.
Division of Cardiology, Department of Medicine, University of Illinois at Chicago, 840 South Wood Street, Suite 920 (MC715), Chicago, IL 60612, USA
* Corresponding author. Division of Cardiology, University of Illinois at Chicago, 840 South Wood Street, 920S (MC 715), Chicago, IL 60612.
E-mail address: darbar@uic.edu

Card Electrophysiol Clin 8 (2016) 481–493
http://dx.doi.org/10.1016/j.ccep.2016.02.009
1877-9182/16/$ – see front matter © 2016 Elsevier Inc. All rights reserved.

Table 1
Clinical risk factors, mechanisms, the magnitude of risk and novel models used to define the underlying mechanisms relating patient characteristics with the development of QT interval prolongation and torsades de pointes

Clinical Risk Factor	Mechanism	Magnitude of Risk	New Models of TdP
Female gender	Estrogen-induced reduction in repolarization reserve	Women at increased risk: 2:1–3:1 vs men	Yang et al,[32] 2012; Gonzalez et al,[34] 2010; Ando et al,[35] 2011; Cheng et al,[36,37] 2012
Bradycardia	Pause-dependent QT prolongation; short-long-short sequence	Typically with heart rates <60 bpm	Cho et al,[39] 2015; Rosso et al,[40] 2014
Hypokalemia	Decreased I_{Kr}	Serum K^+ <3.5 mg/dL	—
Hypomagnesemia	Modulation of $I_{Ca,L}$	Serum Mg^{2+} <1.5 mg/dL	—
Conversion from AF to sinus	Increased QT interval variation	1%–3% incidence of TdP associated with diLQTS	Choy et al,[68] 1999; Darbar et al,[69] 2007; Kannankeril et al,[4] 2010
Pharmacotherapy	Prolongation of QT interval by direct modification of ion channel function	QT-prolonging drugs may increase QT interval by up to 50 ms in clinically prescribed doses	Johannesen et al,[89] 2014; Sugrue et al,[53] 2015

predispose patients with inherited potassium channelopathies to life-threatening ventricular arrhythmias and sudden arrhythmic death are then detailed.

A HISTORY OF PROARRHYTHMOGENIC POTENTIAL OF POTASSIUM CHANNEL BLOCKERS

The first description of the LQTS was reported as far back as the 1800s.[5] By contrast, diLQTS was described by Levy[6] in 1922 when he explained clinical outcomes of abrupt syncope and sudden death in patients undergoing treatment for AF with quinidine. Selzer and Wray,[7] who considered ECG tracings to represent "paroxysmal ventricular fibrillation," described arrhythmia-associated syncope several decades later. This pattern, consisting of polymorphic ventricular tachycardia (**Fig. 1**), was observed and subsequently coined "torsades de pointes" by Dessertenne.[8] The oscillating waveform of TdP runs the risk of progressing to ventricular fibrillation if not stabilized and predisposes the patient to arrhythmic sudden death. Although several mechanisms have been proposed, the underlying pathophysiology of LQTS-triggered polymorphic ventricular tachycardia remains poorly understood. Current efforts at uncovering the mechanisms underlying TdP include in silico modeling of cellular repolarization reserve, evaluation of hormonal effects on potassium channel function, induced pluripotent stem cell (iPSC) modeling of TdP, and mathematical modeling of T-wave properties associated with risk of the arrhythmia (see **Table 1**).

RELATING RISK FACTORS TO PHARMACOLOGIC MECHANISMS

Initial case reports of diLQTS were associated with hypokalemia and atrioventricular block (AVB) as primary risk factors for the development of TdP.[8] However, as this phenomenon became a more clinically appreciated entity in the 1970s and 1980s, underlying clinical risk factors, for example, hypokalemia and female gender, became increasingly recognized as key contributors in determining TdP susceptibility.[4] The observation that TdP may have a clinical and an environmental trigger and also genetic susceptibility led to the hypothesis that normal cardiac rhythm is supported by multiple, redundant mechanisms for the repolarization of ventricular myocardium.[3] The term "repolarization reserve" was first coined by Roden[9] to describe the inherent variability of arrhythmic response to QT interval prolongation with the relationship between perturbations of one ion channel (such as I_{Kr}) in relation to the sum total repolarizing currents. In other words, clinical and genetic risk factors affect cellular repolarization reserve, which modulates susceptibility to TdP.

Of the plasma membrane ion channels that contribute to myocardial repolarization reserve,

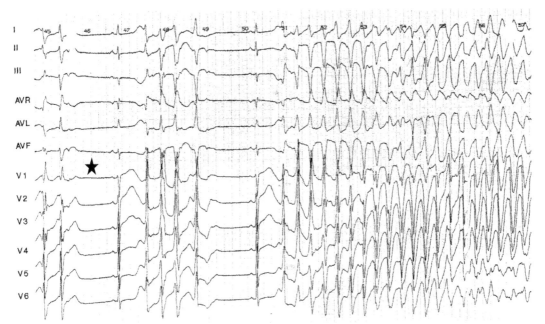

Fig. 1. A 12-lead ECG demonstrating induction of TdP. The 12-lead ECG was taken from a 79-year-old patient with advanced heart failure, who recently began taking dofetilide. The long QT interval is followed by a long pause (as indicated by a *star*), followed by 4 beats of TdP, and then sustained TdP. (*From* Kannankeril P, Roden DM, Darbar D. Drug-induced long QT syndrome. Pharmacol Rev 2010;62:760–81. *Courtesy of* American Society for Pharmacology and Experimental Therapeutics, Bethesda (MD), with permission.)

the rapidly rectifying inward potassium current, I_{Kr}, has been most widely recognized to be responsible for TdP risk.[10–17] In contrast, the slow delayed rectifier potassium current (I_{Ks}) contribution to TdP formation has been more controversial,[18] because the effects of selective I_{Ks}-blocking drugs on action potential duration (APD) have been variable.[19–22] However, recent genetic evidence from whole exome sequencing of 65 diLQTS patients suggests that the *KCNE1* gene is responsible for the risk of life-threatening TdP, thus implicating an I_{Ks}-mediated risk.[23] Other ion channel currents implicated in repolarization reserve include I_{Na}, $I_{Ca,L}$, I_{to}, $I_{Na/K}$, and I_{NCX} and are detailed by Varró and colleagues,[3] in an excellent review of the ionic contributors to cellular repolarization reserve.

Measurement of repolarization reserve in whole animal models has provided additional insights into clinical risk factors for TdP. These models highlight the importance of Triangulation, Reverse use-dependence, Instability (of repolarization current), and Dispersion of Refractoriness, together known as the TRIaD model.[2] Haraguchi and colleagues,[24] who modeled transmural dispersion of repolarization (TDR) during ventricular tachycardia, provide a good example of applying this approach to TdP.[16] They found that arrhythmia risk in TdP is related to scroll wave stability and

is not directly associated with QT interval width. In a rabbit heart model of TdP, Wu and colleagues[25] found that reverse use-dependence of I_{Kr}-blocking drugs, such as sotalol, is directly associated with endogenous late sodium current (I_{Na-L}); this contributes to increases in APD and beat-to-beat variability of repolarization, both independent risk factors for TdP.

Attempts to use the TRIaD model to screen and predict torsadogenic risk associated with pharmaceutical agents have been met with variable success. Yang and colleagues[26] found that some but not all I_{Kr}-blocking drugs (such as dofetilide) augment I_{Na-L} through the phosphoinositide 3-kinase pathway and thus directly contribute to proarrhythmia through a novel mechanism that is distinct from I_{Kr}-related APD prolongation that is used by regulatory agencies to stratify TdP risk. Likewise, iPSC models for screening TdP risk have been described, which can model patient-specific genetic variants and link this variation to diLQTS risk,[27,28] directly aligning with the Precision Medicine Initiative of the National Institutes of Health.[29] With improved understanding of the underlying mechanisms of both genetic and acquired forms of TdP, the opportunity to personalize selection of AAD therapy based on individual risk factors may become a reality (see **Table 1**).

FEMALE GENDER

Female gender has long been recognized as an independent risk factor for prolongation of the QT interval, congenital LQTS, diLQTS, and TdP.[30] Women have a higher resting heart rate than men with QT intervals on average that are 20 milliseconds longer.[31,32] Adult women are 2 to 3 times more likely than men to experience episodes of TdP. However, the underlying mechanism or mechanisms for this differential effect in women remain poorly understood.[33] Yang and colleagues[32] used the O'Hara-Rudy model, an established in silico model of ventricular repolarization, to create simulated "male" and "female" cells and tissues to explore reduced repolarization reserve in women. The model incorporated reduced repolarizing potassium currents and connexin-43 expression, both observed in human women, and showed that such differences were sufficient to predict prolongation of APD in epicardial and endocardial cells in women. In addition, Gonzalez and colleagues[34] used a related Luo-Rudy in silico model to show that adult female myocytes have reduced ventricular repolarization reserve, and that simulated exposure to dofetilide is associated with decreased I_{Ks}, steeper APD to basic cycle length relationship, and increased susceptibility to early afterdepolarizations (EAD) when compared with adult male cells under the same conditions. Interestingly, these investigators found that this difference was age-dependent; there were essentially no differences between in silico models of young male and young female ventricular myocytes. One significant difference in TdP risk between young girls and adult women may be due to the effects of hormone-related changes in ventricular repolarization. Ando and colleagues[35] showed that the contribution of I_{Kr}, encoded by KCNH2, is significantly affected by β-estradiol when stably expressed in human embryonic kidney (HEK)- 239 cells in vitro. KCNH2 currents were inhibited to 62% of control at baseline; when combined with erythromycin, a known I_{Kr}-blocking antibiotic, there was additional KCNH2-mediated current inhibition to 42%, suggesting that, in some cases, women may be more susceptible to diLQTS. However, these findings need to be confirmed with additional in vitro experiments.

Sex hormone experiments in rabbit hearts, which unlike mice or rats express I_{Kr}, have yielded several informative observations regarding risk of TdP. In Langendorff-perfused rabbit hearts, estradiol prolongs monophasic APD in a concentration-dependent manner.[36] In contrast, progesterone prolongs APD at lower concentrations (1–3 μm), but shortens the monophasic APD at higher, more physiologic conditions (10–30 μm), suggesting a biphasic pattern.[37] In addition, progesterone protected against sotalol-induced proarrhythmic events, suggesting that hormone-based APD prolongation may mediate risk of TdP. In a related study, Cheng and colleagues[37] showed in a chronic model of female hormone modulation (ovariectomy followed by hormone replacement therapy with either estrogen, progesterone, or both) that estradiol may potentiate the QTc prolonging effects of d,l-sotalol, whereas progesterone protects against QT prolongation and related arrhythmias by accelerating the process of repolarization. Tisdale and colleagues[38] showed a similar protective effect of progesterone (vs estrogen) in female rabbits ovariectomized and implanted with estrogen, progesterone, and testosterone. Thus, there is strong evidence to support sex hormones as a significant contributor to APD, QT prolongation, and risk of ventricular arrhythmias including TdP.

BRADYCARDIA

Bradycardia and bradyarrhythmias are risk factors for the development of life-threatening arrhythmias, including TdP. However, it is not possible to fully predict TdP risk from QT interval duration and/or AVB alone.[39] In a study of 20 patients (15 women, aged 65.9 ± 15.6 years), Cho and colleagues[39] characterized specific 12-lead ECG patterns in patients diagnosed with atrioventricular (AV) block and displaying TdP waves and compared these ECGs with 80 age- and sex-matched controls without TdP. The development of TdP was typically induced by premature ventricular complexes and all TdP ECGs displayed significant differences in phase 4 repolarization parameters, including increased mean QT interval (716.4 ± 98.9 ms vs 523.2 ± 91.3 ms, $P = .001$), mean T peak to end interval (334.2 ± 59.1 ms vs 144.0 ± 73.7 ms, $P = .001$), and a higher T peak to end interval/QT ratio (0.49 ± 0.09 ms vs 0.27 ± 0.11 ms, $P = .001$). The following additional T-wave parameters also proved to be more prevalent in TdP-displaying AV block patients compared with non-TdP controls: notched T waves (ie, $T_2 > T_1$); triphasic T waves; reversed asymmetry; and T-wave alternans ($P = .001$). A combination of these wave parameters allowed delineation of TdP cases from non-TdP cases with high sensitivity (85%) and specificity (98%).

Rosso and colleagues[40] realized comparable results when examining arrhythmogenic effects of cardiac memory in patients with LQTS complicating AV block. The concept of cardiac memory purports that T waves that were once abnormal secondary to irregular QRS waves (eg, AV block) possess a memory of the vectors of the altered QRS waves and continue to behave under those abnormal conditions. During AV block, the magnitude of the QT prolongation in response to the bradycardia is a determining risk factor for TdP. Rosso and colleagues assessed patients with similar bradycardic profiles and sought to answer why some patients experience more QT prolongation than others, and if this variation in magnitude predisposes to TdP. They examined 91 patients with either 2:1 or high-degree/complete AV block (mean age of 77 $\pm$ 12 years, 53% men). On average, patients with complete AV block presented with longer R-R interval and QT interval duration than those with 2:1 block. Specifically, the analysis focused on alterations in 3 parameters: change in QRS (ΔQRS) morphology, ΔQRS axis, and both ΔQRS morphology and axis together, in the setting of AV block and effect on QT prolongation. Despite similar age, sex, and ECG parameters, including R-R intervals during AV block, subjects with positive ΔQRS morphology showed significantly longer QT and corrected-QT interval (QTc), using Bazett's Formula to assess risk for TdP, compared with cases without ΔQRS morphology (229 $\pm$ 84 ms vs 51 $\pm$ 86 ms, $P<.001$; and 46 $\pm$ 80 ms vs -6 ± 74 ms, $P = .001$). Eight cases of AVB-related TdP were recorded for patients with ΔQRS morphology versus 4 in those without ($P = .026$). Spearman correlation showed a significant correlation between ΔQRS axis and ΔQT ($r = 0.218$; $P = .025$) as well as ΔQTc ($r = 0.308$; $P = .001$). A similar number of cases were recorded for TdP in ΔQRS axis versus no changes (8 vs 4; $P = .023$, respectively). AV block presented the greatest QT prolongation (250 $\pm$ 100 ms; $P<.001$) when changes in both QRS morphology and axis were present. Topilski and colleagues[41] showed that a change in ΔQRS morphology during AV block independently predicted LQTS and was strongly associated with TdP. They think this analysis supports cardiac memory playing a vital role in enhancing QT prolongation, which can further predict TdP during bradycardic events. Moreover, the longer the period of irregular ventricular QRS complexes, the more likely it is that T waves will display a longer period of abnormal behavior. Interestingly, Obreztchikova and colleagues[42] claimed that the morphology of abnormally transcribed I_{Kr} leads to reduction of myocyte potassium channels, which can further potentiate QT prolongation. In addition, in a canine model, the heterogeneity of transmural repolarization gradients were attributed to the induction of cardiac memory T-wave morphology, increasing epicardial left ventricular repolarization gradients.[43]

HYPOKALEMIA AND HYPOMAGNESEMIA

Approximately 28% of TdP reports in the literature are associated with either hypokalemia or hypomagnesemia.[44] Hypokalemia is strongly associated with TdP and has been shown to play a significant role in diLQTS.[45] Drug-induced hypokalemia occurs primarily through 3 recognized mechanisms: (1) transcellular potassium shift (β_2-agonists, insulin, caffeine); (2) increased renal potassium loss (diuretics, mineralocorticoids, penicillins, glucocorticoids); and (3) excess potassium loss in stool (phenolphthalein, sodium polystyrene sulfonate).[46] Recent reports of the effects of hypokalemia on myocardial repolarization currents have implicated I_{Kr} and I_{Ks} in the pathogenesis of TdP. Heterogeneity of potassium channel concentration may partially explain reduction in repolarization reserve in hypokalemia. Guo and colleagues[47] showed in HEK-293 cells that extracellular (serum) $[K^+]_o$ is directly associated with expression of the KCNH2 gene and I_{Kr}. Reduction of $[K^+]_o$ was associated with accelerated internalization and degradation of KCNH2- channels within hours through ubiquitinization. Later work from this group showed that in HEK-293 cells coexpression of I_{Kr} and I_{Ks} may delay hypokalemia-induced KCNH2 degradation through a direct protein-protein interaction; this was not seen by single channel expression of either channel alone.[48] Heterogeneity in TDR may also partially explain TdP susceptibility in hypokalemia. Killeen and colleagues[49] showed, in isolated mouse hearts, that hypokalemia reduces ΔAPD_{90} between epicardium and endocardium, resulting in EADs and nonsustained ventricular tachycardia and sustained ventricular tachycardia on programmed electrical stimulation. Likewise, Melgari and colleagues[50] performed whole-cell patch-clamp measurements of HEK-293 cells stably expressing KCNH2- channels and showed that under conditions of hypokalemia (4 to 1 mmol/L potassium) there is a significant reduction in the I_{Kr} contribution to ventricular repolarization, resulting in pathologic premature extra stimuli. Thus, there is a direct link between extracellular potassium concentration $[K^+]_o$ and the function and expression of I_{Kr} and I_{Ks}.

In addition to the direct effects on $[K^+]_o$, hypokalemia is known to worsen repolarization reserve in patients who have drug-related or genetic alterations in ventricular repolarization. Common drugs known to induce QT interval prolongation and resultant TdP include citalopram, escitalopram, methadone, ondansetron, and azithromycin. For a more complete list and accompanying discussion, Trinkley and colleagues[51] offer an excellent overview (**Box 1**). Each one of these drug categories may have increased TdP risk by the presence of hypokalemia due to partial inhibition of I_{Kr}. Of interest, licorice is a known cause of hypokalemia because of inhibition of the 11β-hydroxysteroid dehydrogenase (type II), which leads to excess cortisol excretion and "pseudohyperaldosteronism," and in extreme cases, may result in TdP.[52] Genetic mutations in *KCNH2* (T473P) and *KCNE1* (G38S) increase susceptibility to hypokalemia-induced TdP by reducing repolarization reserve and QT interval prolongation, demonstrating a drug-independent, genetic predisposition to hypokalemia-related TdP risk.[14,53] These findings underscore the importance of pharmacogenetic mechanism in the determination of TdP risk (See Roden DM: Pharmacogenetics of Potassium Channel Blockers, in this issue).

Although hypomagnesemia has been implicated in the risk for TdP, the underlying mechanism has been less well described. Hypomagnesemia primarily occurs through chronic use of loop diuretics, thiazide diuretics, or alcohol; other causes include intestinal malabsorption and reduced dietary intake.[54] Although Mg^{2+} flux is not a direct contributor to repolarization current, extracellular $[Mg^{2+}]$ has a membrane-stabilizing effect by facilitating normal function of the Na/K pump; without sufficient Mg^{2+} available to this membrane channel, there is depletion of intracellular $[K^+]$, reducing transmembrane K^+ gradient and leading to membrane depolarization and TdP.[54] Hypomagnesemia has been linked to an increase in patient mortality[55] and arrhythmia risk; although the link between hypomagnesemia and TdP-related mortality is yet unproven.[56–58] Recently, there has been some controversy regarding the arrhythmic risk of proton pump inhibitor (PPI)-related hypomagnesemia. It is currently unknown whether PPIs contribute to TdP risk in patients with gastrointestinal disease and electrolyte disturbances.[59–61] Because the mechanism of this observation is currently unknown, further translational studies and controlled prospective trials are necessary to determine the contribution of PPIs toward TdP risk.

ATRIAL FIBRILLATION

AF is the most common sustained cardiac arrhythmia, and its incidence steadily increases.[62] Currently, the lifetime risk of AF is 1:4 for men and women, and by the year 2050, more than 12 million Americans will be affected.[62,63] AF remains an independent risk factor for the development of stroke, thromboembolism, heart failure, and impaired quality of life. Likewise, conversion of

---

Box 1
Potassium channel blocking antiarrhythmics and common drugs that block I_{Kr} and lead to QT prolongation and increased susceptibility to torsades de pointes

Antiarrhythmic drugs

Disopyramide

Dofetilide

Sotalol

Procainamide

Ibutilide

Bepridil

Amiodarone

Common drugs

Arsenic trioxide

Cisapride

Calcium-channel blockers: lidoflazine

Anti-infective agents: Clarithromycin, erythromycin, halofantrine, pentamidine, sparfloxacin

Antiemetics: domperidone, droperidol

Antipsychotic agents: chlorpromazine, haloperidol, mesoridazine, thioridazine, pimozide

Methadone

AF to sinus rhythm is associated with modest long-term improvements in cardiac function, stroke risk, and quality of life.[64] Dispersion of refractoriness of atrial tissue contributes to the mechanism of AF, and thus, I_{Kr}-blocking AADs are prominent antiarrhythmic therapies to treat patients with AF. However, many AADs used to treat AF block I_{Kr} and may result in toxicity that includes QT prolongation and TdP.[65]

Conversely, there is evidence to support the idea that AF in and of itself protects against TdP risk, and that after conversion from AF to sinus rhythm, risk of TdP actually increases.[4] For example, TdP has been noted to occur immediately after conversion of AF to sinus rhythm.[6,66,67] Although this may reflect a reduction in the heart rate that often accompanies restoration of sinus rhythm, recent studies suggest that the underlying mechanisms are likely to be more complicated. In an elegant study, Choy and colleagues[68] examined the extent of QT prolongation by intravenous dofetilide during AF and immediately after restoration of sinus rhythm. Surprisingly, there was minimal change in the QT interval during AF after intravenous dofetilide. However, shortly after return of sinus rhythm, the QT interval prolonged markedly despite dofetilide not changing the heart rate (**Fig. 2**). This group has subsequently

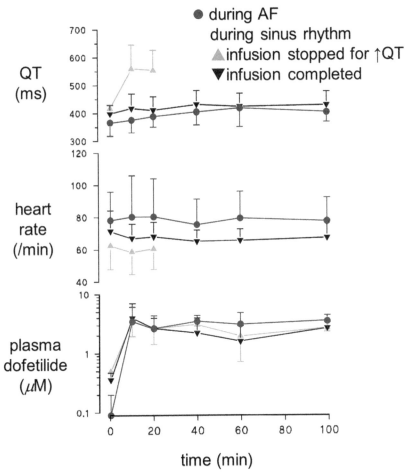

Fig. 2. Evidence for abnormal QT control revealed by infusion of dofetilide before and following conversion of AF. This study compared the effect of dofetilide on QT interval when the drug was administered as a bolus and maintenance infusions greater than 100 minutes during AF, and again within 24 hours of conversion to sinus. There was no major effect of dofetilide on QT when the underlying rhythm was AF (*top panel*). When the same infusion, reaching the same concentrations (*bottom panel*), was administered during sinus rhythm (SR), 2 groups of responses were delineated: group I had marked QT interval prolongation (requiring premature cessation of the infusion), while group II responded as in AF, with no major change in QT, and received the whole infusion. Note that dofetilide produced no change in heart rate from predrug baseline in any group, and that baseline heart rates differed by less than 10 bpm in groups I and II during SR. Thus, heart rate slowing by cardioversion cannot be the sole explanation for the marked drug sensitivity seen here.

shown that QT-RR slopes are very flat during AF even after long pauses and steepen markedly after restoration of sinus rhythm, supporting the hypothesis that AF itself modulates the QT interval both during AF and shortly after conversion to normal rhythm.[69,70]

The mechanism whereby AF may reduce TdP risk is currently unknown. However, AF-related cellular remodeling may be related to preservation of TDR, which in turn, may lead to reduced susceptibility of TdP in patients with diLQTS.[4] In addition, the authors' group postulated that AF generates mechanisms rendering the QT interval resistant to marked prolongation, despite variable R-R intervals and short-long-short cycles. In ongoing studies, detailed phenotyping of a large cohort of patients undergoing elective direct

current (DC) cardioversion for AF is being performed, and the extent of QT interval change is being related to measures of candidate QT modulators, such as inflammation, oxidant stress, catecholamines, and atrial natriuretic factor (ANF) (**Fig. 3**).[71] Furthermore, the development of reliable methods of measuring the QT interval during AF allows the assessment of QT during AF and can be compared to QT in sinus rhythm, taking into account changes in rate.[69] The QT intervals during and following atrial pacing will also be assessed and related to pacing rate, duration, and measures of candidate QT modulators. Other groups are also relating atrial rate to molecular changes underlying ventricular function and rhythm maintenance in order to further dissect this mechanism.[72]

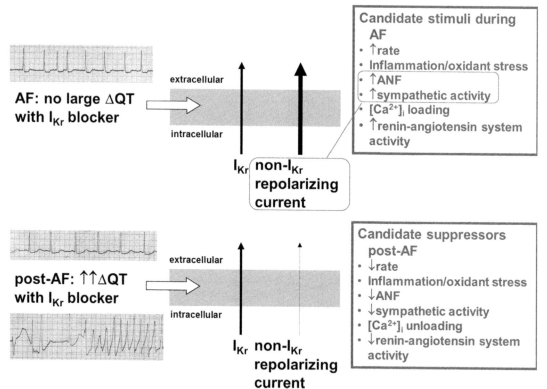

Fig. 3. Potential mechanisms by which the QT interval is modulated before and following cardioversion in patients with AF. As described in the text, challenge with an I_{Kr}-blocking drug when the underlying rhythm is AF generates little change in QT interval, whereas the same challenge shortly after SR is restored can produce marked QT prolongation and TdP (see **Fig. 2**). The rhythm strips show such a result with dofetilide; note the heart rates during AF and SR are similar, and that the drug did not change heart rate. These and other data described in the text suggest that AF generates mechanisms rendering the QT resistant to marked prolongation, despite variable RR intervals and short-long-short cycles. In ongoing studies, detailed phenotyping of a large cohort of patients undergoing elective DC-cardioversion for AF is being conducted and changes in QT will be related to measures of candidate QT modulators, such as inflammation, oxidant stress, catecholamines, and ANF. The development of reliable methods to assess QT interval during AF will permit the evaluation of QT intervals during AF and in SR taking into account changes in heart rate. In addition, comparison of QT intervals during and following atrial pacing, and relating the pacing rate, duration, and measures of candidate QT modulators will be performed.

THE ROLE OF VARIABLE DRUG CONCENTRATIONS IN TORSADES DE POINTES RISK

Initial reports with quinidine noted that the adverse effect often occurred within 24 hours of starting the drug, at a time when excessive accumulation of drug (or potentially active metabolites) would not be expected. Indeed, with routine plasma concentration monitoring came the frequent observations of "subtherapeutic" quinidine concentrations in patients developing TdP.[6,73,74] Studies as early as the 1940s[75,76] identified multiple quinidine metabolites, raising the possibility that variability in response to the drug might reflect variable activity or accumulation of metabolite or metabolites. However, subsequent studies established that the multiple metabolites demonstrate less *in vitro* electrophysiologic activity than the parent drug[77] and that plasma concentrations at the time of TdP were generally lower for the metabolite compared with the parent drug.[78] The lack of a relationship between plasma quinidine concentrations and TdP risk likely reflects the drug's inhibition of multiple ion currents with a range of potencies: block of I_{Kr} at low concentrations[79] to prolong action potentials; at higher concentrations block of other potassium currents to prolong action potentials,[80,81] and block of sodium current (in a frequency-dependent fashion) to shorten action potentials.[82,83]

By contrast, TdP developing during therapy with most other AADs (sotalol, dofetilide) and noncardiovascular therapies (thioridazine, methadone) appears to be dose or concentration related.[84,85] Thus, conditions leading to accumulation of QT-prolonging agents in plasma are in general risk factors for TdP. Sotalol and dofetilide undergo renal excretion and therefore require dose reductions in patients with reduced renal function to avoid TdP.[84,86] This concept extends to drug metabolism: thioridazine is a CYP2D6 substrate, and some data suggest that the drug accumulates in plasma in poor metabolizers with more marked QT prolongation.[87] Similarly, the QT prolonging S-enantiomer of methadone is eliminated by CYP2B6-mediated metabolism, and individuals with reduction-of-function alleles in this gene may therefore be at increased risk for methadone-induced TdP.[88]

EFFECTS OF DRUG CONCENTRATION ON QT INTERVAL AND ARRHYTHMIA RISK

The treatment of arrhythmias with traditional antiarrhythmics has long been known to be beneficial, but also to carry proarrhythmic and protorsadogenic side effects. Blockade of the KCNH2 channel, specifically I_{Kr}, and subsequent QT prolongation as observed on surface ECG can predict TdP.[52] However, QTc prolongation alone could not be attributed to either pure I_{Kr}-blockade from multichannel blockade. In order to differentiate the effects in a prospective, randomized controlled trial with 22 patients (mean age of 26.9 ± 5.5 years, 11 women), Johannesen and colleagues[89] administered dofetilide (pure I_{Kr}-blocker) along with 3 other antiarrhythmics: quinidine (Na^+ channel blockade), ranolazine (Na^+ channel blockade; commonly used as an antianginal), and verapamil (cardiac specific L-type Ca^{2+} channel blockade), each exhibiting varying degrees of I_{Kr}-channel blockade as well. Direct blockade of the K^+ channel by class III antiarrhythmic dofetilide prolonged both early ($J - T_{peak}$) and late ($T_{peak} - T_{end}$) repolarization currents, whereas multichannel blockade from the other antiarrhythmic classes primarily resulted in shortening of early repolarization ($J - T_{peak}$) segment. This observation allowed differentiation of the effects of antiarrhythmics during repolarization. This has clinical significance, of course; the ability to track changes in $J - T_{peak}$ and $T_{peak} - T_{end}$ offers more precise observations in cardiac drug safety evaluation. Specifically, in understanding the triggers for arrhythmias and TdP, it has been shown that blockade of I_{Kr} can potentiate TdP due to increased Na^+ and Ca^{2+} inward current, EAD. Thus, inhibition of this inward ion flux through multichannel blockade may minimize EADs and reduce the risk of arrhythmogenesis and subsequent TdP. Although the direct I_{Kr} blockade by the class III antiarrhythmic dofetilide has been shown to prolong both early and late repolarization currents, the effect of drugs from other classes on I_{Kr} channels (in addition to their respective target channel) appear to alter either the Ca^{2+} or the Na^+ inward currents, resulting in prolongation of early repolarization.

Sugrue and colleagues[53] examined 13 cases of drug-induced TdP secondary to administration of either dofetilide (5 cases, 80% women) or sotalol (8 cases, 75% women), both known to affect cardiac K^+ channels with proarrhythmogenic and protorsadogenic properties.[59,60] Compared with 26 age- and sex-matched controls, the accuracy in predicting TdP risk improved by 9% in cases receiving class III AADs when QTc and T-wave right slope measurements during phase 4 repolarization were combined (QTc, 79%; QTc and T-wave right slope, 88%).[53] QTc in lead V6 and the T-wave right wave slope in aVR were most prominent T-wave parameters, contributing to a strong correlation with TdP (QTc in V6, mean case vs control: 500 ± 44 vs 410 ± 38 milliseconds, $P<.001$, $r = 0.77$; T-wave right wave slope in aVR, mean case vs control: −682.88 ± 38 vs −1509.53 ± 44 mV/s, $P<.001$, $r = 0.56$). ECG analysis showed comparable correlations with QTc in lead V3 and T-wave right slope in lead I. Of the parameters, this analysis showed that T-wave right slope in Lead I possessed high correlation to risk of arrhythmias and allowed delineation of TdP risk from the control groups. Specifically, the characteristics of the slope of the T wave in Lead I were of focus, amplitude, and duration of the terminal portion of the wave. The results suggest that the TdP cases (13/39) presented with shallower right slopes, possibly implicating substantial dispersion of the refractoriness in both the transmural and the apicobasal gradients. Sugrue and colleagues[53] further investigated alterations in index center of gravity (COG), comprising mean x and y coordinates during T-wave progression. They suggest COGx accounted for subtle differences in T waves in TdP cases compared with the control cases. This finding indicates that in cases with T-wave abnormalities, particularly the amplitude and duration, COGx interpretations have the potential to predict those most likely at risk for arrhythmogenesis and TdP.

SUMMARY

Torsadogenic and ventricular arrhythmic risk from ion channelopathies do not occur in isolation and involve underlying clinical risk factors that represent stressors to the homeostasis of potassium repolarization currents. Risk factors such as female gender, bradycardia, hypokalemia, hypomagnesemia, restoration of sinus rhythm from AF, drugs, and genetic variants encoding KCNH2-mediated currents that affect QT interval all figure prominently in the assessment of a patient's overall risk for developing a malignant ventricular arrhythmia. Through the evaluation of clinical risk factors and relating this data to knowledge of drug-induced or genetically determined alterations in potassium channel current (such as I_{Kr}), it is possible to more accurately stratify and then ameliorate their torsadogenic risk. Further research into improved understanding of the underlying mechanisms by which I_{Kr}-blocking drugs mediate QT interval prolongation and TdP is necessary to bridge the clinical and basic factors of arrhythmia risk and prediction scores. Furthermore, incorporating data from both realms will help to prevent these lethal arrhythmias before they happen, thus fulfilling the promise of predictive and precision medicine.

REFERENCES

1. Ponte ML, Keller GA, Di Girolamo G. Mechanisms of drug induced QT interval prolongation. Curr Drug Saf 2010;5:44–53.
2. Sauer AJ, Newton-Cheh C. Clinical and genetic determinants of torsade de pointes risk. Circulation 2012;125:1684–94.
3. Varró A, Baczko I. Cardiac ventricular repolarization reserve: a principle for understanding drug-related proarrhythmic risk. Br J Pharmacol 2011;164:14–36.
4. Kannankeril P, Roden DM, Darbar D. Drug-induced long QT syndrome. Pharmacol Rev 2010;62:760–81.
5. Tranebjaerg L, Bathen J, Tyson J, et al. Jervell and Lange-Nielsen syndrome: a Norwegian perspective. Am J Med Genet 1999;89:137–46.
6. Levy RL. Clinical studies of quinidine. IV. The clinical toxicology of quinidine. JAMA 1922;79:1108–13.
7. Selzer A, Wray HW. Quinidine syncope. Paroxysmal ventricular fibrillation occurring during treatment of chronic atrial arrhythmias. Circulation 1964;30:17–26.
8. Dessertenne F. La tachycardie ventriculaire a dex foyers opposes variables. Arch Mal Coeur Vaiss 1966;59:263–72.
9. Roden DM. Repolarization reserve: a moving target. Circulation 2008;118:981–2.
10. Amoros I, Jimenez-Jaimez J, Tercedor L, et al. Functional effects of a missense mutation in HERG associated with type 2 long QT syndrome. Heart Rhythm 2011;8:463–70.
11. Donner BC, Marschall C, Schmidt KG. A presumably benign human ether-a-go-go-related gene mutation (R176W) with a malignant primary manifestation of long QT syndrome. Cardiol Young 2012;22:360–3.
12. Friemel A, Zunkler BJ. Interactions at human ether-a-go-go-related gene channels. Toxicol Sci 2010;114:346–55.
13. DI Veroli GY, Davies MR, Zhang H, et al. hERG inhibitors with similar potency but different binding kinetics do not pose the same proarrhythmic risk: implications for drug safety assessment. J Cardiovasc Electrophysiol 2014;25:197–207.
14. Liu L, Hayashi K, Kaneda T, et al. A novel mutation in the transmembrane nonpore region of the KCNH2 gene causes severe clinical manifestations of long QT syndrome. Heart Rhythm 2013;10:61–7.
15. Nishimoto O, Matsuda M, Nakamoto K, et al. Peripartum cardiomyopathy presenting with syncope due to Torsades de pointes: a case of long QT syndrome with a novel KCNH2 mutation. Intern Med 2012;51:461–4.
16. Qu Y, Fang M, Gao B, et al. BeKm-1, a peptide inhibitor of human ether-a-go-go-related gene potassium currents, prolongs QTc intervals in isolated rabbit heart. J Pharmacol Exp Ther 2011;337:2–8.

17. Sato A, Chinushi M, Suzuki H, et al. Long QT syndrome with nocturnal cardiac events caused by a KCNH2 missense mutation (G604S). Intern Med 2012;51:1857–60.

18. Jost N, Papp JG, Varro A. Slow delayed rectifier potassium current (IKs) and the repolarization reserve. Ann Noninvasive Electrocardiol 2007;12:64–78.

19. Emori T, Antzelevitch C. Cellular basis for complex T waves and arrhythmic activity following combined I(Kr) and I(Ks) block. J Cardiovasc Electrophysiol 2001;12:1369–78.

20. Sun ZQ, Thomas GP, Antzelevitch C. Chromanol 293B inhibits slowly activating delayed rectifier and transient outward currents in canine left ventricular myocytes. J Cardiovasc Electrophysiol 2001;12: 472–8.

21. Bauer A, Becker R, Karle C, et al. Effects of the I(Kr)-blocking agent dofetilide and of the I(Ks)-blocking agent chromanol 293b on regional disparity of left ventricular repolarization in the intact canine heart. J Cardiovasc Pharmacol 2002;39:460–7.

22. Burashnikov A, Antzelevitch C. Prominent I(Ks) in epicardium and endocardium contributes to development of transmural dispersion of repolarization but protects against development of early afterdepolarizations. J Cardiovasc Electrophysiol 2002;13: 172–7.

23. Weeke P, Mosley JD, Hanna D, et al. Exome sequencing implicates an increased burden of rare potassium channel variants in the risk of drug-induced long QT interval syndrome. J Am Coll Cardiol 2014;63:1430–7.

24. Haraguchi R, Ashihara T, Namba T, et al. Transmural dispersion of repolarization determines scroll wave behavior during ventricular tachyarrhythmias. Circulation 2011;75:80–8.

25. Wu L, Ma J, Li H, et al. Late sodium current contributes to the reverse rate-dependent effect of IKr inhibition on ventricular repolarization. Circulation 2011; 123:1713–20.

26. Yang T, Chun YW, Stroud DM, et al. Screening for acute IKr block is insufficient to detect torsades de pointes liability: role of late sodium current. Circulation 2014;130:224–34.

27. Fermini B, Hancox JC, Abi-Gerges N, et al. A new perspective in the field of cardiac safety testing through the comprehensive in vitro proarrhythmia assay paradigm. J Biomol Screen 2015;21(1):1–11.

28. Nozaki Y, Honda Y, Tsujimoto S, et al. Availability of human induced pluripotent stem cell-derived cardiomyocytes in assessment of drug potential for QT prolongation. Toxicol Appl Pharmacol 2014;278: 72–7.

29. Mehta A, Chung Y, Sequiera GL, et al. Pharmacoelectrophysiology of viral-free induced pluripotent stem cell-derived human cardiomyocytes. Toxicol Sci 2013;131:458–69.

30. Li G, Cheng G, Wu J, et al. Drug-induced long QT syndrome in women. Adv Ther 2013;30:793–802.

31. O'Hara T, Virag L, Varro A, et al. Simulation of the undiseased human cardiac ventricular action potential: model formulation and experimental validation. PLoS Comput Biol 2011;7:e1002061.

32. Yang T, Atack TC, Stroud DM, et al. Blocking Scn10a channels in heart reduces late sodium current and is antiarrhythmic. Circ Res 2012;111:322–32.

33. Ciaccio EJ. Torsades, sex hormones, and ventricular repolarization. J Cardiovasc Electrophysiol 2011;22: 332–3.

34. Gonzalez R, Gomis-Tena J, Corrias A, et al. Sex and age related differences in drug induced QT prolongation by dofetilide under reduced repolarization reserve in simulated ventricular cells. Conf Proc IEEE Eng Med Biol Soc 2010;2010: 3245–8.

35. Ando F, Kuruma A, Kawano S. Synergic effects of beta-estradiol and erythromycin on hERG currents. J Membr Biol 2011;241:31–8.

36. Cheng J, Ma X, Zhang J, et al. Diverse modulating effects of estradiol and progesterone on the monophasic action potential duration in Langendorff-perfused female rabbit hearts. Fundam Clin Pharmacol 2012;26:219–26.

37. Cheng J, Su D, Ma X, et al. Concurrent supplement of estradiol and progesterone reduces the cardiac sensitivity to D,L-sotalol-induced arrhythmias in ovariectomized rabbits. J Cardiovasc Pharmacol Ther 2012;17:208–14.

38. Tisdale JE, Overholser BR, Wroblewski HA, et al. The influence of progesterone alone and in combination with estradiol on ventricular action potential duration and triangulation in response to potassium channel inhibition. J Cardiovasc Electrophysiol 2011;22:325–31.

39. Cho MS, Nam GB, Kim YG, et al. Electrocardiographic predictors of bradycardia-induced torsades de pointes in patients with acquired atrioventricular block. Heart Rhythm 2015;12:498–505.

40. Rosso R, Adler A, Strasberg B, et al. Long QT syndrome complicating atrioventricular block: arrhythmogenic effects of cardiac memory. Circ Arrhythm Electrophysiol 2014;7:1129–35.

41. Topilski I, Rogowski O, Rosso R, et al. The morphology of the QT interval predicts torsade de pointes during acquired bradyarrhythmias. J Am Coll Cardiol 2007;49:320–8.

42. Obreztchikova MN, Patberg KW, Plotnikov AN, et al. I(Kr) contributes to the altered ventricular repolarization that determines long-term cardiac memory. Cardiovasc Res 2006;71:88–96.

43. Coronel R, Opthof T, Plotnikov AN, et al. Long-term cardiac memory in canine heart is associated with the evolution of a transmural repolarization gradient. Cardiovasc Res 2007;74:416–25.

44. Abo-Salem E, Fowler JC, Attari M, et al. Antibiotic-induced cardiac arrhythmias. Cardiovasc Ther 2014;32:19–25.

45. Darbar D, Kimbrough J, Jawaid A, et al. Persistent atrial fibrillation is associated with reduced risk of torsades de pointes in patients with drug-induced long QT syndrome. J Am Coll Cardiol 2008;51:836–42.

46. Gennari FJ. Hypokalemia. N Engl J Med 1998;339: 451–8.

47. Guo J, Massaeli H, Xu J, et al. Extracellular K+ concentration controls cell surface density of IKr in rabbit hearts and of the HERG channel in human cell lines. J Clin Invest 2009;119:2745–57.

48. Guo J, Wang T, Yang T, et al. Interaction between the cardiac rapidly (IKr) and slowly (IKs) activating delayed rectifier potassium channels revealed by low K+-induced hERG endocytic degradation. J Biol Chem 2011;286:34664–74.

49. Killeen MJ, Thomas G, Gurung IS, et al. Arrhythmogenic mechanisms in the isolated perfused hypokalaemic murine heart. Acta Physiol (Oxf) 2007;189: 33–46.

50. Melgari D, Du C, El Harchi A, et al. Suppression of the hERG potassium channel response to premature stimulation by reduction in extracellular potassium concentration. Physiol Rep 2014;2.

51. Trinkley KE, Page RL 2nd, Lien H, et al. QT interval prolongation and the risk of torsades de pointes: essentials for clinicians. Curr Med Res Opin 2013;29: 1719–26.

52. Panduranga P, Al-Rawahi N. Licorice-induced severe hypokalemia with recurrent torsade de pointes. Ann Noninvasive Electrocardiol 2013;18:593–6.

53. Yamaguchi Y, Mizumaki K, Hata Y, et al. Abnormal repolarization dynamics in a patient with KCNE1(G38S) who presented with torsades de pointes. J Electrocardiol 2016;49(1):94–8.

54. Efstratiadis G, Sarigianni M, Gougourelas I. Hypomagnesemia and cardiovascular system. Hippokratia 2006;10:147–52.

55. Fairley J, Glassford NJ, Zhang L, et al. Magnesium status and magnesium therapy in critically ill patients: a systematic review. J Crit Care 2015;30:1349–58.

56. Hoorn EJ, van der Hoek J, de Man RA, et al. A case series of proton pump inhibitor-induced hypomagnesemia. Am J Kidney Dis 2010;56:112–6.

57. Khan AM, Lubitz SA, Sullivan LM, et al. Low serum magnesium and the development of atrial fibrillation in the community: the Framingham Heart Study. Circulation 2013;127:33–8.

58. Scherr J, Schuster T, Pressler A, et al. Repolarization perturbation and hypomagnesemia after extreme exercise. Med Sci Sports Exerc 2012;44:1637–43.

59. Bansal T, Abeygunasekara S, Ezzat V. An unusual presentation of primary renal hypokalemia-hypomagnesemia (Gitelman's syndrome). Ren Fail 2010;32:407–10.

60. Chen KP, Lee J, Mark RG, et al. Proton pump inhibitor use is not associated with cardiac arrhythmia in critically ill patients. J Clin Pharmacol 2015;55:774–9.

61. El-Charabaty E, Saifan C, Abdallah M, et al. Effects of proton pump inhibitors and electrolyte disturbances on arrhythmias. Int J Gen Med 2013;6: 515–8.

62. Savage N. Physiology: beating stroke. Nature 2013; 493:S12–3.

63. Lip GY, Tse HF, Lane DA. Atrial fibrillation. Lancet 2012;379:648–61.

64. Ezekowitz MD. Maintaining sinus rhythm–making treatment better than the disease. N Engl J Med 2007;357:1039–41.

65. Lafuente-Lafuente C, Valembois L, Bergmann JF, et al. Antiarrhythmics for maintaining sinus rhythm after cardioversion of atrial fibrillation. Cochrane Database Syst Rev 2015;(3):CD005049.

66. Motte G, Coumel P, Abitbol G, et al. The long QT syndrome and syncope caused by spike torsades. Arch Mal Coeur Vaiss 1970;63:831–53 [in French].

67. Stambler BS, Wood MA, Ellenbogen KA, et al. Efficacy and safety of repeated intravenous doses of ibutilide for rapid conversion of atrial flutter or fibrillation. Ibutilide Repeat Dose Study Investigators. Circulation 1996;94:1613–21.

68. Choy AM, Darbar D, Dell'Orto S, et al. Exaggerated QT prolongation after cardioversion of atrial fibrillation. J Am Coll Cardiol 1999;34:396–401.

69. Darbar D, Hardin B, Harris P, et al. A rate-independent method of assessing QT-RR slope following conversion of atrial fibrillation. J Cardiovasc Electrophysiol 2007;18:636–41.

70. Roden DM, Kannankeril P, Darbar D. On the relationship among QT interval, atrial fibrillation, and torsade de pointes. Europace 2007;9:iv1–3.

71. Kolek M, Parvez B, Song Y, et al. Comprehensive evaluation of QT interval during abrupt changes in heart rate and associated neurohormonal and inflammatory markers. Circulation 2014;130:A864.

72. Gopinathannair R, Etheridge SP, Marchlinski FE, et al. Arrhythmia-induced cardiomyopathies: mechanisms, recognition, and management. J Am Coll Cardiol 2015;66:1714–28.

73. Jenzer HR, Hagemeijer F. Quinidine syncope: torsade de pointes with low quinidine plasma concentrations. Eur J Cardiol 1976;4:447–51.

74. Roden DM, Woosley RL, Primm RK. Incidence and clinical features of the quinidine-associated long QT syndrome: implications for patient care. Am Heart J 1986;111:1088–93.

75. Brodie BB, Udenfriend S. Estimation of quinidine in human plasma, with note of estimation of quinidine. J Pharmacol Exp Ther 1943;78:154.

76. Brodie BB, Baer JE, Craig LC. Metabolic products of the cinchona alkaloids in human urine. J Biol Chem 1951;188:567–81.

77. Thompson KA, Blair IA, Woosley RL, et al. Comparative in vitro electrophysiology of quinidine, its major metabolites and dihydroquinidine. J Pharmacol Exp Ther 1987;241:84–90.

78. Thompson KA, Murray JJ, Blair IA, et al. Plasma concentrations of quinidine, its major metabolites, and dihydroquinidine in patients with torsades de pointes. Clin Pharmacol Ther 1988;43:636–42.

79. Yang T, Roden DM. Extracellular potassium modulation of drug block of IKr. Implications for torsades de pointes and reverse use-dependence. Circulation 1996;93:407–11.

80. Hiraoka M, Sawada K, Kawano S. Effects of quinidine on plateau currents of guinea-pig ventricular myocytes. J Mol Cell Cardiol 1986;18:1097–106.

81. Imaizumi Y, Giles WR. Quinidine-induced inhibition of transient outward current in cardiac muscle. Am J Physiol 1987;253:H704–8.

82. Johnson EA, McKinnon MG. The differential effect of quinidine and pyrilamine on the myocardial action potential at various rates of stimulation. J Pharmacol Exp Ther 1957;120:460–8.

83. Roden DM, Iansmith DH, Woosley RL. Frequency-dependent interactions of mexiletine and quinidine on depolarization and repolarization in canine Purkinje fibers. J Pharmacol Exp Ther 1987;243:1218–24.

84. Reiffel JA, Appel G. Importance of QT interval determination and renal function assessment during antiarrhythmic drug therapy. J Cardiovasc Pharmacol Ther 2001;6:111–9.

85. Krantz MJ, Lewkowiez L, Hays H, et al. Torsade de pointes associated with very-high-dose methadone. Ann Intern Med 2002;137:501–4.

86. Anderson JL, Prystowsky EN. Sotalol: an important new antiarrhythmic. Am Heart J 1999;137:388–409.

87. Llerena A, Berecz R, de la Rubia A, et al. Use of the mesoridazine/thioridazine ratio as a marker for CYP2D6 enzyme activity. Ther Drug Monit 2000;22:397–401.

88. Eap CB, Crettol S, Rougier JS, et al. Stereoselective block of hERG channel by (S)-methadone and QT interval prolongation in CYP2B6 slow metabolizers. Clin Pharmacol Ther 2007;81:719–28.

89. Johannesen L, Vicente J, Mason JW, et al. Differentiating drug-induced multichannel block on the electrocardiogram: randomized study of dofetilide, quinidine, ranolazine, and verapamil. Clin Pharmacol Ther 2014;96(5):549–58.

Guidelines for Potassium Channel Blocker Use

Anne M. Gillis, MD, FRCPC, FHRS

KEYWORDS

- Atrial fibrillation • Atrial flutter • Potassium channel blockers • Practice guidelines
- Ventricular arrhythmias

KEY POINTS

- The choice of antiarrhythmic drug is based on the efficacy and safety profile and influenced by the presence or absence of structural heart disease.
- Because of its adverse side-effect profile, amiodarone is recommended for the management of atrial fibrillation only when other agents have failed or are contraindicated.
- Antiarrhythmic drugs do not improve survival in those with ventricular arrhythmias or at risk of sudden cardiac arrest.
- For treatment of symptomatic ventricular arrhythmias in the setting of coronary artery disease or cardiomyopathy, amiodarone is generally the preferred agent, although sotalol may be considered in patients with mild ventricular dysfunction.

INTRODUCTION

This article summarizes recommendations for the clinical use of antiarrhythmic drugs for the treatment and prevention of atrial and ventricular arrhythmias based on the current guideline and consensus documents. By the nature and process of guideline/consensus document development, the role of the novel potassium channel blockers that are currently under clinical investigation, some of which are discussed in earlier articles, have not yet been determined. It is also important to emphasize that many of the antiarrhythmic drugs currently available for clinical use have effects on multiple ion channels, including potassium ion channels, which contribute to their efficacy.

ATRIAL FIBRILLATION/ATRIAL FLUTTER

Guidelines for the management of atrial fibrillation (AF) and atrial flutter have recently been updated by the Canadian Cardiovascular Society,[1–3] the European Society of Cardiology[4,5] and the American College of Cardiology/American Heart Association/Heart Rhythm Society (ACC/AHA/HRS).[6] Randomized clinical trials have failed to show a superiority of a rhythm control strategy compared with a heart rate control strategy on survival or stroke prevention.[7–9] Accordingly, the choice of a rhythm control strategy should be individualized based on the severity of symptoms, the impact on patients' quality of life, the desire to improve clinical outcomes, as well as patient preferences.[1–6] Choices of antiarrhythmic drug therapy are based on the presence or absence of significant structural heart disease and a history of congestive heart failure as well as the safety and efficacy profile of the drugs.

PHARMACOLOGIC CARDIOVERSION OF RECENT-ONSET ATRIAL FIBRILLATION

The choice of antiarrhythmic drugs for pharmacologic cardioversion of recent-onset AF are shown

Disclosures: Dr A.M. Gillis receives research support from Medtronic as local principal investigator of a device registry.
Department of Cardiac Sciences, Libin Cardiovascular Institute of Alberta, University of Calgary, 3280 Hospital Drive Northwest, Calgary, Alberta T2N 4Z6, Canada
E-mail address: amgillis@ucalgary.ca

Card Electrophysiol Clin 8 (2016) 495–501
http://dx.doi.org/10.1016/j.ccep.2016.02.010

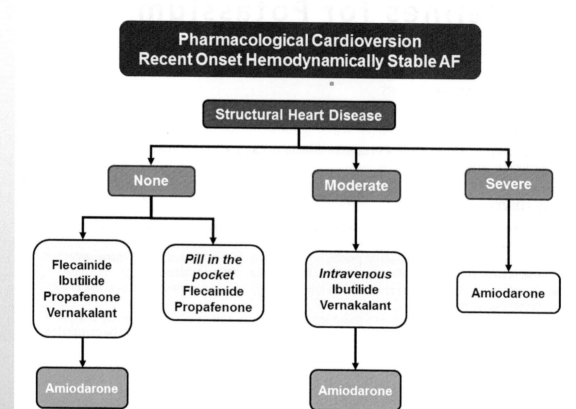

Fig. 1. Drug choices for pharmacologic conversion of recent-onset AF are based on the presence or absence and severity of structural heart disease.

in **Fig. 1** and **Table 1**. The ACC/AHA/HRS' guidelines recommend the use of flecainide, dofetilide, propafenone, or intravenous ibutilide for cardioversion of AF or atrial flutter if contraindications for the selected drug are absent.[6] It is also recommended that dofetilide therapy should be initiated in hospital under continuous electrocardiogram (ECG) monitoring because of the risk of marked QT interval prolongation. The European Society of Cardiology's guidelines recommend

Table 1 Drugs for pharmacologic cardioversion of atrial fibrillation	
Intravenous Drugs	**Dose**
Flecainide	2 mg/kg
Ibutilide	1 mg over 10 min may repeat once (0.001 mg/kg if weight <60 kg)
Propafenone	2 mg/kg
Amiodarone[a]	150 mg over 10 min then 1 mg/min × 6 h then 0.5 mg/min for 18 h or switch to oral dose
Vernakalant	3 mg/kg over 10 min; 2 mg/kg after 10 min if AF persists
Oral Drugs	**Dose**
Amiodarone	400–800 mg in divided doses to a total of 10 g then 100–200 mg/d
Flecainide	200–300 mg single dose
Propafenone	450–600 mg single dose
Dofetilide	125–500 mg bid based on creatinine clearance and QT interval

[a] Amiodarone is less effective for early termination of AF.

the initial choice of intravenous flecainide, propafenone, ibutilide, or vernakalant for pharmacologic cardioversion of recent-onset AF in the setting of no or minimal structural heart disease, the use of intravenous ibutilide or vernakalant in the presence of moderately severe structural heart disease, and the use intravenous amiodarone in the setting of severe structural heart disease.[5] Intravenous flecainide, propafenone, and vernakalant are not available in North America.

Practical tips

- The risk of torsade de pointes ventricular tachycardia following administration of ibutilide can be reduced by pretreatment with magnesium sulfate administered intravenously.

- When compared over 6 hours, intravenous amiodarone is not as effective as intravenous flecainide, ibutilide, propafenone, or vernakalant for termination of AF.

- All guidelines indicate that flecainide or propafenone may be considered as a pill in the pocket approach in the absence of significant structural heart disease if observed to be safe in a monitored setting.

- Adding a rapidly acting beta-blocker or calcium channel blocker in conjunction with flecainide or propafenone may be considered for prevention of atrial flutter with 1:1 atrioventricular conduction particularly if this approach has been demonstrated to be safe in a monitored setting.

In current clinical practice, a trial of longer-term antiarrhythmic drug therapy (2–4 weeks) chosen based on clinical factors for pharmacologic cardioversion is frequently considered before a planned electrical cardioversion if AF persists.[1,6]

MAINTENANCE OF SINUS RHYTHM

The choices of antiarrhythmic drugs for a rhythm control strategy are summarized in **Fig. 2** and **Table 2**. Antiarrhythmic drug choices are guided by the presence or absence of structural heart disease as well as their safety profile. The European Society of Cardiology's guidelines consider the presence of left ventricular hypertrophy as a contraindication for the use of flecainide, propafenone, or sotalol,[5] whereas the current Canadian guidelines do not.[1] The decision to eliminate left ventricular hypertrophy as a discriminating factor for some antiarrhythmic drug choices was based on a lack of compelling clinical evidence of harm in this setting.[1,10] The American guidelines do not recommend the use of dofetilide, flecainide, propafenone, or sotalol in the presence of severe left ventricular hypertrophy defined as a wall thickness greater than 1.5 cm.[6]

The recommendation of dronedarone, dofetilide, flecainide, propafenone, or sotalol as first-line choices for treatment of AF in the absence of significant structural heart disease is based on their side-effect profile compared with amiodarone. Over the long-term, these drugs individually have a modest efficacy for suppression of AF compared with amiodarone (30%–50% at 1 year vs 60%–70% at 1 year for amiodarone).[1] However, the higher incidence of significant adverse effects associated with amiodarone use has led to this hierarchical recommendation that its use be considered when other drugs have failed or are contraindicated.[1,5,6]

Dronedarone is the only drug reported to reduce hospitalizations and improve survival as reported in the ATHENA trial (A Placebo-Controlled, Double-Blind, Parallel Arm Trial to Assess the Efficacy of Dronedarone 400 mg bid for the Prevention of Cardiovascular Hospitalization or Death from Any Cause in Patients with Atrial Fibrillation/Atrial Flutter).[11] However, dronedarone has been reported to increase mortality in patients with recently decompensated heart failure[12] and in patients with permanent AF and significant cardiovascular risk factors.[13] Consequently, the updated AF guidelines recommend that dronedarone is contraindicated in patients with a history of heart failure or in patients in permanent AF.[2,5,6] Sotalol may be used with caution in patients with a mild reduction in systolic function.[1,6] Dofetilide has been reported to be safe in the setting of systolic dysfunction, but it must be initiated in hospital under continuous ECG monitoring for detection of significant QT interval prolongation and detection of torsade de pointes ventricular tachycardia.[6] Dofetilide is not included in the Canadian or European guidelines, as it has not been approved by regulatory agencies. Amiodarone remains the only agent recommended for use in patients with severe left ventricular systolic dysfunction.[1–6]

Practical tips

- Flecainide and propafenone are contraindicated in the setting of coronary artery disease and prior myocardial infarction.

- Class IC drugs should be combined with atrioventricular nodal blocking drugs.

- These drugs are contraindicated in the setting of long QT syndrome.

- Other drugs that prolong the QT interval should be avoided or used with caution.
- Sotalol and dofetilide should be used with caution in patients at risk for QT interval prolongation, for example, women and patients on diuretics.
- Dronedarone should be used with caution in combination with digoxin.
- Dronedarone should not be used in permanent AF.
- Dronedarone should be avoided in patients with a history of heart failure.

Despite the widespread dissemination of these guidelines, survey data from multiple geographies identify nonadherence to the current guidelines.[14,15] Amiodarone is often prescribed as first-line therapy for patients with minimal structural heart disease. Furthermore, in as many as 20% of patients, the prescription of class IC antiarrhythmic drugs did not conform to the guidelines.

TREATMENT OF VENTRICULAR ARRHYTHMIAS AND PREVENTION OF SUDDEN CARDIAC DEATH

Recommendations on the management of ventricular arrhythmias and prevention of sudden cardiac death have recently been published.[16,17] In randomized clinical trials, the currently available membrane active antiarrhythmic drugs have not been shown to improve survival.[16–22] Indeed class IC antiarrhythmic drugs have been shown to be harmful in patients with ventricular premature beats following a myocardial infarction,[18] and d-sotalol increased mortality in patients with left ventricular dysfunction following myocardial infarction.[21] Clinical trials have demonstrated the superiority of implantable cardioverter defibrillators (ICD) compared with antiarrhythmic drug therapy in primary and secondary prevention trials.[23–28] Thus, the role of antiarrhythmic therapy is primarily adjunctive and limited to specific situations. The choice of antiarrhythmic drug therapy is frequently limited to amiodarone because of the presence of severely depressed left ventricular dysfunction and the known proarrhythmic effects

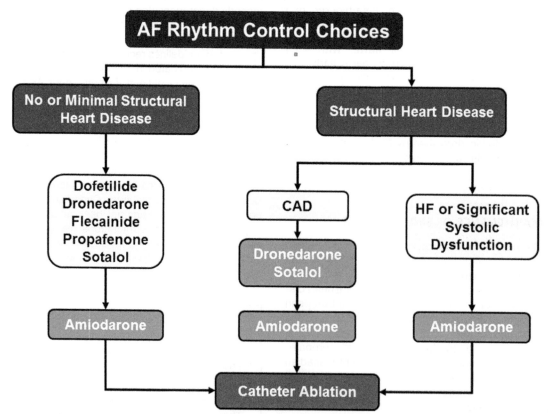

Fig. 2. Drug choices for maintenance of sinus rhythm are based on drug safety profile and presence of structural heart disease. CAD, coronary artery disease; HF, heart failure.

Table 2
Antiarrhythmic drugs for rhythm control

Class	Drug	Dosage	Efficacy	Adverse Effects
IC	Flecainide	50–200 mg bid	30%–50% at 1 y	Bradycardia Rapid ventricular response to AF or atrial flutter (1:1 conduction) Ventricular proarrhythmia
	Propafenone	150–300 mg tid	30%–50% at 1 y	Abnormal taste Bradycardia Rapid ventricular response to AF or atrial flutter (1:1 conduction) Ventricular proarrhythmia
III	Amiodarone	100–200 mg once daily (after 10 g loading)	60%–70% at 1 y	Bradycardia GI upset Hepatic toxicity Neuropathy, tremor Photosensitivity Thyroid dysfunction Pulmonary toxicity Torsades de pointes (rare)
	Dronedarone	400 mg bid	40% at 1 y	Bradycardia GI upset
	Sotalol	40–160 mg bid	30%–50%	Torsades de pointes Bradycardia Beta-blocker side effects

Abbreviations: AV, atrioventricular; CAD, coronary artery disease; EF, ejection fraction; GI, gastrointestinal; ICD, implantable cardioverter defibrillator; VT, ventricular tachycardia.

of other class I or class III antiarrhythmic drugs in this setting.

Sotalol and amiodarone have been used to suppress atrial and ventricular arrhythmias in the ICD population with the aim of reducing shock therapy.[29,30] However, sotalol should not be used in the setting of severe left ventricular dysfunction.

Practical tips

- Amiodarone is recommended for the treatment of polymorphic ventricular tachycardia in the setting of acute coronary syndromes.
- Amiodarone may be considered for the treatment of symptomatic ventricular arrhythmias following myocardial infarction or in the setting of left ventricular dysfunction, but it has no impact on survival.
- Class IC drugs are contraindicated for the treatment of ventricular arrhythmias following myocardial infarction and in patients with left ventricular dysfunction.
- Amiodarone or catheter ablation is recommended for ICD patients to prevent recurrent shocks due to sustained ventricular arrhythmias.
- Sotalol is useful for prevention of shocks in ICD patients with mild to moderate left ventricular dysfunction.

REFERENCES

1. Gillis AM, Verma A, Talajic M, et al, CCS Atrial Fibrillation Guidelines Committee. Canadian Cardiovascular Society atrial fibrillation guidelines 2010: rate and rhythm management. Can J Cardiol 2011;27: 47–59.
2. Skanes AC, Healey JS, Cairns JA, et al, Canadian Cardiovascular Society Atrial Fibrillation Guidelines Committee. Focused 2012 update of the Canadian Cardiovascular Society atrial fibrillation guidelines: recommendations for stroke prevention and rate/rhythm control. Can J Cardiol 2012;28:125–36.
3. Verma A, Cairns JA, Mitchell LB, et al, CCS Atrial Fibrillation Guidelines Committee. 2014 focused update of the Canadian Cardiovascular Society Guidelines for the management of atrial fibrillation. Can J Cardiol 2014;30:114–30.
4. Camm AJ, Kirchhof P, Lip GY, et al, ESC Committee for Practice Guidelines.; European Heart Rhythm Association, European Association for Cardio-Thoracic Surgery. Guidelines for the management of atrial fibrillation: the Task Force for the Management of Atrial Fibrillation of the European Society of Cardiology (ESC). Eur Heart J 2010;31:2369–429.
5. Camm AJ, Lip GY, De Caterina R, et al, ESC Committee for Practice Guidelines-CPG, ESC Committee for Practice Guidelines (CPG). 2012 focused update

of the ESC guidelines for the management of atrial fibrillation: an update of the 2010 ESC guidelines for the management of atrial fibrillation. Eur Heart J 2012;33:2719–47.

6. January CT, Wann LS, Alpert JS, et al, American College of Cardiology/American Heart Association Task Force on Practice Guidelines. 2014 AHA/ACC/HRS guideline for the management of patients with atrial fibrillation: a report of the American College of Cardiology/American Heart Association Task Force on Practice Guidelines and the Heart Rhythm Society. J Am Coll Cardiol 2014;64:e1–76.

7. Wyse DG, Waldo AL, DiMarco JP, et al, Atrial Fibrillation Follow-up Investigation of Rhythm Management (AFFIRM) Investigators. A comparison of rate control and rhythm control in patients with atrial fibrillation. N Engl J Med 2002;347:1825–33.

8. Van Gelder IC, Hagens VE, Bosker HA, et al, Rate Control versus Electrical Cardioversion for Persistent Atrial Fibrillation Study Group. A comparison of rate control and rhythm control in patients with recurrent persistent atrial fibrillation. N Engl J Med 2002;347: 1834–40.

9. Roy D, Talajic M, Nattel S, et al, Atrial Fibrillation and Congestive Heart Failure Investigators. Rhythm control versus rate control for atrial fibrillation and heart failure. N Engl J Med 2008;358:2667–77.

10. Chung R, Houghtaling PL, Tchou M, et al. Left ventricular hypertrophy and antiarrhythmic drugs in atrial fibrillation: impact on mortality. Pacing Clin Electrophysiol 2014;37:1338–48.

11. Hohnloser SH, Crijns HJ, van Eickels M, et al, ATHENA Investigators. Effect of dronedarone on cardiovascular events in atrial fibrillation. N Engl J Med 2009;360:668–78.

12. Køber L, Torp-Pedersen C, McMurray JJ, et al, Dronedarone Study Group. Increased mortality after dronedarone therapy for severe heart failure. N Engl J Med 2008;358:2678–87.

13. Connolly SJ, Camm AJ, Halperin JL, et al, PALLAS Investigators. Dronedarone in high-risk permanent atrial fibrillation. N Engl J Med 2011;365:2268–76.

14. Kowey PR, Breithardt G, Camm J, et al. Physician stated atrial fibrillation management in light of treatment guidelines: data from an international, observational prospective survey. Clin Cardiol 2010;33: 172–8.

15. Chiang CE, Goethals M, O'Neill JO, et al, on behalf of the RealiseAF survey investigators. Inappropriate use of antiarrhythmic drugs in paroxysmal and persistent atrial fibrillation in a large contemporary international survey: insights from RealiseAF. Europace 2013;15:1733–40.

16. Priori SG, Blomström-Lundqvist C, Mazzanti A, et al, Authors/Task Force Members, Document Reviewers. 2015 ESC guidelines for the management of patients with ventricular arrhythmias and the prevention of sudden cardiac death: the Task Force for the Management of Patients with Ventricular Arrhythmias and the Prevention of Sudden Cardiac Death of the European Society of Cardiology (ESC) Endorsed by: Association for European Paediatric and Congenital Cardiology (AEPC). Eur Heart J 2015;36:2793–867.

17. Pedersen CT, Kay GN, Kalman J, et al, EP-Europace,UK. EHRA/HRS/APHRS expert consensus on ventricular arrhythmias. Heart Rhythm 2014;11: e166–96.

18. Echt DS, Liebson PR, Mitchell LB, et al. Mortality and morbidity in patients receiving encainide, flecainide, or placebo. The Cardiac Arrhythmia Suppression Trial. N Engl J Med 1991;324:781–8.

19. Singh SN, Fletcher RD, Fisher SG, et al. Amiodarone in patients with congestive heart failure and asymptomatic ventricular arrhythmia. Survival Trial of Antiarrhythmic Therapy in Congestive Heart Failure. N Engl J Med 1995;333:77–82.

20. Amiodarone Trials Meta Analysis Investigators. Effect of prophylactic amiodarone on mortality after acute myocardial infarction and in congestive heart failure: meta-analysis of individual data from 6500 patients in randomised trials. Amiodarone Trials Meta-Analysis Investigators. Lancet 1997;350: 1417–24.

21. Waldo AL, Camm AJ, deRuyter H, et al. Effect of d-sotalol on mortality in patients with left ventricular dysfunction after recent and remote myocardial infarction. The SWORD Investigators. Survival with Oral d-Sotalol. Lancet 1996;348:7–12.

22. Piccini JP, Berger JS, O'Connor CM. Amiodarone for the prevention of sudden cardiac death: a meta-analysis of randomized controlled trials. Eur Heart J 2009;30:1245–53.

23. The Antiarrhythmics versus Implantable Defibrillators (AVID) Investigators. A comparison of antiarrhythmic-drug therapy with implantable defibrillators in patients resuscitated from near-fatal ventricular arrhythmias. N Engl J Med 1997;337: 1576–83.

24. Connolly SJ, Gent M, Roberts RS, et al. Canadian implantable defibrillator study (CIDS): a randomized trial of the implantable cardioverter defibrillator against amiodarone. Circulation 2000;101: 1297–302.

25. Kuck KH, Cappato R, Siebels J, et al. Randomized comparison of antiarrhythmic drug therapy with implantable defibrillators in patients resuscitated from cardiac arrest: the Cardiac Arrest Study Hamburg (CASH). Circulation 2000;102: 748–54.

26. Connolly SJ, Hallstrom AP, Cappato R, et al. Meta-analysis of the implantable cardioverter defibrillator secondary prevention trials. AVID, CASH and CIDS studies. Antiarrhythmics vs Implantable Defibrillator

study. Cardiac Arrest Study Hamburg. Canadian Implantable Defibrillator Study. Eur Heart J 2000; 21:2071–8.

27. Moss AJ, Zareba W, Hall WJ, et al. Prophylactic implantation of a defibrillator in patients with myocardial infarction and reduced ejection fraction. N Engl J Med 2002;346:877–83.

28. Bardy GH, Lee KL, Mark DB, et al, Sudden Cardiac Death in Heart Failure Trial (SCD-HeFT) Investigators. Amiodarone or an implantable cardioverter-defibrillator for congestive heart failure. N Engl J Med 2005;352:225–37.

29. Pacifico A, Hohnloser SH, Williams JH, et al. Prevention of implantable-defibrillator shocks by treatment with sotalol. d,l-Sotalol Implantable Cardioverter-Defibrillator Study Group. N Engl J Med 1999;340:1855–62.

30. Connolly SJ, Dorian P, Roberts RS, et al, Optimal Pharmacological Therapy in Cardioverter Defibrillator Patients (OPTIC) Investigators. Comparison of beta-blockers, amiodarone plus beta-blockers, or sotalol for prevention of shocks from implantable cardioverter defibrillators: the OPTIC Study: a randomized trial. JAMA 2006;295:165–71.

Moving?

Make sure your subscription moves with you!

To notify us of your new address, find your **Clinics Account Number** (located on your mailing label above your name), and contact customer service at:

Email: journalscustomerservice-usa@elsevier.com

800-654-2452 (subscribers in the U.S. & Canada)
314-447-8871 (subscribers outside of the U.S. & Canada)

Fax number: 314-447-8029

Elsevier Health Sciences Division
Subscription Customer Service
3251 Riverport Lane
Maryland Heights, MO 63043

Printed and bound by CPI Group (UK) Ltd, Croydon, CR0 4YY

03/10/2024

01040302-0005